Introductory Applied Biostatistics
Volume II for Boston University

Ralph B. D'Agostino, Sr. | Lisa M. Sullivan | Alexa S. Beiser

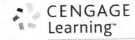
CENGAGE
Learning™

Australia • Brazil • Japan • Korea • Mexico • Singapore • Spain • United Kingdom • United States

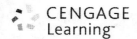
CENGAGE
Learning™

Introductory Applied Biostatistics for Boston University

D'Agostino, Sr. | Sullivan | Beiser

Executive Editor:
Maureen Staudt
Michael Stranz

Senior Project Development Manager:
Linda de Stefano

Marketing Specialist:
Sara Mercurio
Lindsay Shapiro

Production/Manufacturing Manager:
Donna M. Brown

PreMedia Supervisor:
Joel Brennecke

Rights & Permissions Specialist:
Kalina Hintz
Todd Osborne

Cover Image:
Getty Images*

For product information and technology assistance, contact us at
Cengage Learning Customer & Sales Support, 1-800-354-9706

For permission to use material from this text or product, submit all requests online at **cengage.com/permissions**
Further permissions questions can be emailed to
permissionrequest@cengage.com

Library of Congress Control Number: 0000000000

ISBN-13: 978-1-4240-7582-9

ISBN-10: 1-4240-7582-3

Cengage Learning
5191 Natorp Boulevard
Mason, Ohio 45040
USA

Cengage Learning is a leading provider of customized learning solutions with office locations around the globe, including Singapore, the United Kingdom, Australia, Mexico, Brazil, and Japan. Locate your local office at:
international.cengage.com/region

Cengage Learning products are represented in Canada by Nelson Education, Ltd.

For your lifelong learning solutions, visit **www.cengage.com/custom**

Visit our corporate website at **www.cengage.com**

Printed in the United States of America
1 2 3 4 5 6 7 12 11 10 09 08

Brief Contents

Descriptive Statistics
(Ch. 2)

Probability
(Ch. 3)

Sampling Distributions
(Ch. 4)

Statistical Inference
(Chapters 5–13)

OUTCOME VARIABLE	GROUPING VARIABLE(S)/ PREDICTOR(S)	ANALYSIS	CHAPTER(S)
Continuous	—	Estimate μ; Compare μ to Known, Historical Value	5/12
Continuous	Dichotomous (2 groups)	Compare Independent Means (Estimate/Test $(\mu_1 - \mu_2)$) or the Mean Difference (μ_d)	6/12
Continuous	Discrete (>2 groups)	Test the Equality of k Means using Analysis of Variance $(\mu_1 = \mu_2 = \cdots = \mu_k)$	9/12
Continuous	Continuous	Estimate Correlation or Determine Regression Equation	10/12
Continuous	Several Continuous or Dichotomous	Multiple Linear Regression Analysis	10
Dichotomous	—	Estimate p; Compare p to Known, Historical Value	7
Dichotomous	Dichotomous (2 groups)	Compare Independent Proportions (Estimate/Test $(p_1 - p_2)$)	7/8
Dichotomous	Discrete (>2 groups)	Test the Equality of k Proportions (Chi-Square Test)	7
Dichotomous	Several Continuous or Dichotomous	Multiple Logistic Regression Analysis	11
Discrete	Discrete	Compare Distributions Among k Populations (Chi-Square Test)	7
Time Event	Several Continuous or Dichotomous	Survival Analysis	13

7

Categorical Data

In Chapter 2 we defined variables as either *continuous* or *discrete*. Continuous (or measurement) variables assume, in theory, any value between the minimum and maximum value on a given measurement scale. Discrete variables take on a limited number of values or categories and can be either *ordinal* or *categorical* (sometimes called *nominal*) variables. Ordinal variables take on a limited number of values or categories and the categories are ordered. For example, socioeconomic status (SES) is an ordinal variable with the following response categories: lower SES, lower-middle, middle, upper-middle, and upper SES. Categorical variables take on a limited number of categories and the categories are unordered. For example, hospital type is a categorical variable with the following response categories: teaching, nonteaching. Statistical inference techniques applied to continuous (and sometimes ordinal) variables are concerned with means (μ) of those variables. Statistical inference techniques applied to discrete variables are concerned, instead, with the proportions of subjects in each response category.

In this chapter, we present statistical inference techniques for categorical variables. We begin the discussion with the case of dichotomous variables from the binomial distribution (i.e., each observation takes on one of two possible values, usually denoted success and failure) and then consider applications involving variables from multinomial distributions (i.e., each observation takes on one of several—more than two—possible values). We discuss one-sample and two-sample techniques for proportions analogous to the techniques presented in Chapters 5 and 6 relative to means.

In Section 7.1, we present statistical inference techniques for the one-sample case in which the analytic variable is dichotomous. In Section 7.2, we discuss cross-tabulation tables and several measures used to compare proportions between two independent populations. In Section 7.3, we discuss the evaluation of diagnostic tests. In Section 7.4, we present statistical inference techniques for the two-sample case in which the analytic variable is dichotomous. In Section 7.5, we consider analytic variables from the multinomial distribution and introduce chi-square tests. In Section 7.6, we discuss power and sample size determination. Key formulas are summarized in Section 7.7 and statistical computing applications are presented in Section 7.8. In Section 7.9, we use data from the Framingham Heart Study to illustrate the applications presented here.

7.1 Statistical Inference Concerning p

Recall the binomial distribution, in which each observation takes on one of two possible values, called success and failure. Suppose for analytic purposes, successes are coded as 1s and failures are coded as 0s. The parameter of interest is the proportion of successes in the population, or the *population proportion*, denoted p. The population proportion is defined as

$$p = \frac{\text{Number of successes}}{\text{Population size}} = \frac{X}{N} \qquad (7.1)$$

The two areas of statistical inference concerning p are estimation and hypothesis testing. The goal in estimation is to make valid inferences about the population proportion based on a single random sample from the population. There are two types of estimates for the population proportion: *the point estimate* and *the confidence interval estimate*. The point estimate is the "best" single-number estimate of the population proportion and is given by the sample proportion, denoted $\hat{p}$ (shown next). The confidence interval estimate is a range of plausible values for the population proportion.

$$\hat{p} = \frac{\text{Number of successes in the sample}}{n} = \frac{X}{n} \qquad (7.2)$$

EXAMPLE 7.1

Point Estimate for Proportion of Patients with Osteoarthritis

Suppose we wish to estimate the proportion of patients in a particular physician's practice with diagnosed osteoarthritis. The medical records of a random sample of 200 patients are reviewed for the diagnosis of osteoarthritis. Suppose that 38 patients are observed with diagnosed osteoarthritis. A point estimate for the proportion of all patients in this physician's practice with osteoarthritis (7.2) is given by: $\hat{p} = 38/200 = 0.19$, or 19%. ▪

As in applications concerning means, it is useful to know the standard error in order to assess the variation in the point estimate—in this case, the sample proportion. The standard error of the sample proportion is given by the following:

$$s.e.(\hat{p}) = \sqrt{\frac{p(1-p)}{n}} \qquad (7.3)$$

where $s.e.$ = standard error
$\quad\quad p$ = the population proportion

In most applications, the population proportion, p, is unknown. For large samples, the following can be used to estimate the standard error of the sample proportion:

$$s.e.(\hat{p}) = \sqrt{\frac{\hat{p}(1-\hat{p})}{n}} \qquad (7.4)$$

For applications involving binomial variables, a large sample is one with at least 5 successes and 5 failures. A large sample is defined as one that satisfies the following: $\min(n\hat{p}, n(1-\hat{p})) \geq 5$ (i.e., the smaller of $n\hat{p}$ and $n(1-\hat{p})$ must be greater than or equal to 5).

In Example 7.1, $\min(n\hat{p}, n(1-\hat{p})) = \min(200(0.19), 200(1-0.19)) = \min(38, 162) = 38 \geq 5$; therefore, the sample is sufficiently large. The standard error of the sample proportion is $\sqrt{0.19 * 0.81/200} = \sqrt{0.0007695} = 0.028$.

Table 7.1 *Statistical Inference Concerning p*

Attributes	Test Statistic*	Confidence Interval†
Simple random sample from binomial population, large sample	$Z = \dfrac{\hat{p} - p_0}{\sqrt{\dfrac{p_0(1 - p_0)}{n}}}$ where p_0 = value specified under H_0	$\hat{p} \pm Z_{1-(\alpha/2)}\sqrt{\dfrac{\hat{p}(1 - \hat{p})}{n}}$

*$\min(np_0, n(1 - p_0)) \geq 5$;
†$\min(n\hat{p}, n(1 - \hat{p})) \geq 5$

Confidence intervals for the population proportion can be generated using the techniques described in previous chapters. For large samples, we can appeal to the Central Limit Theorem for the derivation of the appropriate confidence interval (and test statistic in the test of hypothesis applications). Table 7.1 contains the formulas for the confidence interval for p and the test statistic for tests concerning p.

Table B.2A in the Appendix contains the values from the standard normal distribution for commonly used confidence levels ($Z_{1-(\alpha/2)}$). When the sample size is large (i.e., if and only if $\min(n\hat{p}, n(1 - \hat{p})) \geq 5$), the confidence interval formula given in Table 7.1 is appropriate. If the sample size is not sufficiently large, alternative formulas are available that are based on the binomial distribution and not the normal approximation, which is given here.

EXAMPLE 7.2

Estimating Proportion of Patients with Osteoarthritis

Consider the data from Example 7.1 and compute a 95% confidence interval for the proportion of all patients in the physician's practice with diagnosed osteoarthritis. The appropriate formula is given in Table 7.1:

$$\hat{p} \pm Z_{1-(\alpha/2)}\sqrt{\frac{\hat{p}(1 - \hat{p})}{n}}$$

Substituting the sample data and the appropriate value from Table B.2A for 95% confidence:

$$0.19 \pm 1.96\sqrt{\frac{0.19(1 - 0.19)}{200}}$$

$$0.19 \pm 1.96(0.028)$$

$$0.19 \pm 0.0549$$

$$(0.135, 0.245)$$

Thus, we are 95% confident that the true proportion of patients in this physician's practice with diagnosed osteoarthritis is between 13.5% and 24.5%. ■

Estimating Proportion of Patients with Osteoarthritis Using SAS

The following output was generated using SAS Proc Freq, which generates a frequency distribution table for a categorical (or ordinal) variable. In this example, we record whether each subject has been diagnosed with osteoarthritis (or not). The usual convention is to assign scores of 1 to successes (i.e., diagnosis of osteoarthritis) and scores of 0 to failures (i.e., free of osteoarthritis). The input data consists of designations (0 or 1) for each subject. A brief interpretation appears after the output.

SAS Output for Example 7.2

```
                 The FREQ Procedure

                                 Cumulative    Cumulative
 x     Frequency      Percent     Frequency      Percent
-----------------------------------------------------------
 0        162          81.00         162          81.00
 1         38          19.00         200         100.00


          Binomial Proportion for x = 1
          -------------------------------
          Proportion                 0.1900
          ASE                        0.0277
          95% Lower Conf Limit       0.1356
          95% Upper Conf Limit       0.2444


          Exact Conf Limits
          95% Lower Conf Limit       0.1381
          95% Upper Conf Limit       0.2513


           Test of H0: Proportion = 0.5

          ASE under H0               0.0354
          Z                         -8.7681
          One-sided Pr <   Z         <.0001
          Two-sided Pr > |Z|         <.0001


             Sample Size = 200
```

Interpretation of SAS Output for Example 7.2

Of interest in the frequency distribution table produced by SAS are the frequencies (i.e., the total numbers) of respondents with 0s and 1s and the percent of respondents with 0s and 1s. There are 38 (out of 200) respondents scored as 1 (success = diagnosis of osteoarthritis). The percent of respondents with the diagnosis is 19%. SAS then provides a 95% confidence interval for the proportion as 13.56% to 24.44%. SAS also provides exact confidence limits, which are used when the sample size is small (i.e., when we do not satisfy $\min(n\hat{p}, n(1 - \hat{p})) \geq 5$). In the last part of the output, SAS provides a test of hypothesis, specifically, the test of H_0: $p = 0.5$, which may or may not be of interest. In the following examples, we illustrate the procedure for a test of hypothesis for a population proportion. ▦

EXAMPLE 7.3

Testing Proportion of Cases with Abnormality Correctly Detected Against a Referent

Suppose that a diagnostic test has been shown to be 80% effective in detecting a genetic abnormality in human cells. An investigator modifies the diagnostic testing protocol and wishes to test if the new protocol has a detection rate that is significantly different from 80% in specimens known to possess the abnormality. The new protocol is applied to 300 independent specimens of human cells known to possess the abnormality. The abnormality is detected in 222 specimens. Run the appropriate test at a 5% level of significance.

1. Set up hypotheses.

$$H_0\text{: } p = 0.80$$
$$H_1\text{: } p \neq 0.80, \quad \alpha = 0.05$$

2. Select the appropriate test statistic.
   First, we check whether or not the sample size is sufficiently large:

$$\min(np_0, n(1 - p_0)) = \min(300(0.8), 300(1 - 0.8))$$
$$= \min(240, 60) = 60 \geq 5 \; ✔$$

The appropriate test statistic is given in Table 7.1:

$$Z = \frac{\hat{p} - p_0}{\sqrt{\dfrac{p_0(1 - p_0)}{n}}}$$

3. Decision rule (see Table B.2B in the Appendix for the appropriate critical value).

$$\text{Reject } H_0 \text{ if } Z \leq -1.960 \text{ or if } Z \geq 1.960$$
$$\text{Do not reject } H_0 \text{ if } -1.960 < Z < 1.960$$

4. Test statistic.

Substituting the sample data and the value of p specified in H_0 (i.e., $p_0 = 0.80$):

$$\hat{p} = \frac{222}{300} = 0.74$$

$$Z = \frac{\hat{p} - p_0}{\sqrt{\dfrac{p_0(1 - p_0)}{n}}}$$

$$Z = \frac{0.74 - 0.80}{\sqrt{\dfrac{0.80(1 - 0.80)}{300}}} = \frac{-0.06}{0.023} = -2.61$$

5. Conclusion.

Reject H_0 since $-2.61 \leq -1.960$. We have significant evidence, $\alpha = 0.05$, to show that the modified protocol has a significantly different detection rate than 80% (the rate for the original diagnostic test). The detection rate is lower with the modified protocol (74%) as compared to the original. For this example, $p < 0.010$ (see Table B.2B). ■

EXAMPLE 7.4

Testing Proportion of Cases with Flu Following Vaccination Against Referent

In the winter of 2002, 15% of all pediatric outpatient visits at a particular clinic were due to a single strain of flu. An investigator hypothesizes that the proportion of visits due to flu will decrease if patients are provided with flu shots. Suppose that flu shots were given to a random sample of 125 pediatric patients in the fall of 2003. These patients were tracked over the following winter to assess whether or not they come to clinic for flu (visits for other illnesses or injuries were not counted). Of these patients, 12% were seen in the winter of 2003–2004 for flu. Based on the data, is there evidence of a significant reduction in the proportion of patients seen in the clinic for flu after receiving the flu shot? Use a 5% level of significance.

1. Set up hypotheses.

$$H_0: p = 0.15$$
$$H_1: p < 0.15, \quad \alpha = 0.05$$

2. Select the appropriate test statistic.

First, check whether or not the sample size is sufficiently large:

$$\min(np_0, n(1 - p_0)) = \min(125(0.15), 125(1 - 0.15))$$
$$= \min(18.75, 106.25) = 18.75 \geq 5 \quad ✔$$

The appropriate test statistic is given in Table 7.1:

$$Z = \frac{\hat{p} - p_0}{\sqrt{\dfrac{p_0(1 - p_0)}{n}}}$$

3. Decision rule (see Table B.2B in the Appendix for the appropriate critical value).

$$\text{Reject } H_0 \text{ if } Z \leq -1.645$$
$$\text{Do not reject } H_0 \text{ if } Z > -1.645$$

4. Test statistic.

$$\hat{p} = 0.12$$

$$Z = \frac{\hat{p} - p_0}{\sqrt{\dfrac{p_0(1 - p_0)}{n}}}$$

Substituting the sample data and the value of p specified in H_0 (i.e., $p_0 = 0.15$):

$$Z = \frac{0.12 - 0.15}{\sqrt{\dfrac{0.15(1 - 0.15)}{125}}} = \frac{-0.03}{0.032} = -0.938$$

5. Conclusion.

Do not reject H_0 since $-0.938 > -1.645$. We do not have significant evidence, $\alpha = 0.05$, to show a reduction in the proportion of patients seen in the clinic for flu after receiving the vaccine. ■

Example 7.4 brings up an important issue of clinical versus statistical significance. In the formal test of hypothesis, we failed to reach statistical significance. However, we may have committed a Type II error (e.g., a larger sample size may be required to detect an effect). In any statistical application it is extremely important to look at the direction and magnitude of the observed effect. In Example 7.4, there is a reduction in the proportion of flu cases seen following the vaccines. The point estimate is 0.12, or 12%. Our test did not indicate that this was statistically significantly lower than 15%; however, there is a reduction and it should be evaluated carefully. Is this reduction clinically important? On a different note, was the study design we used optimal to address the question of effectiveness of the flu shots in pediatric patients? A concurrent comparison group might have provided a better comparison than historical data (i.e., $p_0 = 0.15$). We will discuss tests with a concurrent comparison group in the following sections.

7.2 Cross-Tabulation Tables

In applications involving discrete variables, *cross-tabulation* tables are often constructed to display the data. Cross-tabulation tables are also called $R \times C$ ("R by C") tables, where R denotes the number of rows in the table and C denotes the number of columns. A 2×2 table is illustrated in Example 7.5.

EXAMPLE 7.5
Cross-Tabulation to Summarize Proportions in Two Populations

A longitudinal study is conducted to evaluate the long-term complications in diabetic patients treated under two competing treatment regimens. Complications are measured by incidence of foot disease, eye disease, *or* cardiovascular disease within a 10-year observation period. The following 2×2 cross-tabulation table summarizes the data:

	Long-Term Complications		
Treatment	*Yes*	*No*	*Total*
Treatment 1	12	88	100
Treatment 2	8	92	100
Total	20	180	200

The estimate of the population proportion of all patients who develop complications under treatment 1 (p_1) is $\hat{p}_1 = 12/100 = 0.12$, by (7.2). This is equivalent to the estimate of the probability that a single patient develops complications under treatment 1. The estimate of the probability that a single patient develops complications under treatment 2 is $\hat{p}_2 = 8/100 = 0.08$. ▪

The probability of success or outcome (in Example 7.5, the outcome of interest is the development of complications) is often called the *risk* of outcome. There are a number of statistics used to compare risks of outcomes between populations (or between treatments). These statistics are called *effect measures* and are described in detail in Chapter 8.

SAS EXAMPLE 7.5
Generating Cross-Tabulations Using SAS

The following output was generated using SAS Proc Freq, which generates a contingency table (or cross-tabulation) when two variables are specified. A brief interpretation appears after the output.

SAS Output for Example 7.5

```
The FREQ Procedure
                      Table of trt by compl
             Frequency|
             Percent  |
             Row Pct  |          compl
             Col Pct  |yes        |z_no       |    Total
             ---------+--------+--------+
             trt_1    |      12 |      88 |      100
                      |    6.00 |   44.00 |    50.00
                      |   12.00 |   88.00 |
                      |   60.00 |   48.89 |
       trt   ---------+--------+--------+
             trt_2    |       8 |      92 |      100
                      |    4.00 |   46.00 |    50.00
                      |    8.00 |   92.00 |
                      |   40.00 |   51.11 |
             ---------+--------+--------+
             Total           20      180      200
                          10.00    90.00   100.00

                    Sample Size = 200
```

Interpretation of SAS Output for Example 7.5

SAS generates a contingency table and in each cell of the table displays the Frequency, the Percent, the Row Percent, and the Column Percent (see legend in top left corner of table). The Frequency is the number of subjects in each cell, and the Percent is the percent of all subjects in each cell. For example, there are 12 patients in the top left cell (i.e., subjects on treatment 1 who also had complications). These patients reflect 6% of the total sample (12/200 = 0.06). The Row Percent is the percent of subjects in the particular row that fall in that cell. For example, there are 100 patients on treatment 1, or 100 patients in the first row of the contingency table. The 12 patients who had complications reflect 12% of all patients on treatment 1 (12/100 = 0.12). The Column Percent is the percent of subjects in the particular column who fall in that cell. For example, there are 20 patients who report complications. These 20 patients appear in the first column of the contingency table. The 12 patients in treatment 1 who had complications reflect 60% of all patients who had complications (12/20 = 0.60). The row total and column total (called the marginal totals) are displayed to the right and at the bottom of the contingency table, respectively. Both row and column frequencies and percents (of total) are displayed.

7.3 Diagnostic Tests: Sensitivity and Specificity

A diagnostic test is a tool used to detect outcomes or events that are not directly observable. For example, an individual may have a condition or disease that is not directly observable by a physician. A diagnostic test designed to detect such a condition can be used as a tool to assist the physician in detection. Desirable properties in diagnostic tests include the following:

- The diagnostic test will indicate an event when the event is present, and
- The diagnostic test will indicate a nonevent when the event is absent.

EXAMPLE 7.6

Estimating Sensitivity and Specificity

A clinical trial is conducted to evaluate a diagnostic screening test designed to detect chromosomal fetal abnormalities. Chromosomal fetal abnormalities are confirmed using amniocentesis. The diagnostic test is performed on a random sample of 200 pregnant women, who later undergo an amniocentesis. The following 2×2 cross-tabulation table summarizes the data:

| | Diagnostic Test | | |
Amniocentesis	*Positive*	*Negative*	*Total*
Abnormal (Disease)	14	6	20
Normal (No Disease)	64	116	180
Total	78	122	200

Based on amniocentesis, the estimate of the population proportion of all women carrying fetuses with chromosomal abnormalities (p) is $\hat{p} = 20/200 = 0.10$, by (7.2). ■

The following statistics are used to describe diagnostic tests: the *sensitivity* of the test, the *specificity* of the test, the *predictive value positive* (PV$^+$) and the *predictive value negative* (PV$^-$). These statistics are defined as follows:

$$Sensitivity = P(\text{Positive test} \mid \text{Disease}) \qquad (7.5)$$
$$Specificity = P(\text{Negative test} \mid \text{No disease})$$
$$Predictive\ value\ positive = P(\text{Disease/Positive test})$$
$$Predictive\ value\ negative = P(\text{No disease/Negative test})$$

In Example 7.6, the estimate of the sensitivity of the test is $14/20 = 0.70$. The estimate of the specificity is $116/180 = 0.64$. The estimate of the predictive value positive is $PV^+ = 14/78 = 0.18$, and the estimate of the predictive negative is $PV^- = 116/122 = 0.95$.

In most cases, higher sensitivities and higher specificities are desirable. There are instances, however, where a better test is determined by only one criterion (e.g., higher sensitivity).

SAS EXAMPLE 7.6 **Estimating Sensitivity and Specificity Using SAS**

The following output was generated using SAS Proc Freq, which generates a contingency table (or cross-tabulation) when two variables are specified. SAS does not produce the estimates of sensitivity, specificity, false positive rate, and false negative rate directly, but these can be extracted from the contingency table. The statistics of interest are described after the output.

SAS Output for Example 7.6

```
                  The FREQ Procedure
               Table of amnio by diagtest
          amnio       diagtest
          Frequency|
          Percent  |
          Row Pct  |
          Col Pct  |positive|negative|  Total
          ---------+--------+--------+
          abnormal |    14 |     6 |     20
                   |  7.00 |  3.00 |  10.00
                   | 70.00 | 30.00 |
                   | 17.95 |  4.92 |
          ---------+--------+--------+
          normal   |    64 |   116 |    180
                   | 32.00 | 58.00 |  90.00
                   | 35.56 | 64.44 |
                   | 82.05 | 95.08 |
          ---------+--------+--------+
          Total         78     122     200
                      39.00   61.00   100.
```

Interpretation of SAS Output for Example 7.6

The sensitivity is the proportion of abnormal cases correctly classified by the test as positive, $14/20 = 0.70$. This is the Row Percent in the top left cell of the table. The specificity is the proportion of normal cases that are correctly classified by the test as negative, $116/180 = 0.644$. This is the Row Percent of the bottom right cell of the table. The predictive positive value is the

proportion of normal cases classified as positive that are, in fact diseased, PV⁺.
This is the Column Percent of the top left cell of the table. The predictive
value Negative is the proportion of cases classified as Negative that are, in fact,
normal, PV⁻ $= 116/122 = 0.95$. This is the Column Percent of the bottom
right cell of the table.

7.4 Statistical Inference Concerning $(p_1 - p_2)$

We often compare two independent populations with respect to the proportion of successes in each. A better study design to evaluate the effectiveness of
flu shots in pediatric patients (Example 7.4) would involve two comparison
groups. One group would receive the flu shots and the other would receive a
placebo shot (to maintain blinding—why is this important?). The analysis
would then compare the groups with respect to the proportions of children
who developed flu. In the two independent samples situation, one parameter
of interest is the difference in proportions, the risk difference: $(p_1 - p_2)$, where
$p_1 = $ the proportion of successes in population 1 and $p_2 = $ the proportion of
successes in population 2.

The point estimate for the risk difference, or difference in independent
proportions, is given by

$$\hat{p}_1 - \hat{p}_2 \qquad\qquad (7.6)$$

where $\hat{p}_i = $ the sample proportion in population i $(i = 1, 2)$

If samples from both populations are sufficiently large (see criteria in
Table 7.2), then the confidence interval formula shown in Table 7.2 can be
used to estimate $(p_1 - p_2)$.

Table B.2A contains the values from the standard normal distribution for
commonly used confidence levels. When the sample sizes are adequate (i.e., if
and only if $\min(n_1 \hat{p}_1, n_1(1 - \hat{p}_1)) \geq 5$ and $\min(n_2 \hat{p}_2, n_2(1 - \hat{p}_2)) \geq 5$), the confidence interval formula given in Table 7.2 is appropriate. If either (or both) sam-
ple size(s) are not adequate, alternative formulas are available that are based on
the binomial distribution and not the normal approximation given here.

Table 7.2 *Confidence Interval for* $(p_1 - p_2)$

Attributes	Confidence Interval
Simple random samples from binomial populations Independent populations Large samples:	$(\hat{p}_1 - \hat{p}_2) \pm Z_{1-(\alpha/2)}\sqrt{\left(\dfrac{\hat{p}_1(1 - \hat{p}_1)}{n_1}\right) + \left(\dfrac{\hat{p}_2(1 - \hat{p}_2)}{n_2}\right)}$
$\min(n_1 \hat{p}_1, n_1(1 - \hat{p}_1)) \geq 5$ *and* $\min(n_2 \hat{p}_2, n_2(1 - \hat{p}_2)) \geq 5$	where $\hat{p}_1 = X_1/n_1$ and $\hat{p}_2 = X_2/n_2$

EXAMPLE 7.7

Estimating Difference in Proportions of Children Who Use the Emergency Room Between Treatments

We want to evaluate the effectiveness of a new treatment for asthma. The new treatment is administered in an inhaler and will be compared to a standard treatment administered in the same way. Because asthma is a serious condition, it would be unethical to use a placebo comparator in this trial. Suppose our outcome variable is emergency room (ER) use for complications of asthma during a 6-month follow-up period. A random sample of 375 asthmatic children are selected from a registry, of which 250 are randomized to the new treatment group and 125 are randomized to the comparison group (standard treatment). Both groups are provided instruction on the proper use of their inhalers. This allocation scheme is called 2-to-1, where twice as many participants are randomized to the investigational treatment as the control. Both groups of children are followed for 6 months and monitored for ER use. Of the children on the new treatment, 60 used the ER during the 6 months for complications of asthma, and 19 of the children on the standard treatment used the ER for complications of asthma during the same period. Construct a 95% confidence interval for the difference in the proportions of asthmatic children on the new and standard treatments who used the ER during the 6-month follow-up period.

The data layout is as follows:

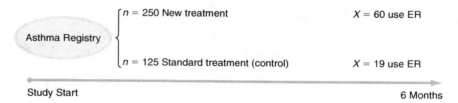

The sample proportions are

$$\hat{p}_1 = \frac{60}{250} = 0.24, \qquad \hat{p}_2 = \frac{19}{125} = 0.15$$

A point estimate for the difference in proportions is given by (7.6):

$$\hat{p}_1 - \hat{p}_2 = 0.24 - 0.15 = 0.09$$

Now, check whether or not the sample sizes are sufficiently large:

$$\min(n_1\hat{p}_1, n_1(1 - \hat{p}_1)) = \min(250(0.24), 250(1 - 0.24))$$
$$= \min(60, 190) = 60 \geq 5 ✔$$

and

$$\min(n_2\hat{p}_2, n_2(1 - \hat{p}_2)) = \min(125(0.15), 125(1 - 0.15))$$
$$= \min(19, 106) = 19 \geq 5 ✔$$

The formula from Table 7.2 is appropriate:

$$(\hat{p}_1 - \hat{p}_2) \pm Z_{1-(\alpha/2)}\sqrt{\left(\frac{\hat{p}_1(1 - \hat{p}_1)}{n_1}\right) + \left(\frac{\hat{p}_2(1 - \hat{p}_2)}{n_2}\right)}$$

Substituting the sample data and the appropriate value from Table B.2A for 95% confidence:

$$0.09 \pm 1.960\sqrt{\frac{0.24(1 - 0.24)}{250} + \frac{0.15(1 - 0.15)}{125}}$$

$$0.09 \pm 1.960(0.042)$$
$$0.09 \pm 0.082$$
$$(0.008, 0.172)$$

Thus, we are 95% confident that the true difference in the population proportions of asthmatic children on the new treatment as compared to children on standard treatment who used the ER during a 6-month period is between 0.8% and 17.2%. Based on the confidence interval estimate, can we say that there is a significant difference in the proportions of asthmatic children on the new treatment as compared to the standard treatment who used the ER during a 6-month period? (*Hint*: Does the confidence interval estimate include 0?) Is the new treatment effective? Notice the direction of the effect. ▪

> NOTE: The two-sample confidence interval concerning $(p_1 - p_2)$ estimates the *difference* in proportions, as opposed to the value of either proportion (as was the case in the one-sample applications).

In some applications, it is of interest to compare two populations on the basis of the proportions of successes in each using a formal test of hypothesis. Table 7.3 contains the test statistic for tests concerning $(p_1 - p_2)$.

Table 7.3 *Test Statistic for* $(p_1 - p_2)$

Attributes	Test Statistic
Large samples* Simple random samples from binomial populations Independent populations	$Z = \dfrac{\hat{p}_1 - \hat{p}_2}{\sqrt{\hat{p}(1 - \hat{p})\left(\dfrac{1}{n_1} + \dfrac{1}{n_2}\right)}}$ where $\hat{p}_1 = X_1/n_1$ and $\hat{p}_2 = X_2/n_2$ $\hat{p} = \dfrac{(X_1 + X_2)}{(n_1 + n_2)}$

*$\min(n_1\hat{p}_1, n_1(1 - \hat{p}_1)) \geq 5$ and $\min(n_2\hat{p}_2, n_2(1 - \hat{p}_2)) \geq 5$

EXAMPLE 7.8

Testing Difference in Proportions of Patients Who Experience Pain Relief Between Treatments

A new drug is being compared to an existing drug for its effectiveness in relieving headache pain. One hundred subjects who suffer from chronic headaches are randomly assigned to either Group 1: Existing Drug, or Group 2: New Drug. Subjects do not know which drug they are taking in this experiment. Subjects are provided with a single dose of the assigned drug and instructed to take the full dose as soon as they experience headache pain and to record whether or not they experience relief from headache pain within 60 minutes. Among the 50 subjects assigned to Group 1: Existing Drug, 28 reported relief from headache pain within 60 minutes. Among the 50 subjects assigned to Group 2: New Drug, 34 reported relief from headache pain within 60 minutes. Based on the data, is the proportion of subjects reporting relief from headache pain within 60 minutes under the New Drug significantly different from the proportion of subjects reporting relief within 60 minutes under the Existing Drug? Use a 5% level of significance.

The data layout is as follows:

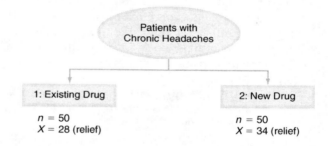

1. Set up hypotheses.

$$H_0: p_1 = p_2$$
$$H_1: p_1 \neq p_2, \quad \alpha = 0.05$$

where p_1 = the proportion of patients who experience relief from headache pain using the Existing Drug
p_2 = the proportion of patients who experience relief from headache pain using the New Drug

2. Select the appropriate test statistic.
   The sample proportions are

$$\hat{p}_1 = \frac{28}{50} = 0.56, \qquad \hat{p}_2 = \frac{34}{50} = 0.68$$

First, check whether or not the sample sizes are sufficiently large:

$$\min(n_1\,\hat{p}_1, n_1(1 - \hat{p}_1)) = \min(50(0.56), 50(1 - 0.56))$$
$$= \min(28, 22) = 22 \geq 5 \ ✔$$

and

$$\min(n_2\,\hat{p}_2, n_2(1 - \hat{p}_2)) = \min(50(0.68), 50(1 - 0.68))$$
$$= \min(34, 16) = 16 \geq 5 \ ✔$$

The appropriate test statistic is given in Table 7.3:

$$Z = \frac{\hat{p}_1 - \hat{p}_2}{\sqrt{\hat{p}(1 - \hat{p})\left(\dfrac{1}{n_1} + \dfrac{1}{n_2}\right)}}$$

3. Decision rule.

$$\text{Reject } H_0 \text{ if } Z \leq -1.960 \text{ or if } Z \geq 1.960$$
$$\text{Do not reject } H_0 \text{ if } -1.960 < Z < 1.960$$

4. Test statistic.

$$Z = \frac{\hat{p}_1 - \hat{p}_2}{\sqrt{\hat{p}(1 - \hat{p})\left(\dfrac{1}{n_1} + \dfrac{1}{n_2}\right)}}$$

We compute the estimate of the common proportion:

$$\hat{p} = \frac{X_1 + X_2}{n_1 + n_2} = \frac{28 + 34}{50 + 50} = 0.62$$

Note that $\hat{p}$ lies between $\hat{p}_1$ and $\hat{p}_2$.
Now substituting the sample data:

$$Z = \frac{0.56 - 0.68}{\sqrt{0.62(1 - 0.62)\left(\dfrac{1}{50} + \dfrac{1}{50}\right)}} = \frac{-0.12}{0.097} = -1.24$$

5. Conclusion.
Do not reject H_0 since $-1.960 < -1.24 < 1.960$. We do not have significant evidence, $\alpha = 0.05$, to show a difference in the proportions of subjects experiencing relief from headache pain with the New Drug within 60 minutes. ▦

7.5 Chi-Square Tests

In the previous sections, we focused attention on variables from the binomial distribution (i.e., observations took on one of two possible values, called success and failure). We now consider variables from the multinomial distribution in which each observation takes on one of several (more than two) possible values. Some of the techniques described in the previous sections can be applied to sample data from a multinomial distribution. For example, instead of estimating the proportion of successes in the population, we estimate the proportion of subjects in response category 1, the proportion of subjects in response category 2, and so on.

Here we describe two tests, called the goodness-of-fit test and the test of independence, which are used for tests of hypotheses in the presence of multinomial data in one-sample and two-or-more sample applications, respectively. Both tests involve a test statistic that follows a chi-square distribution (χ^2).

7.5.1 Goodness-of-Fit Test

We begin with the case of a categorical variable measured in a single sample. The following example illustrates the goodness-of-fit test.

EXAMPLE 7.9

Goodness of Fit Test for Patient Preferences

Following coronary artery bypass graft (CABG) surgery, patients are encouraged to participate in a cardiac rehabilitation program. The program lasts approximately 14 weeks and includes exercise training, nutritional information, and general lifestyle guidelines. One particular hospital is offering three cardiac rehabilitation programs that are identical in content but are offered at three different times. The administration is interested in whether the three time slots are equally popular or convenient for the patients. A total of 100 patients are involved in the investigation, and each patient is asked to select the one day and time (from three options) that is most convenient. The following data are observed:

	Mondays 6:00–7:30 PM	Thursdays 4:00–5:30 PM	Saturdays 8:00–9:30 AM
Time slot:			
Number of patients:	47	32	21

The day and time variable follows a multinomial distribution with three response categories, denoted $k = 3$ (i.e., Mon. 6:00–7:30 PM, Thurs. 4:00–5:30 PM, Sat. 8:00–9:30 AM). The proportions of patients in the sample selecting each day and time are given by (7.2): $\hat{p}_1 = 47/100 = 0.47$, $\hat{p}_2 = 32/100 = 0.32$, and $\hat{p}_3 = 21/100 = 0.21$.

We wish to use the data to test the hypothesis that the three day and time options are equally popular. Mathematically, this is represented as follows:

1. Set up hypotheses.

H_0: $p_1 = p_2 = p_3$, $\alpha = 0.05$ (Population proportions are equal)
H_1: H_0 is false   (Population proportions are not all equal)

NOTE: We do not write H_1: $p_1 \neq p_2 \neq p_3$, as we will reject H_0 in favor of H_1 if *any* of the three proportions are not equal, not only if *all* three are not equal (e.g., we will reject H_0 if $p_1 \neq p_2$, regardless of whether p_3 is equal to either p_1 or p_2).

The following are equivalent to the preceding hypotheses:

H_0: $p_1 = 0.33, p_2 = 0.33, p_3 = 0.33$
H_1: H_0 is false

2. Select the appropriate test statistic.
   In tests involving multinomial distributions, the test statistic is no longer based on the sample proportion, but on the *observed frequencies*, or numbers of subjects in each response category. In this example, we observed 47 patients in the first response category, 32 in the second, and 21 in the third. If the null hypothesis were true—that is, if the true proportions of patients in each response category were equal (i.e., if $p_1 = p_2 = p_3 = 0.33$)—then we would have *expected* approximately 33 patients to select each time slot (since $n = 100$).
   χ^2 tests are based on the agreement between expected (under H_0) *and observed (sample) frequencies.* The χ^2 statistic for testing whether the distribution of a single multinomial variable is as specified under H_0 is given by

$$\chi^2 = \sum \frac{(O - E)^2}{E} \tag{7.7}$$

where $\sum$ indicates summation over the k response categories
O = observed frequencies
E = expected frequencies (i.e., if H_0 is true, or under H_0)

The statistic follows a χ^2 distribution and has df $= k - 1$, where $k =$ the number of response categories. The general form of the χ^2 distribution is shown in Figure 7.1.
   Notice that all of the values in the χ^2 distribution are greater than or equal to zero. In order to test the hypotheses of interest, we need to determine an appropriate critical value. In χ^2 tests, we reject the null hypothesis in favor of the alternative hypothesis if the value of the test statistic is large. The test statistic (7.7) is large when the observed and expected frequencies are not similar. In such a case, we reject H_0.

Figure 7.1 *Chi-Square Distribution*

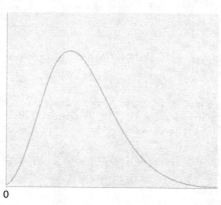

0

3. Decision rule.

   In order to select the appropriate critical value, we first determine the degrees of freedom.

$$df = k - 1 = 3 - 1 = 2$$

The appropriate critical value of χ^2 is $\chi^2 = 5.99$ from Table B.5 in the Appendix. The decision rule is

$$\text{Reject } H_0 \text{ if } \chi^2 \geq 5.99$$
$$\text{Do not reject } H_0 \text{ if } \chi^2 < 5.99$$

4. Test statistic.

   To organize the computations of the test statistic (7.7), the following table is used:

Time Slot:	Mondays 6:00–7:30 PM	Thursdays 4:00–5:30 PM	Saturdays 8:00–9:30 AM	Total
O = observed frequency:	47	32	21	100
E = expected frequency:	33.3	33.3	33.3	100
(O − E):	13.7	−1.3	−12.3	0
(O − E)²/E:	$(13.7)^2/33.3$ $= 5.64$	$(-1.3)^2/33.3$ $= 0.05$	$(-12.3)^2/33.3$ $= 4.54$	10.23

NOTE: The sum of the expected frequencies is equal to the sum of the observed frequencies ($n = 100$).

The test statistic is $\chi^2 = 10.23$.

5. Conclusion.

Reject H_0 since $10.23 \geq 5.99$. We have significant evidence, $\alpha = 0.05$, to show that the three time slots are not equally popular or convenient for the patients. In fact, almost half (47%) of the patients selected the Monday 6:00–7:30 PM slot. For this example, $p < 0.01$ (see Table B.5). ◾

SAS EXAMPLE 7.9 **Goodness of Fit Test for Patient Preferences Using SAS**

The following output was generated using SAS Proc Freq with an option to run a goodness-of-fit test. Specifically, the user specifies the distribution of responses under the null hypothesis (see Section 7.9 for the SAS code).

SAS Output for Example 7.9

The FREQ Procedure

day	Frequency	Percent	Test Percent	Cumulative Frequency	Cumulative Percent
Mon	47	47.00	33.00	47	47.00
Sat	21	21.00	33.00	68	68.00
Thurs	32	32.00	33.00	100	100.00

Chi-Square Test
for Specified Proportions

Chi-Square	10.3333
DF	2
Pr > ChiSq	0.0057

Sample Size = 100

Interpretation of SAS Output for Example 7.9

SAS first generates a frequency distribution table and provides the number and percent of respondents in each response category. SAS then lists the Test Percent in each category (these are supplied by the user and reflect the expected proportions). The last two columns contain the cumulative frequencies and cumulative percents for the sample data. SAS then produces the chi-square statistic for the goodness-of-fit test along with degrees of freedom (df $= k - 1$) and a p value. Here $\chi^2 = 10.33$ and $p = 0.0057$. We therefore reject H_0 because $p = 0.0057 < 0.05$ and conclude that the three time slots are not equally popular or convenient for the patients. ◾

EXAMPLE 7.10

Goodness of Fit Test for Teen Issues

Volunteers at a teen hotline have been assigned based on the assumption that 40% of all calls are drug related, 25% are sex related (e.g., date rape), 25% are stress related, and 10% concern educational issues. For this investigation, each call is classified into one category based on the primary issue raised by the caller. To test the hypothesis, the following data are collected from 120 randomly selected calls placed to the teen hotline. Based on the data, is the assumption regarding the distribution of topic issues appropriate?

Topic Issue:	Drugs	Sex	Stress	Education
Number of calls:	52	38	21	9

1. Set up hypotheses.

H_0: $p_1 = 0.40$, $p_2 = 0.25$, $p_3 = 0.25$, $p_4 = 0.10$
H_1: H_0 is false

or

H_0: Distribution across categories is 0.40, 0.25, 0.25, 0.10
H_1: H_0 is false, $\alpha = 0.05$

2. Select the appropriate test statistic.

$$\chi^2 = \sum \frac{(O - E)^2}{E}$$

where $\sum$ indicates summation over the k response categories
 O = observed frequencies
 E = expected frequencies (i.e., if H_0 is true, or under H_0)

3. Decision rule.

   In order to select the appropriate critical value, we first determine the degrees of freedom.

$$df = k - 1 = 4 - 1 = 3$$

The appropriate critical value of χ^2 is $\chi^2 = 7.815$ from Table B.5. The decision rule is

Reject H_0 if $\chi^2 \geq 7.815$
Do not reject H_0 if $\chi^2 < 7.815$

4. Test statistic.

To organize the computations of the test statistic (7.7), the following table is used:

Topic Issue:	Drugs	Sex	Stress	Education	TOTAL
O = observed frequency:	52	38	21	9	120
E = expected frequency:	48	30	30	12	120
(O − E):	4	8	−9	−3	0
$(O − E)^2/E$:	$(4)^2/48 =$ 0.33	$(8)^2/30 =$ 2.13	$(−9)^2/30 =$ 2.70	$(−3)^2/12 =$ 0.75	5.913

NOTE: The expected frequencies are computed assuming that H_0 is true, or under H_0: $120(0.40) = 48$, $120(0.25) = 30$, $120(0.25) = 30$, and $120(0.10) = 12$.

The test statistic is $\chi^2 = 5.913$.

5. Conclusion.

Do not reject H_0 since $5.913 < 7.815$. We do not have significant evidence, $\alpha = 0.05$, to show that the distribution of topic issues in the calls placed to the teen hotline is not as assumed (i.e., 40% drug related, 25% sex related, 25% stress related, and 10% education related). ▪

EXAMPLE 7.11

Goodness of Fit Test for Genetic Abnormalities

Genetic counselors work with pregnant women (usually women at high risk of fetal abnormalities or those who might not be at high risk but screen positive for abnormalities based on standard screening tests) and hypothesize that about one-half of all abnormalities are trisomy 21, one-third are trisomy 18, and the remainder are trisomy 13. (Trisomy indicates three copies of a particular chromosome, e.g., 21, and reflects a particular abnormality associated with that chromosome.) To test the hypothesis, a sample of 200 pregnant women who deliver babies with abnormalities are studied. The specific abnormalities are recorded and are summarized here. Based on the data, is the assumption regarding the distribution of abnormalities appropriate?

	Trisomy 21	Trisomy 18	Trisomy 13	Total
Number of women:	107	70	23	200

1. Set up hypotheses.

$$H_0: p_1 = 0.50, \ p_2 = 0.33, \ p_3 = 0.17$$
$$H_1: H_0 \text{ is false}, \quad \alpha = 0.05$$

2. Select the appropriate test statistic.

$$\chi^2 = \sum \frac{(O - E)^2}{E}$$

where $\sum$ indicates summation over the k response categories
   O = observed frequencies
   E = expected frequencies (i.e., if H_0 is true, or under H_0)

3. Decision rule.

In order to select the appropriate critical value, we first determine the degrees of freedom:

$$\text{df} = k - 1 = 3 - 1 = 2$$

The appropriate critical value of χ^2 is $\chi^2 = 5.99$ from Table B.5. The decision rule is

Reject H_0 if $\chi^2 \geq 5.99$
Do not reject H_0 if $\chi^2 < 5.99$

4. Test statistic.

To organize the computations of the test statistic (7.7), the following table is used:

	Trisomy 21	Trisomy 18	Trisomy 13	TOTAL
O = observed frequency:	107	70	23	200
E = expected frequency:	100	66	34	200
$(O - E)$:	7	4	−11	0
$(O - E)^2/E$:	$(7)^2/100 = 0.49$	$(4)^2/66 = 0.24$	$(-11)^2/34 = 3.55$	4.29

NOTE: The expected frequencies are computed assuming that H_0 is true.

The test statistic is $\chi^2 = 4.29$.

5. Conclusion.

Do not reject H_0 since $4.29 < 5.99$. We do not have significant evidence, $\alpha = 0.05$, to show that the distribution of abnormalities is not as assumed (i.e., 50% trisomy 21, 33% trisomy 18, and 17% trisomy 13).

7.5.2 Tests of Independence

We now consider applications involving two or more samples or two categorical variables, where interest lies in evaluating whether these two categorical variables are related (dependent) or unrelated (independent). The following example illustrates the use of the χ^2 test of independence.

EXAMPLE 7.12

Testing Independence Between Site and Treatment Regimen

The following data were collected in a multisite observational study of medical effectiveness in Type II diabetes. Three sites were involved: a health maintenance organization (HMO), a university teaching hospital (UTH), and an independent practice association (IPA). Type II diabetic patients were enrolled in the study from each site and monitored over a 3-year observation period. The data shown display the treatment regimens of patients measured at baseline by site.

Site	Treatment Regimen			
	Diet & Exercise	Oral Hypoglycemics	Insulin	TOTAL
HMO:	294	827	579	1700
UTH:	132	288	352	772
IPA:	189	516	404	1109
TOTAL:	615	1631	1335	3581

The table is a 3×3 *cross-tabulation table* or a *contingency table*. Both site and treatment regimen are categorical variables. Site is called the *row variable* and treatment regimen is called the *column variable*. The number of rows in the table is denoted R and the number of columns is denoted C. In this example, $R = 3$ and $C = 3$. The *row totals* are shown on the right side of the table, and the *column totals* are shown at the bottom of the table. The row and column totals are called the *marginal totals*. The 9 combinations of site and treatment regimen are called the *cells* of the table (e.g., patients in the HMO treated by diet and exercise denote one cell of the table, patients in the HMO treated by oral hypoglycemics denote another, and so on).

We wish to use the data to test the hypothesis that the two variables (site and treatment regimen) are independent (i.e., no difference in treatment regimens across sites). The hypotheses are written as follows:

1. Set up hypotheses.

H_0: Site and Treatment Regimen are independent   (No relationship between site and treatment regimen)

H_1: H_0 is false, $\alpha = 0.05$ (Site and treatment regimen are related)

NOTE: In the test of independence, the hypotheses are generally expressed in words as opposed to mathematical symbols.

2. Select the appropriate test statistic.

The test statistic in the test of independence is similar to the test statistic used in the goodness-of-fit test illustrated in the previous section. It is based on the *observed frequencies,* or numbers of subjects in each cell of the contingency table. In this example, we involved 1700 patients from the HMO, 772 from the UTH, and 1109 from the IPA. If the null hypothesis, H_0, is true (i.e., if there is no relationship between site and treatment regimen), we would expect the distribution of patients by treatment regimen to be similar across sites (i.e., the proportions of patients in each treatment regimen would be approximately equal in each of the sites).

Again, χ^2 tests are based on the agreement between expected (under H_0) and observed (sample) frequencies. Recall from probability theory, that when two events are independent, the probability of their intersection is given by

$$P(A \text{ and } B) = P(A) \cdot P(B) \tag{7.8}$$

For example, if site and treatment regimen are independent, then the probability that a patient is in the HMO *and* treated by diet and exercise is given by

$$P(\text{HMO and Diet/Exercise}) = P(\text{HMO}) \cdot P(\text{Diet/Exercise})$$
$$= (1700/3581)(615/3581) = (0.4747)(0.1717) = 0.0815$$

Similarly, if site and treatment regimen are independent, then the probability that a patient is in the UTH and treated by insulin is given by

$$P(\text{UTH and Insulin}) = P(\text{UTH}) \cdot P(\text{Insulin})$$
$$= (772/3581)(1335/3581) = (0.216)(0.373) = 0.0806$$

Therefore, if site and treatment regimen are independent, the probabilities (or proportions) of patients in each cell of the table can be computed using (7.8). To compute the test statistic, we must compute the *expected frequencies* (i.e., the *expected numbers* of patients in each cell of the table if site and treatment regimen are independent). Formula (7.8) yields the proportions of patients in each cell. To convert these proportions to frequencies, we use the following:

$$\text{Expected cell frequency} = n \cdot P(\text{cell}) \qquad (7.9)$$

This is equivalent to

$$\text{Expected cell frequency} = (\text{Row total} \cdot \text{Column total})/n \qquad (7.10)$$

For example, if site and treatment regimen are independent, then the expected number of patients in the HMO and treated by diet and exercise is given by (7.9) as

$$\text{Expected frequency (HMO and Diet/Exercise)} = 3581(0.0815) = 291.9$$

Equivalent to this by (7.10) is

$$\begin{aligned}\text{Expected frequency (HMO and Diet/Exercise)} \\ = (1700)(615)/3581 = 291.9\end{aligned}$$

The χ^2 statistic for tests of independence is given by

$$\chi^2 = \sum \frac{(O - E)^2}{E} \qquad (7.11)$$

where $\sum$ indicates summation over all cells of the contingency table
$\quad O$ = observed frequencies
$\quad E$ = expected frequencies (i.e., if H_0 is true, or under H_0)

The statistic follows a χ^2 distribution and has df $= (R - 1)(C - 1)$, where R = the number of rows in the contingency table and C = the number of columns in the contingency table.

Similar to the goodness-of-fit tests, we reject the null hypothesis in favor of the alternative hypothesis if the value of the test statistic is large. The test statistic (7.11) is large when the observed and expected frequencies are not similar.

3. Decision rule.

In order to select the appropriate critical value, we first determine the degrees of freedom:

$$\text{df} = (R - 1)(C - 1) = (3 - 1)(3 - 1) = 2(2) = 4$$

The appropriate critical value of χ^2 is $\chi^2 = 9.49$ from Table B.5. The decision rule is

$$\text{Reject } H_0 \text{ if } \chi^2 \geq 9.49$$
$$\text{Do not reject } H_0 \text{ if } \chi^2 < 9.49$$

4. Test statistic.

To organize the computations of the test statistic (7.11), we use the contingency table given earlier. The observed frequencies in each cell are shown. We compute the expected frequencies for each cell using (7.10) and display expected frequencies in parentheses to distinguish them from the observed frequencies. The computations are shown in detail for a few sample cells.

| *Site* | *Diet & Exercise* | *Treatment Regimen* | | *TOTAL* |
		Oral Hypoglycemics	*Insulin*	
HMO:	294 ((1700*615)/ 3581 = 291.9)	827 ((1700*1631)/ 3581 = 774.3)	579 ((1700*1335)/ 3581 = 633.8)	1700
UTH:	132 ((772*615/ 3581 = 132.6)	288 (351.6)	352 (287.8)	772
IPA:	189 (190.5)	516 (505.1)	404 (413.4)	1109
TOTAL:	615	1631	1335	3581

NOTE: The marginal totals of the expected frequencies = the marginal totals of the observed frequencies. For example, 291.9 + 774.3 + 633.8 = 1700. Similarly, 291.9 + 132.6 + 190.5 = 615.

Using the observed and expected frequencies, we compute the test statistic (7.11):

$$\chi^2 = \sum \frac{(O-E)^2}{E} = \frac{(294 - 291.9)^2}{291.9} + \frac{(827 - 774.3)^2}{774.3} + \frac{(579 - 633.8)^2}{633.8}$$

$$+ \frac{(132 - 132.6)^2}{132.6} + \frac{(288 - 351.6)^2}{351.6} + \frac{(352 - 287.8)^2}{287.8}$$

$$+ \frac{(189 - 190.5)^2}{190.5} + \frac{(516 - 505.1)^2}{505.1} + \frac{(404 - 413.3)^2}{413.4}$$

$$\chi^2 = 0.014 + 3.359 + 4.732 + 0.003 + 11.509 + 14.320$$
$$+ 0.011 + 0.235 + 0.215 = 34.629$$

5. Conclusion.

Reject H_0 since $34.629 \geq 9.49$. We have significant evidence, $\alpha = 0.05$, to show that site and treatment regimen are not independent (i.e., they are related). For this example, $p < 0.005$ (see Table B.5). Notice in the table that there are discrepancies between the observed and expected frequencies, particularly among the university teaching hospital patients.

SAS EXAMPLE 7.12 **Testing Independence Between Site and Treatment Regimen Using SAS**

The following output was generated using SAS Proc Freq. We requested a chi-square test of independence. In this example, we also requested some additional statistics, which are described following the output.

SAS Output for Example 7.12

```
                    The FREQ Procedure
                  Table of site by trt
        site            trt
        Frequency       |
        Expected        |
        Cell Chi-Square|
        Percent         |
        Row Pct         |
        Col Pct         |diet     |insulin |oral     |  Total
        ---------------+--------+--------+--------+
        hmo             |    294 |    579 |    827 |   1700
                        | 291.96 | 633.76 | 774.28 |
                        | 0.0143 | 4.7318 | 3.5895 |
                        |   8.21 |  16.17 |  23.09 |  47.47
                        |  17.29 |  34.06 |  48.65 |
                        |  47.80 |  43.37 |  50.71 |
        ---------------+--------+--------+--------+
        ipa             |    189 |    404 |    516 |   1109
                        | 190.46 | 413.44 | 505.1  |
                        | 0.0112 | 0.2154 | 0.235  |
                        |   5.28 |  11.28 |  14.41 |  30.97
                        |  17.04 |  36.43 |  46.53 |
                        |  30.73 |  30.26 |  31.64 |
        ---------------+--------+--------+--------+
        uth             |    132 |    352 |    288 |    772
                        | 132.58 | 287.8  | 351.61 |
                        | 0.0026 | 14.32  | 11.509 |
                        |   3.69 |   9.83 |   8.04 |  21.56
                        |  17.10 |  45.60 |  37.31 |
                        |  21.46 |  26.37 |  17.66 |
        ---------------+--------+--------+--------+
        Total               615     1335     1631     3581
                          17.17    37.28    45.55   100.00
```

```
              Statistics for Table of site by trt
    Statistic                           DF        Value          Prob
    ---------------------------------------------------------------
    Chi-Square                           4       34.6291        <.0001
    Likelihood Ratio Chi-Square          4       34.4975        <.0001
    Mantel-Haenszel Chi-Square           1       10.5953        0.0011
    Phi Coefficient                               0.0983
    Contingency Coefficient                       0.0979
    Cramer's V                                    0.0695
                      Sample Size = 3581
```

Interpretation of SAS Output for Example 7.12

SAS generates a contingency table and in each cell of the table displays a number of statistics. We requested some additional statistics here (compare this output with the outputs of SAS Examples 7.5 and 7.6). In each cell, SAS produces the Frequency, the Expected frequency (computed by formula (7.10)), the Cell Chi-Square (computed by formula (7.11) in each cell), the Percent, the Row Percent, and the Column Percent. (See legend in top left corner of the table.)

SAS generates a number of statistics that can be used to assess relationships between variables in a contingency table. We are concerned with the test of H_0: Site and Treatment Regimen are independent versus H_1: H_0 is false. SAS produces the χ^2 statistic $= 34.629$ and the associated p value, $p < 0.0001$. Assuming $\alpha = 0.05$, we reject H_0 since $p = 0.0001 < \alpha = 0.05$. We have significant evidence, $\alpha = 0.05$, to show that site and treatment regimen are not independent (i.e., they are related).

To understand the nature of the relationship, we evaluate the Row Percents. For example, among HMO patients, 17% are on Diet, 34% on Insulin, and 49% on Oral Hypoglycemics. Among the IPA patients, 17% are on Diet, 36% on Insulin, and 47% on Oral Hypoglycemics. There is little difference between the treatment regimens of patients at these two sites. The difference appears to be with the UTH patients. Among the UTH patients, 17% are on Diet, 46% on Insulin, and 37% on Oral Hypoglycemics. A higher proportion of IPA patients are on Insulin as compared to the other sites. This resulted in a statistically significant difference. Is it clinically meaningful? ■

EXAMPLE 7.13   ## Testing Independence Between Gender and Treatment Regimen

Consider the study described in Example 7.12. Suppose an investigator is interested in evaluating whether or not treatment regimens differ by gender. Restricting our analyses to the HMO patients, the following table displays the numbers of male and female patients according to their treatment regimens. Based on the data, is there evidence of a significant relationship between gender and treatment regimen among the HMO patients?

Gender	Treatment Regimen			
	Diet & Exercise	Oral Hypoglycemics	Insulin	TOTAL
Female:	147	435	256	838
Male:	147	392	323	862
TOTAL:	294	827	579	1700

In this contingency table, gender is the row variable ($R = 2$) and treatment regimen is the column variable ($C = 3$).

1. Set up hypotheses.

H_0: Gender and Treatment Regimen are independent   (No relationship between gender and treatment regimen)

H_1: H_0 is false, $\alpha = 0.05$ (Gender and treatment regimen are related)

2. Select the appropriate test statistic.

$$\chi^2 = \sum \frac{(O - E)^2}{E}$$

where $\sum$ indicates summation over all cells of the contingency table
O = observed frequencies
E = expected frequencies (i.e., if H_0 is true, or under H_0)

3. Decision rule.
In order to select the appropriate critical value, we first determine the degrees of freedom:

$$\text{df} = (R - 1)(C - 1) = (2 - 1)(3 - 1) = 1(2) = 2$$

The appropriate critical value of χ^2 is $\chi^2 = 5.99$ from Table B.5. The decision rule is

Reject H_0 if $\chi^2 \geq 5.99$
Do not reject H_0 if $\chi^2 < 5.99$

4. Test statistic.

To organize the computations of the test statistic (7.11), we use the contingency table given previously. The observed frequencies in each cell are shown along with the expected frequencies computed by (7.10) and displayed in parentheses.

		Treatment Regimen		
Gender	*Diet & Exercise*	*Oral Hypoglycemics*	*Insulin*	TOTAL
Female:	147 (144.9)	435 (407.7)	256 (285.4)	838
Male:	147 (149.1)	392 (419.3)	323 (293.6)	862
TOTAL:	294	827	579	1700

Using the observed and expected frequencies, we compute the test statistic (7.11):

$$\chi^2 = \sum \frac{(O-E)^2}{E} = \frac{(147-144.9)^2}{144.9} + \frac{(435-407.7)^2}{407.7}$$

$$+ \frac{(256-285.4)^2}{285.4} + \frac{(147-149.1)^2}{149.1}$$

$$+ \frac{(392-419.3)^2}{419.3} + \frac{(323-293.6)^2}{293.6}$$

$$\chi^2 = 0.030 + 1.833 + 3.031 + 0.029 + 1.782 + 2.947 = 9.652$$

5. Conclusion.

Reject H_0 since $9.652 \geq 5.99$. We have significant evidence, $\alpha = 0.05$, to show that gender and treatment regimen are not independent (i.e., they are related) in the sample of HMO patients. For this example, $p < 0.01$ (see Table B.5).

SAS EXAMPLE 7.13 **Testing Independence Between Gender and Treatment Regimen Using SAS**

The following output was generated using SAS Proc Freq. Again, we requested a chi-square test of independence but not as many statistics as were requested for SAS Example 7.12. A brief interpretation appears after the output.

SAS Output for Example 7.13

```
                    The FREQ Procedure
                  Table of gender by trt
       gender       trt
       Frequency|
       Percent  |
       Row Pct  |
       Col Pct  |diet     |insulin |oral     |   Total
       ---------+---------+--------+---------+
       female   |    147  |   256  |    435  |    838
                |   8.65  | 15.06  |  25.59  |  49.29
                |  17.54  | 30.55  |  51.91  |
                |  50.00  | 44.21  |  52.60  |
       ---------+---------+--------+---------+
       male     |    147  |   323  |    392  |    862
                |   8.65  | 19.00  |  23.06  |  50.71
                |  17.05  | 37.47  |  45.48  |
                |  50.00  | 55.79  |  47.40  |
       ---------+---------+--------+---------+
       Total         294      579      827     1700
                   17.29    34.06    48.65   100.00
```

```
          Statistics for Table of gender by trt
Statistic                         DF      Value        Prob
------------------------------------------------------------
Chi-Square                         2      9.6519      0.0080
Likelihood Ratio Chi-Square        2      9.6684      0.0080
Mantel-Haenszel Chi-Square         1      2.6751      0.1019
Phi Coefficient                           0.0753
Contingency Coefficient                   0.0751
Cramer's V                                0.0753
```

```
            Sample Size = 1700
```

Interpretation of SAS Output for Example 7.13

SAS generates a contingency table and in each cell of the table displays the Frequency, the Percent, the Row Percent, and the Column Percent. (See legend in top left corner of table.) The Frequency is the number of subjects in each cell; the Percent is the percent of all subjects in each cell. For example, there are 147 patients in the top left cell (i.e., females on diet and exercise treatment). These patients reflect 8.65% of the total sample (i.e., 147/1700 = 0.0865). The Row Percent is the percent of subjects in the particular row that fall in that cell. For example, there are 838 female patients or 838 patients in the first row of the contingency table. The 147 female patients on diet and exercise treatment reflect 17.54% of all female patients (i.e., 147/838 = 0.1754). The Column Percent is the percent of subjects in the particular column that fall in that cell. For example, there are 294 patients treated by diet and exercise. These 294 patients appear in the first column of the contingency table. The 147 female patients on diet and exercise treatment reflect 50% of all patients treated by diet and exercise (i.e., 147/294 = 0.50). The row total and column total (called the marginal totals) are displayed to the right and at the bottom of the contingency table, respectively. Both row and column frequencies and percents (of total) are displayed.

SAS generates a number of statistics that can be used to assess relationships between variables in a contingency table. We are concerned with the test of H_0: Gender and Treatment Regimen are independent versus H_1: H_0 is false. SAS produces the χ^2 statistic = 9.652 and the associated p value, $p = 0.008$. Assuming $\alpha = 0.05$, we reject H_0 since $p = 0.008 < \alpha = 0.05$. We have significant evidence, $\alpha = 0.05$, to show that gender and treatment regimen are not independent (i.e., they are related) in the sample of HMO patients. What is the nature of the relationship between gender and treatment? ■

NOTE: Chi-square tests are valid when the expected frequencies in each cell (or response category) are greater than or equal to 5. If an expected frequency falls below 5, then alternative techniques should be used.

EXAMPLE 7.14

Testing Independence Between Center and Genetic Abnormalities

Consider the study described in Example 7.11 involving the distribution of abnormalities among women who deliver babies with abnormalities. Suppose we wish to test if there is a difference in the distribution of abnormalities among clinical centers. Based on the following data, is there evidence of a significant relationship between the types of abnormalities and clinical center?

	Type of Abnormality			
	Trisomy 21	*Trisomy 18*	*Trisomy 13*	*Total*
Center A:	107	70	23	200
Center B:	65	62	23	150
Center C:	60	32	8	100
Total:	232	164	54	450

1. Set up hypotheses.

   H_0: Center and Type of Abnormality are independent
   H_1: H_0 is false, $\alpha = 0.05$

2. Select the appropriate test statistic.

$$\chi^2 = \sum \frac{(O - E)^2}{E}$$

3. Decision rule.

In order to select the appropriate critical value, we first determine the degrees of freedom:

$$df = (R - 1)(C - 1) = (3 - 1)(3 - 1) = 2(2) = 4$$

The appropriate critical value of χ^2 is $\chi^2 = 9.49$ from Table B.5. The decision rule is

Reject H_0 if $\chi^2 \geq 9.49$

Do not reject H_0 if $\chi^2 < 9.49$

4. Test statistic.

To organize the computations of the test statistic (7.11), we use the contingency table given earlier. The observed frequencies in each cell are shown. We compute the expected frequencies for each cell using (7.10) and display expected frequencies in parentheses to distinguish them from the observed frequencies.

	Treatment Regimen			
Center:	Trisomy 21	Trisomy 18	Trisomy 13	TOTAL
Center A:	107 (103.1)	70 (72.9)	23 (24)	200
Center B:	65 (77.3)	62 (54.7)	23 (18)	150
Center C:	60 (51.6)	32 (36.4)	8 (12)	100
TOTAL:	232	164	54	450

Using the observed and expected frequencies, we compute the test statistic (7.11). Only the results are shown here.

$$\chi^2 = 0.15 + 0.12 + 0.04 + 1.96 + 0.97 + 1.39 + 1.37 + 0.53 + 1.33$$
$$= 7.86$$

5. Conclusion.

Do not reject H_0 since $7.86 < 9.49$. We do not have significant evidence, $\alpha = 0.05$, to show that there is an association between clinical center and type of trisomy.

7.6 Precision, Power, and Sample Size Determination

In Section 7.2, we illustrated estimation techniques for the population proportion p. The following formula is used to determine the sample size requirements to produce an estimate for p with a certain level of precision:

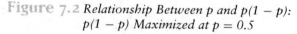

$$n = p(1 - p)\left(\frac{Z_{1-(\alpha/2)}}{E}\right)^2 \tag{7.12}$$

where $Z_{1-(\alpha/2)}$ reflects the desired level of confidence (e.g., 95%)
p = the population proportion
E = margin of error

Equation (7.12) produces the *minimum* number of subjects required to ensure a margin of error equal to E in the confidence interval for p with the specified level of confidence. Recall that in estimating the sample size to make an inference about μ, an estimate of σ was required. Several alternatives were suggested to estimate σ. In the binomial case, our goal is to make an inference about p. However, the formula for estimating the sample size (7.12) involves p. An estimate from a previous study or an estimate based on pilot data may be used in (7.12). If such an estimate is not available, it can be shown that $p(1 - p)$ is maximized at $p = 0.50$ (see Figure 7.2). Therefore, the most

Figure 7.2 *Relationship Between p and p(1 − p): p(1 − p) Maximized at p = 0.5*

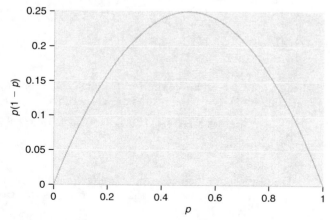

conservative estimate of n is produced by substituting $p = 0.5$ into the formula (7.12):

$$n = 0.5(1 - 0.5) \left(\frac{Z_{1-(\alpha/2)}}{E} \right)^2 \tag{7.13}$$

which is equivalent to

$$n = 0.25 \left(\frac{Z_{1-(\alpha/2)}}{E} \right)^2 \tag{7.14}$$

where $Z_{1-(\alpha/2)}$ reflects the desired level of confidence (e.g., 95%)
E = margin of error

EXAMPLE 7.15

Sample Size Determination to Estimate Proportion of Patients Who Favor New Policy

An investigator wishes to estimate the proportion of patients in a particular health plan in favor of a new policy (e.g., reimbursement for services) and wants the estimate to be within 3% of the true proportion of patients in favor of the new policy. How many subjects would be required to produce such an estimate with 95% confidence?

Suppose that there is no available data on the issue, that is, no estimate for p that can be used in (7.12). Therefore (7.14) is used:

$$n = 0.25 \left(\frac{Z_{1-(\alpha/2)}}{E} \right)^2$$

Substituting $E = 0.03$ (the margin of error in the estimate of the proportion) and the appropriate value for 95% confidence:

$$n = 0.25 \left(\frac{1.96}{0.03} \right)^2 = 1067.1$$

Since (7.14) produces the minimum number of subjects to satisfy our criteria, 1068 patients must be sampled in order to produce a 95% confidence interval estimate for the proportion of patients in favor of the new policy with a margin of error of 3%.

SAS EXAMPLE 7.15

Sample Size Determination to Estimate Proportion of Patients Who Favor New Policy Using SAS

SAS does not have a procedure to generate sample size requirements. However, we can program formulas (7.12) and (7.14) as we did in previous chapters. In the following, we generated sample size requirements for various scenarios, including the one described in Example 7.15. A brief interpretation appears after the output.

SAS Output for Example 7.15

Obs	c_level	z	p	e	n
1	0.95	1.95996	0.5	0.03	1068
2	0.95	1.95996	0.1	0.03	385
3	0.95	1.95996	0.2	0.03	683
4	0.95	1.95996	0.3	0.03	897
5	0.95	1.95996	0.4	0.03	1025
6	0.95	1.95996	0.5	0.03	1068
7	0.95	1.95996	0.6	0.03	1025
8	0.95	1.95996	0.7	0.03	897
9	0.95	1.95996	0.8	0.03	683
10	0.95	1.95996	0.9	0.03	385

Interpretation of SAS Output for Example 7.15

We considered several scenarios. The first scenario reflects the situation in Example 7.15 where p is not known and we use the most conservative $p = 0.5$. SAS estimates that $n = 1068$ subjects are required. To illustrate the effect of the estimate of p on the computations, we considered various values of p in scenarios 2–10. Specifically, we considered $p = 0.10, 0.20, \ldots, 0.90$. Notice that the sample size estimate is largest when $p = 0.5$. ■

EXAMPLE 7.16

Sample Size Determination to Estimate Proportion of High School Seniors Who Smoke

A study is run to estimate the proportion of high school seniors who smoke. The study involved a random sample of 100 high school seniors, and 28 reported that they were smokers. A 95% confidence interval for the true proportion of all high school seniors who smoke was computed as 0.28 ± 0.088. Suppose that we wanted to estimate the true proportion with a margin of error not exceeding 0.05 (the analysis based on the sample of size 100 had a margin of error of 0.088). How many subjects would be required to ensure a margin of error of 0.05 with 95% confidence?

Because we have data from the initial study, we use (7.12):

$$n = p(1 - p)\left(\frac{Z_{1-(\alpha/2)}}{E}\right)^2 = 0.28(1 - 0.28)\left(\frac{1.96}{0.05}\right)^2 = 309.8$$

In order to estimate the true proportion of high school seniors who smoke with a margin of error of 0.05, we need a sample of at least 310 high school seniors. ■

In Chapter 5, we introduced the concepts of precision (in estimation) and statistical power (in hypothesis testing). We now present formulas for determining sample size to achieve a specified power in the two-sample test for proportions. Recall, power (Power $= 1 - \beta = P(\text{Reject } H_0 | H_0 \text{ false})$) depends on three components:

1. n_i = sample sizes $(i = 1, 2)$
2. α = level of significance = $P(\text{Type I error})$
3. ES = the effect size = the standardized difference in proportions specified under H_0 and H_1

In the two-sample applications the hypotheses are

$$H_0\text{: } p_1 = p_2$$
$$H_1\text{: } p_1 \neq p_2$$

or equivalently,

$$H_0\text{: } p_1 - p_2 = 0$$
$$H_1\text{: } p_1 - p_2 \neq 0$$

where p_1 = proportion of successes in population 1
p_2 = proportion of successes in population 2

The effect size (ES) is defined as the difference in the proportions under H_0 and H_1. In the two-sample applications, the parameter of interest is $(p_1 - p_2)$. The ES is defined as follows:

$$ES = |p_2 - p_1| \tag{7.15}$$

In many applications, the number of subjects (i.e., n_1 and n_2) that can be involved depends on financial, logistic, and/or time constraints. In other cases, the sample size required to ensure a certain level of power can be determined relative to alternative hypotheses of importance. The sample size required to ensure a specific level of power in a *two-sided, two independent samples test for proportions* is

$$n_i = \left(\frac{\sqrt{\overline{p}\,\overline{q}\,2}\;Z_{1-(\alpha/2)} + \sqrt{p_1 q_1 + p_2 q_2}\;Z_{1-\beta}}{ES} \right)^2 \tag{7.16}$$

where n_i is the minimum number of subjects required in sample
$i\ (i = 1, 2)$
$Z_{1-(\alpha/2)}$ is the value from the standard normal distribution with lower-tail area equal to $1 - \alpha/2$
$Z_{1-\beta}$ is the value from the standard normal distribution with lower-tail area equal to $1 - \beta$
ES is the effect size (7.15)

In addition, p_1 = proportion of successes in population 1, $q_1 = 1 - p_1$
p_2 = proportion of successes in population 2, $q_2 = 1 - p_2$

$$\overline{p} = \frac{p_1 + p_2}{2}, \qquad \overline{q} = 1 - \overline{p}$$

The following example illustrates the use of formula (7.16).

EXAMPLE 7.17

Sample Size Determination in Tests for Differences in Proportions

Suppose we wish to design a study to compare two treatments with respect to the proportion of successes in each. A two-sided test is planned at a 5% level of significance. Based on a review of the literature, $p_1 = 0.20$. How many subjects would be required per group to detect $p_2 = 0.10$ with 90% power?

The formula to determine sample sizes is given by (7.16):

$$n_i = \left(\frac{\sqrt{\overline{p}\,\overline{q}\,2}\ Z_{1-(\alpha/2)} + \sqrt{p_1 q_1 + p_2 q_2}\ Z_{1-\beta}}{ES} \right)^2$$

The *ES* is (7.15)

$$ES = |p_2 - p_1| = |0.10 - 0.20| = 0.10$$

Since $\alpha = 0.05$, $Z_{1-(\alpha/2)} = Z_{0.975} = 1.96$. Similarly, for power $= 0.90$, $\beta = 0.10$; therefore, $Z_{1-\beta} = 1.282$.

$$\overline{p} = \frac{0.10 + 0.20}{2} = 0.15, \qquad \overline{q} = 1 - 0.15 = 0.85$$

Substituting,

$$n_i = \left(\frac{\sqrt{0.15(0.85)2}(1.96) + \sqrt{0.20(0.80) + (0.10)(0.90)}(1.282)}{0.10} \right)^2 = 265.9$$

Thus, $n_1 = n_2 = 266$ subjects (532 total) are needed.   ▪

SAS does not have a procedure to generate sample size requirements. We can program formulas (7.15) and (7.16) as we did in previous chapters. In the following, we generated sample size requirements for various scenarios, including the one described in Example 7.17. A brief interpretation appears after the output.

SAS Output for Example 7.17

Obs	alpha	beta	z_alpha2	z_beta	p1	p2	power	es	n_2
1	0.05	0.1	1.95996	1.28155	0.2	0.1	0.9	0.1	266
2	0.05	0.1	1.95996	1.28155	0.2	0.3	0.9	0.1	392
3	0.05	0.2	1.95996	0.84162	0.2	0.1	0.8	0.1	199
4	0.05	0.2	1.95996	0.84162	0.2	0.3	0.8	0.1	294

Interpretation of SAS Output for Example 7.17

We considered several scenarios. The first scenario reflects the situation in Example 7.17. SAS estimates that 266 subjects are required per group to detect the specified difference with 90% power. In scenario 2, we specify $p_2 = 0.3$. Notice that the effect size is the same as the effect size in scenario 1. However, SAS estimates that 392 subjects are required per group. The values of p_1 and p_2 affect the sample size computation (and not just the difference between them). In the last two scenarios, we specify power = 80%. Notice that fewer cases are required to detect the same differences with lower power. ▪

7.7 Key Formulas

Application	Notation/Formula	Description
Confidence interval estimate for p	$\hat{p} \pm Z_{1-(\alpha/2)} \sqrt{\dfrac{\hat{p}(1-\hat{p})}{n}}$	See Table 7.1 for necessary conditions (find Z in Table B.2A)
Test $H_0: p = p_0$	$Z = \dfrac{\hat{p} - p_0}{\sqrt{\dfrac{p_0(1-p_0)}{n}}}$	See Table 7.1 for necessary conditions
Confidence interval estimate for $(p_1 - p_2)$	$(\hat{p}_1 - \hat{p}_2) \pm Z_{1-(\alpha/2)} \sqrt{\dfrac{\hat{p}_1(1-\hat{p}_1)}{n_1} + \dfrac{\hat{p}_2(1-\hat{p}_2)}{n_2}}$	See Table 7.2 for necessary conditions (find Z in Table B.2A)
Test $H_0: p_1 = p_2$	$Z = \dfrac{\hat{p}_1 - \hat{p}_2}{\sqrt{\hat{p}(1-\hat{p})\left(\dfrac{1}{n_1} + \dfrac{1}{n_2}\right)}}$	See Table 7.3 for necessary conditions and definitions of components of Z
Test H_0: distribution of responses follows specified pattern	$\chi^2 = \sum \dfrac{(O - E)^2}{E}, \ df = k - 1$	Chi-square goodness-of-fit test
Test H_0: two variables are independent	$\chi^2 = \sum \dfrac{(O - E)^2}{E}, \ df = (r - 1) * (c - 1)$	Chi-square test of independence
Find n to estimate p	$n = p(1-p) \left[\dfrac{Z_{1-(\alpha/2)}}{E}\right]^2$	Sample size to estimate p with margin of error E
Find n_1, n_2 to test $H_0: p_1 = p_2$	$n_i = \left(\dfrac{\sqrt{\bar{p}\bar{q}\,2}\,Z_{1-(\alpha/2)} + \sqrt{p_1 q_1 + p_2 q_2}\,Z_{1-\beta}}{ES}\right)^2$	Sample sizes to detect effect size ES with power $1 - \beta$

7.8 Statistical Computing

Following are the SAS programs that were used to generate the frequency distribution tables, confidence interval estimates for the proportion of successes in a population, the contingency tables, and the chi-square goodness-of-fit and tests of independence and to determine the required sample size to estimate *p* and to compare to proportions using a test of hypothesis. The SAS procedures used and brief descriptions are noted in the header to each example. Notes are provided to the right of the SAS programs (in blue) for orientation purposes and are not part of the programs. In addition, there are blank lines in the programs that are solely to accommodate the notes. Blank lines and spaces can be used throughout SAS programs to enhance readability. A summary of the SAS procedures used in the examples is provided at the end of this section.

SAS EXAMPLE 7.2 **Frequency Distribution Table for Single Categorical Variable, CI for *p*** *Estimate Proportion of Patients with Osteoarthritis (Example 7.2)*

Suppose we wish to estimate the proportion of patients in a particular physician's practice with diagnosed osteoarthritis. A random sample of 200 patients is selected and each patient's medical record is reviewed for the diagnosis of osteoarthritis. Suppose that 38 patients are observed with diagnosed osteoarthritis. Generate a frequency distribution table and determine a point estimate and 95% confidence interval using SAS for the proportion of all patients with diagnosed osteoarthritis.

Program Code

```
options ps=62 ls=80;
```
Formats the output page to 62 lines in length and 80 columns in width

```
data in;
  input x count;
```
Beginning of Data Step
Inputs two variables *x* and *count*, here $x = 0$ if the patient does not have osteoarthritis and $x = 1$ if the patient has osteoarthritis. Count reflects the number of patients in each category.

```
cards;
0 162
1 38
run;
```
Beginning of Raw Data section.
actual observations (value of *x* and *count* on each line)

```
proc freq;
```
Procedure call. Proc Freq generates a frequency distribution table for a categorical (or ordinal) variable.

```
  tables x/binomial
    (level='1');
```
Specification of analytic variable *x*. The binomial option requests a confidence interval for the proportion and the level='1' indicates that a success is coded as 1.

```
  weight count;
```
Specification of variable containing the number of subjects in each category. *count*.

```
run;
```
End of procedure section.

SAS EXAMPLE 7.5 **Cross-Tabulation Table**

Cross-Tabulation of Treatment by Long-Term Complications (Example 7.5)

A longitudinal study is conducted to evaluate the long-term complications in diabetic patients treated under two competing treatment regimens. Complications are measured by incidence of foot disease, eye disease, *or* cardiovascular disease within a 10-year observation period. The following 2×2 cross-tabulation table summarizes the data. Estimate the relative risk and odds ratio using SAS.

	Long-Term Complications		
Treatment	YES	NO	Total
Treatment 1	12	88	100
Treatment 2	8	92	100
Total	20	180	200

Program Code

```
options ps=62 ls=80;
```
Formats the output page to 62 lines in length and 80 columns in width.

```
data in;
  input trt $ compl $ count;
```
Beginning of Data Step

Inputs three variables *trt* (treatment 1 or 2), *compl* (complications yes or no) and *count*, where count reflects the number of patients in each cell of the table. Here we input both trt and compl using character labels, and we indicate this to SAS using the "$" symbol.

```
cards;
trt_1 z_no 88
trt_1 yes 12
trt_2 z_no 92
trt_2 yes 8
run;
```
Beginning of Raw Data section.

actual observations (value of *trt*, *compl* and *count* on each line)

Because SAS alphabetizes labels. we use z_no to ensure that the yes response is in column 1.

```
proc freq;
```
Procedure call. Proc Freq generates a contingency table for two categorical (or ordinal) variables.

```
  tables trt*compl;
  weight count;
```
Specification of analytic variables *trt* and *compl*.

Specification of variable containing the number of subjects in each cell of the table, *count*.

```
run;
```
End of procedure section.

SAS EXAMPLE 7.9 **Frequency Distribution Table and Chi-Square Goodness-of-Fit Test**
Chi-Square Goodness-of-Fit Test (Example 7.9)

Following coronary artery bypass graft (CABG) surgery, patients are encouraged to participate in a cardiac rehabilitation program. The program lasts approximately 14 weeks and includes exercise training, nutritional information, and general lifestyle guidelines. One particular hospital is offering three cardiac rehabilitation programs that are identical in content but are offered at three different times. The administration is interested in whether the three time slots are equally popular among or convenient for the patients. A total of 100 patients are involved in the investigation, and each patient is asked to select the one day and time (from three options) that is most convenient. The following data are observed:

	Mondays 6:00–7:30 PM	Thursdays 4:00–5:30 PM	Saturdays 8:00–9:30 AM
Time slot:			
Number of patients:	47	32	21

Program Code

```
options ps=62 ls=80;

data in;
  input day $ count;




cards;
Mon 47
Thurs 32
Sat 21
run;

proc freq;

  tables day/chisq
    testp=(0.33 0.33 0.33);

  weight count;

run;
```

Formats the output page to 62 lines in length and 80 columns in width

Beginning of Data Step

Inputs two variables *day* (which contains the 3 options) and *count*, which contains the number of patients in each response category. Here we input *day* using character data, and we indicate this to SAS using the "$" symbol

Beginning of Raw Data section.

actual observations (value of *day* and *count* on each line)

Procedure call. Proc Freq generates a frequency distribution table for a categorical (or ordinal) variable.

Specification of the analytic variable *day* and the chisq option along with the expected proportions (under H_0) in parentheses following the testp option.

Specification of variable containing the number of subjects in each cell of the table, *count*.

End of procedure section.

SAS EXAMPLE 7.12 **Contingency Table and Chi-Square Test of Independence**

*Test If There Is a Relationship Between Site and Treatment Regimen
(Example 7.12)*

The following data were collected in a multisite observational study of medical effectiveness in Type II diabetes. Three sites were involved in the study: a health maintenance organization (HMO), a university teaching hospital (UTH), and an independent practice association (IPA). Type II diabetic patients were enrolled in the study from each site and monitored over a 3-year observation period. The data shown display the treatment regimens of patients measured at baseline by site. Test if there is a relationship between site and treatment regimen using the chi-square test of independence in SAS.

	Treatment Regimen			
Site	*Diet & Exercise*	*Oral Hypoglycemics*	*Insulin*	TOTAL
HMO:	294	827	579	1700
UTH:	132	288	352	772
IPA:	189	516	404	1109
TOTAL:	615	1631	1335	3581

Program Code

```
options ps=62 ls=80;


data in;
  input site $ trt $ count;
```

Formats the output page to 62 lines in length and
  80 columns in width
Beginning of Data Step
Inputs three variables *site* (HMO, UTH, or IPA), *trt* (diet,
  oral hypoglycemics, or insulin) and *count*, where count
  reflects the number of patients in each cell of the table.
  Here we input both site and *trt* using character labels,
  and we indicate this to SAS using the "$" symbol.

```
cards;
hmo diet 294
hmo oral 827
hmo insulin 579
uth diet 132
uth oral 288
uth insulin 352
ipa diet 189
ipa oral 516
ipa insulin 404
run;
```

Beginning of Raw Data section.
actual observations (value of *site*,
trt and *count* on each line)

```
proc freq;
```
Procedure call. Proc Freq generates a contingency table for two categorical (or ordinal) variables.

```
 tables site*trt/expected cellchi2 chisq;
```
Specification of analytic variables *site* and *trt*. We also request that SAS produce expected frequencies in each cell, the chi-square statistic for each cell and run a chi-square test of independence with the expected, cellchi2, and chisq options, respectively.

```
 weight count;
```
Specification of variable containing the number of subjects in each cell of the table, *count*.

```
run;
```
End of procedure section.

SAS EXAMPLE 7.13 **Contingency Table and Chi-Square Test of Independence**

Test If There Is a Relationship Between Gender and Treatment Regimen (Example 7.13)

Suppose an investigator is interested in evaluating whether or not treatment regimens differ by gender. Restricting our analyses to the HMO patients, the following table displays the numbers of male and female patients according to their treatment regimens. Based on the data, is there evidence of a significant relationship between gender and treatment regimen among the HMO patients? Test if there is a relationship between site and treatment regimen using the chi-square test of independence in SAS.

	Treatment Regimen			
Gender	Diet & Exercise	Oral Hypoglycemics	Insulin	TOTAL
Female:	147	435	256	838
Male:	147	392	323	862
TOTAL:	294	827	579	1700

Program Code

```
options ps=62 ls=80;
```
Formats the output page to 62 lines in length and 80 columns in width

```
data in;
 input gender $ trt $ count;
```
Beginning of Data Step

Inputs three variables gender (male or female), *trt* (diet, oral hypoglycemics or insulin), and *count*, where count reflects the number of patients in each cell of the table. Here we input both gender and trt using character labels, and we indicate this to SAS using the "$" symbol

```
cards;
male diet 147
male oral 392
male insulin 323
female diet 147
female oral 435
female insulin 256
run;

proc freq;

  tables gender*trt/chisq;



  weight count;

run;
```

Beginning of Raw Data section.

actual observations (value of *gender*, *trt*, and *count* on each line)

Procedure call. Proc Freq generates a contingency table for two categorical (or ordinal) variables.

Specification of analytic variables *gender* and *trt*. We request that SAS runs a chi-square test of independence with the chisq option.

Specification of variable containing the number of subjects in each cell of the table, *count*.

End of procedure section.

SAS EXAMPLE 7.15 **Determine the Number of Subjects Required to Generate a Confidence Interval for p**

Patients in Favor of a New Policy (Example 7.15)

An investigator wishes to estimate the proportion of patients in a particular health plan in favor of a new policy (e.g., reimbursement for services) and wants the estimate to be within 3% of the true proportion of patients in favor of the new policy. How many subjects would be required to produce such an estimate with 95% confidence?

Program Code

```
options ps=62 ls=80;
data in;
  input c_level e p;
z=probit((1-c_level)/2);

if p=. then p=0.5;

tempn=(p*(1-p))*(z/e)**2;

n=ceil(tempn);
```

Formats the output page to 55 lines in length and 80 columns in width

Beginning of Data Step

Inputs 3 variables *c_level*, *e*, and *p*.

Determines the value from the standard normal distribution (*z*) with lower-tail area (1-*c_level*)/2

If *p* is not available (input as missing), then SAS recodes *p* to 0.5 (see (7.13))

Creates a temporary variable, called *tempn*, determined by formula (7.12)

Computes a variable *n* using the ceil function, which computes the smallest integer greater than *tempn* (i.e., rounds up)

```
/*    Input the following information (required)          Beginning of comment section
    c_level: Confidence Level: range 0.0 to 1.0 (e.g., 0.95),
    e: Margin of Error, and
    p  Proportion of Successes: range 0.0 to 1.0
    NOTE: p may not be available, in which case enter . to indicate
        p is missing
*/                                                        End of comment
cards;                                                    Beginning of Raw Data section
0.95   0.03    .                                          actual observations
0.95   0.03  0.10                                         values of c_level, e, and p
0.95   0.03  0.20                                         on each line
0.95   0.03  0.30
0.95   0.03  0.40
0.95   0.03  0.50
0.95   0.03  0.60
0.95   0.03  0.70
0.95   0.03  0.80
0.95   0.03  0.90
run;


proc print;                                              Procedure call. Print to display
  var c_level z p e n;                                   input and computed variables.
run;                                                     End of procedure section.
```

SAS EXAMPLE 7.17 **Determine the Number of Subjects Required to Detect a Specific Effect Size in a Test of Hypothesis About $(p_1 - p_2)$**

Sample Size Requirements (Example 7.17)

Suppose we wish to design a study to compare two treatments with respect to the proportion of successes in each. A two sided test is planned at a 5% level of significance. Based on a review of the literature, $p_1 = 0.20$. How many subjects would be required per group to detect $p_2 = 0.10$ with 90% power?

Program Code

```
options ps=62 ls=80;          Formats the output page to 62 lines in length and 80 columns in width
data in;                      Beginning of Data Step.
  input alpha power p1 p2;    Inputs 4 variables alpha, power, p1, and p2.
z_alpha2=probit(1-alpha/2);   Determines the value from the standard normal distribution with
                                lower-tail area 1-alpha/2.

beta=1-power;                 Computes beta.
z_beta=probit(1-beta);        Determines the value from the standard normal distribution with
                                lower-tail area 1-beta
```

```
q1=1-p1;
q2=1-p2;
pbar=(p1+p2)/2;
qbar=1-pbar;
es=abs(p2-p1);

tempn_2=(sqrt(pbar*qbar*2)*z_alpha2+sqrt(p1*q1+p2*q2)*z_beta)**2/
        (es)**2;

n_2=ceil(tempn_2);


/*

   Input the following information (required)
   alpha: Level of Significance: range 0.0 to 1.0 (e.g., 0.05),
   power: Power: range 0.0 to 1.0 (e.g., 0.80),
   p1: Proportion of Successes in Group 1, and
   p2: Proportion of Successes in Group 2.

*/
cards;
0.05 0.90 0.20 0.10
0.05 0.90 0.20 0.30
0.05 0.80 0.20 0.10
0.05 0.80 0.20 0.30
run;

proc print;
   var alpha beta z_alpha2 z_beta p1 p2
       power es n_2;
run;
```

Compute components for (7.16)

Computes the effect size (es)
Compute (7.16)

Computes a variable n_2 using the ceil function, which computes the smallest integer greater than tempn_2 (i.e., rounds up).

Beginning of comment section

End of comment section
Beginning of Raw Data section
actual observations

Procedure call. Print to display computed variables.

End of procedure section

7.8.1 Summary of SAS Procedures

The SAS Freq Procedure is used to generate a frequency distribution table and to generate contingency tables. Specific options can be requested to produce estimates of relative risks and odds ratios, and to run a chi-square test of independence. The specific options are shown in italics below. Users should refer to the examples in this section for complete descriptions of the procedure and specific options. A general description of the procedure and options is provided in the table on the next page.

Procedure	Sample Procedure Call	Description
proc freq	proc freq; tables x/*binomial (level = '1')*; *weight count*;	Generates a frequency distribution table for a categorical (or ordinal) variable. When x is dichotomous, the binomial option can be specified to generate a CI for the proportion. The level = '1' statement indicates that a success is coded as 1. The weight option indicates that summary data are input and the variable count contains the numbers of subjects in each response category.
	proc freq; tables x/*chisq testp=(p0 p1 p2 ... pk)*;	Generates a frequency distribution table for a categorical (or ordinal) variable. The chisq option is used to request a goodness-of-fit test and the values following the testp option indicate the expected proportions for the k response categories
	proc freq; tables a*b;	Generates a contingency table (*a* by *b*).
	proc freq; tables a*b/expected cellchi2 chisq;	Generates a contingency table and produces the expected frequency in each cell, the value of the chi-square statistic in each cell, and runs the chi-square test of independence.

7.9 Analysis of Framingham Heart Study Data

The Framingham data set includes data collected from the original cohort. Participants contributed up to three examination cycles of data. Here we analyze data collected in the first examination cycle (called the period = 1 examination) and use SAS Proc Freq to generate frequency distribution tables and 95% confidence intervals for several dichotomous variables. We then run a goodness-of-fit test and a test of independence. For the last two illustrations, we created an ordinal variable with four levels from the continuous BMI variable as follows: BMI < 18.5 (underweight), 18.5–24.9 (normal weight), 25.0–29.9 (overweight), and ≥ 30.0 (obese). The SAS code to create this variable and to attach a format for better interpretability is given next.

Framingham Data Analysis—SAS Code

```
proc format;
 value bmifmt 1='<18.5      '2='18.5-24.9' 3='25.0-29.9' 4='30.0+';
run;
```

```
data fhs;
 set in.frmgham;
 if period=1;

if 0 le mbi lt 18.5 then bmi_grp=1;
else if 18.5 le bmi lt 25.0 then bmi_grp=2;
else if 25.0 le bmi lt 30.0 then bmi_grp=3;
else if bmi ge 30.0 then bmi_grp=4;
format bmi_grp bmifmt.;
run;

proc freq data=fhs;
 tables bpmeds cursmoke diabetes/binomial (level='1');
run;

proc freq data=fhs;
 tables bmi_grp/chisq testp=(0.01 0.39 0.40 0.20);
run;

proc freq data=fhs;
 tables sex*bmi_grp/chisq;
run;
```

Framingham Data Analysis—SAS Output

The FREQ Procedure

Anti-hypertensive meds Y/N

BPMEDS	Frequency	Percent	Cumulative Frequency	Cumulative Percent
0	4229	96.71	4229	96.71
1	144	3.29	4373	100.00

Frequency Missing = 61

Binomial Proportion
for BPMEDS = 1

Proportion	0.0329
ASE	0.0027
95% Lower Conf Limit	0.0276
95% Upper Conf Limit	0.0382

```
              Exact Conf Limits
              95% Lower Conf Limit        0.0278
              95% Upper Conf Limit        0.0387

                Test of H0: Proportion = 0.5

              ASE under H0                0.0076
              Z                          -61.7735
              One-sided Pr <  Z           <.0001
              Two-sided Pr > |Z|          <.0001

                Effective Sample Size = 4373
                  Frequency Missing = 61
```

Current Cig Smoker Y/N

CURSMOKE	Frequency	Percent	Cumulative Frequency	Cumulative Percent
0	2253	50.81	2253	50.81
1	2181	49.19	4434	100.00

The SAS System   9

The FREQ Procedure

```
                Binomial Proportion
                  for CURSMOKE = 1
           ---------------------------------
           Proportion                 0.4919
           ASE                        0.0075
           95% Lower Conf Limit       0.4772
           95% Upper Conf Limit       0.5066

           Exact Conf Limits
           95% Lower Conf Limit       0.4771
           95% Upper Conf Limit       0.5067

             Test of H0: Proportion = 0.5

           ASE under H0               0.0075
           Z                          -1.0813
           One-sided Pr <  Z          0.1398
           Two-sided Pr > |Z|         0.2796

                 Sample Size = 4434
                  Diabetic Y/N
```

DIABETES	Frequency	Percent	Cumulative Frequency	Cumulative Percent
0	4313	97.27	4313	97.27
1	121	2.73	4434	100.00

The SAS System   10

The FREQ Procedure

Binomial Proportion
for DIABETES = 1

Proportion   0.0273
ASE   0.0024
95% Lower Conf Limit   0.0225
95% Upper Conf Limit   0.0321

Exact Conf Limits
95% Lower Conf Limit   0.0227
95% Upper Conf Limit   0.0325

Test of H0: Proportion = 0.5

ASE under H0   0.0075
Z   -62.9540
One-sided Pr < Z   <.0001
Two-sided Pr > |Z| <.0001

Sample Size = 4434

For presentation, the preceding data could be summarized as follows:

	Percent	*95% CI*
Antihypertensive medication:	3.3%	(2.8%–3.9%)
Current smoking:	49.1%	(47.7%–50.7%)
Diabetes:	2.7%	(2.3%–3.3%)

Suppose that national data are reported to suggest that 1% of Americans are underweight, 39% are in the normal BMI range, 40% are overweight and 20% are obese. We are interested in whether the Framingham data follow that distribution. Using SAS, we perform a goodness-of-fit with that referent distribution and produce the following:

```
                    The FREQ Procedure
                                 Test    Cumulative   Cumulative
bmi_grp   Frequency    Percent  Percent   Frequency    Percent
-----------------------------------------------------------------
<18.5           76       1.71     1.00         76        1.71
18.5-24.9     1936      43.66    39.00       2012       45.38
25.0-29.9     1845      41.61    40.00       3857       86.99
30.0+          577      13.01    20.00       4434      100.00
```

```
                    Chi-Square Test
               for Specified Proportions
               --------------------------
               Chi-Square        158.4245
               DF                       3
               Pr > ChiSq         <.0001

               Sample Size = 4434
```

Do the Framingham data follow the reported distribution? How do the Framingham data line up with the national figures?

Using the same BMI categories, we now use SAS to test for a difference in the distribution of weight categories by sex.

```
                    The FREQ Procedure
                  Table of SEX by bmi_grp

SEX(SEX)       bmi_grp

Frequency|
Percent  |
Row Pct  |
Col Pct  |<18.5   |18.5-24.|25.0-29.|30.0+   |   Total
         |        |9       |9       |        |
---------+--------+--------+--------+--------+
M        |    17  |   703  |   992  |   232  |   1944
         |  0.38  |  15.85 |  22.37 |   5.23 |  43.84
         |  0.87  |  36.16 |  51.03 |  11.93 |
         |  22.37 |  36.31 |  53.77 |  40.21 |
---------+--------+--------+--------+--------+
F        |    59  |  1233  |   853  |   345  |   2490
         |  1.33  |  27.81 |  19.24 |   7.78 |  56.16
         |  2.37  |  49.52 |  34.26 |  13.86 |
         |  77.63 |  63.69 |  46.23 |  59.79 |
---------+--------+--------+--------+--------+
Total          76     1936     1845      577     4434
             1.71    43.66    41.61    13.01   100.00
```

```
              Statistics for Table of SEX by bmi_grp

Statistic                          DF        Value         Prob
------------------------------------------------------------------
Chi-Square                          3      135.7296       <.0001
Likelihood Ratio Chi-Square         3      136.8781       <.0001
Mantel-Haenszel Chi-Square          1       43.7383       <.0001
Phi Coefficient                               0.1750
Contingency Coefficient                       0.1723
Cramer's V                                    0.1750


                    Sample Size = 4434
```

Is there a significant difference in the distribution of weight categories by sex? If so, what is the nature of the difference?

7.10 Problems

1. Recent attention has focused on the health care system, particularly on managed care plans. A study was undertaken within one managed care plan to assess whether patients' reports of satisfaction with the plan were related to their leaving the plan within 1 year. In a random sample of 120 patients who reported that they were satisfied with the plan, 30 left that plan within 1 year. In a second random sample of 150 patients who reported that they were not satisfied with the plan, 62 left within 1 year. Compute a 95% confidence interval for the difference in the proportions of patients who left the plan within 1 year relative to their satisfaction reports.

2. An investigator wishes to estimate the proportion of Type II diabetic patients who take insulin to manage their diabetes. A large, national database of Type II diabetic patients is used to generate the estimate. The database involves a random sample of 1200 Type II diabetic patients, 423 of whom report taking insulin to manage their diabetes.
   a. Compute a point estimate for the proportion of all Type II diabetics who take insulin to manage their diabetes.
   b. Compute the standard error of the point estimate.
   c. Compute a 95% confidence interval for the proportion of all Type II diabetics who take insulin to manage their diabetes.

3. Recent studies have investigated the relationship between gender and career advancement. The following data represent a random sample of

mathematicians classified by gender and academic rank. Using the following data, test for a relationship between gender and academic rank.

	Instructor	Academic Rank Assistant Professor	Associate Professor	Full Professor
Female:	12	15	18	7
Male:	21	25	30	22

4. An investigator wishes to test if patients tend to use the middle response in 5-point ordinal scales more frequently than other response options. Scales such as these are used in health status and satisfaction measures. One hundred patients were asked to rate their own health on the following 5-point ordinal scale. Based on the data, is there evidence that the distribution of responses is 10%, 20%, 40%, 20%, 10%, respectively? Use $\alpha = 0.05$.

Health status:	Excellent	Very Good	Good	Fair	Poor
# Patients:	12	18	50	10	10

5. A manufacturer of medical devices has two plants and wants to compare them on the proportion of defective items produced. In a random sample of 250 items from plant I, 28 were defective. In a random sample of 220 items from plant II, 38 were defective. Is there any significant evidence to support the claim that plant II produces more defective items? Use a 5% level of significance.

6. As the first step in a study to evaluate highway fatalities, the traffic department wants to evaluate whether the left-hand lane of a three-lane highway services twice the traffic volume as the other two lanes. The following data were collected, reflecting the numbers of vehicles traveling each of the three lanes during the rush hour. Use the data to test the claim that twice as many vehicles travel the left lane as compared to the other two lanes ($\alpha = 0.05$).

	Right Lane	Center Lane	Left Lane
# Vehicles:	205	220	575

7. A corporation offers six different health plans to its employees. Each year the corporation offers them an opportunity to switch plans. In 2002, 15% of all employees switched from one plan to another. With all of the emphasis on health plans this year, the corporation thinks that a higher proportion of employees will switch. A random sample of 125 employees is selected, and 25 indicate that they will switch plans in 2003. Based on the data, is the proportion of employees who switch plans significantly higher in 2003? Run the appropriate test at a 5% level of significance.

8. A study is conducted over 10 years to investigate long-term complication rates in patients treated with two different therapies. The data are shown here:

Therapy	Complications	
	No	Yes
1:	911	89
2:	873	127

   a. Generate a point estimate for the difference in proportions.
   b. Compute a 95% confidence interval for the difference in proportions.
   c. Based on (a) and (b), is there a significant difference in the therapies?

9. A study is conducted comparing two experimental treatments to a control treatment with respect to their effectiveness in reducing joint pain in patients with arthritis. One hundred and fifty patients are randomly assigned to one of the three treatments, and the following data are collected, representing the numbers of patients reporting improvement in joint pain after the assigned treatment is administered:

	Control	Experimental 1	Experimental 2
Number of subjects:	50	50	50
Number reporting improvement:	21	28	34

   Is there a significant difference in the proportions of patients reporting improvement in joint pain among the treatments? Run the appropriate test at the 5% level of significance.

10. Using the data in Problem 9,

   a. Construct a 95% confidence interval for the difference in the proportions of patients reporting improvement in joint pain between the Control and Experimental 1 treatments.

   b. Based on (a), is there a significant difference in the proportions of patients reporting improvement in joint pain between the Control and Experimental 1 treatments? Justify your answer (be brief but complete).

11. An investigator wished to design a study to estimate the proportion of patients in a particular hospital whose primary insurance coverage is Medicaid.

   a. How many subjects would be required to estimate the true proportion within 4% with 95% confidence?

   b. Suppose a similar study was conducted in 2003 and produced the following 95% confidence interval for the proportion of patients in the same hospital whose primary insurance coverage was Medicaid: 27% ± 6%. If the point estimate from the 2003 study is used, how does that affect the answer given in (a)?

   c. Which answer is more appropriate, (a) or (b)? Be brief.

12. Prior to being randomized to one of two competing therapies, the severity of participants' migraines is clinically assessed. The following table displays the severity classifications for patients assigned to the medical and nontraditional therapies. Is there a significant association between severity and assigned therapy? Run the appropriate test at $\alpha = 0.05$.

	Severity Classification			
Therapy	*Minimal*	*Moderate*	*Severe*	*Total*
Medical	90	60	50	200
Nontraditional	50	60	90	200
Total	140	120	140	400

13. A survey is conducted among current MPH students to assess their knowledge of safe (alcohol) drinking limits. Two hundred students are randomly selected for the investigation, and 60% correctly identified safe drinking limits.

   a. Construct a 95% confidence interval for the proportion of all MPH students who could correctly identify safe drinking limits.

b. It has been reported that 70% of practicing clinicians can correctly identify safe drinking limits when asked in a survey format. One hundred of the MPH students involved in the survey are former or current practicing clinicians, and 72% of these individuals correctly identified safe drinking limits in the survey. Is the proportion of current MPH students who are former or current practicing clinicians significantly different from the proportion reported in the literature? Run the appropriate test at $\alpha = 0.05$.

14. Suppose we wish to design a study to estimate the proportion of patients who received pain therapy following a particular surgical procedure in a local hospital. How many subjects would be required in the study to ensure that the estimate was within 4 percentage points of the true proportion with 95% confidence?

15. The following table was derived from a study of HIV patients, and the data reflect the numbers of subjects classified by their primary HIV risk factor and gender. Test if there is a relationship between HIV risk factor and gender using a 5% level of significance.

	Gender	
HIV Risk Factor	Male	Female
IV drug user:	24	40
Homosexual:	32	18
Other:	15	25

16. Under standard care, 10% of all patients suffering their first MI are readmitted to the hospital within 6 weeks. A new protocol for care following the first MI is proposed and evaluated. Two hundred patients receive the new protocol following an MI and 12 are readmitted to the hospital within 6 weeks. Is there a significant reduction in the proportion of patients readmitted to the hospital within 6 weeks under the new protocol? Run the appropriate test at the 5% level of significance.

17. Suppose that the data in Problem 16 are criticized based on the use of a 10% readmission rate under standard care. A new study is mounted to directly compare standard care to the new protocol using a randomized trial. Based on the following data, is there a significant reduction in the readmission rate under the new protocol? Run the appropriate test at the 5% level of significance.

Treatment	Number of Patients	Number Readmitted Within 6 Weeks
Standard care	125	16
New protocol	125	11

18. Some investigators suggest that medication adherence exceeding 85% is sufficient to classify a patient as "adherent" and medication adherence below 85% suggests that the patient is "not adherent." Suppose in a clinical trial that each patient is classified as either adherent or not based on this definition.

a. Construct a 95% confidence interval for the difference in proportions of adherent patients between the intervention and control groups using the data shown here.

	Intervention	Control
Number of patients:	75	75
Number with medication adherence ≥ 85%:	47	36

b. Based on (a), is there a significant difference in proportions of adherent patients between the intervention and control groups? Justify your answer briefly.

19. Patients were enrolled into the study described in Problem 18 from three clinical centers. Based on the following data, is there a significant difference in the proportions of adherent patients among the clinical centers? Run the appropriate test at $\alpha = 0.05$.

	Enrollment Sites		
	Center 1	Center 2	Center 3
Adherent (>85%):	28	30	25
Not adherent (<85%):	21	29	17

20. Suppose an observational study is conducted to investigate the smoking behaviors of male and female patients with a history of coronary heart disease. Among 220 men surveyed, 80 were smokers. Among 190 women surveyed, 95 were smokers.

a. Construct a 95% confidence interval for the difference in the proportions of males and females who smoke.

b. Based on (a), would you reject $H_0: p_1 = p_2$ in favor of $H_1: p_1 \neq p_2$? Justify your answer briefly.

21. Suppose we wish to estimate what proportion of patients in an HMO spend more than $500 on prescription medications over 12 months. In a random sample of 150 patients, 34% spent more than $500.

a. Construct a 95% confidence interval for the true proportion of patients who spend more than $500 on prescription medications per year.

b. How many subjects would be required to estimate the true proportion who spend more than $500 on prescription medications per year with a margin of error no more than 2%, with 95% confidence?

22. Suppose a cross-sectional study is conducted to investigate cardio-vascular risk factors among a sample of patients seeking medical care at one of two local hospitals. A total of 200 patients are enrolled. Construct a 95% confidence interval for the difference in proportions of patients with a family history of cardiovascular disease (CVD) between hospitals.

	Enrollment Site	
Family History of CVD	Hospital 1	Hospital 2
Yes:	24	14
No:	76	86
Total:	100	100

23. The following table was constructed based on a comparison of various sociodemographic characteristics between men and women enrolled in a study of cardiovascular risk factors:

Characteristic	Men (n = 160)	Women (n = 140)	p
Mean age (SD)	45 (7.8)	46 (8.6)	0.7256
% High school graduate	78	64	0.0245
Mean annual income (SD)	47,345 (8,456)	31.987 (9,645)	0.0001
% with no insurance	8	9	0.9876

a. Which, if any, of the characteristics shown are significantly different between men and women? Assume $\alpha = 0.05$. Justify your answer.

b. Write the hypotheses tested and show the formula of the test statistic used to compare educational levels between men and women.

c. Suppose we wish to test whether the study population (men and women combined) had a significantly higher-than-average proportion of patients with no insurance. The reported proportion is 7%. Write the hypotheses we would test, and show the formula of the test statistic we would use to conduct such a test.

24. Investigators want to use a self-reported measure of pain to evaluate the effectiveness of a new medication designed to reduce postoperative pain. Before using the measure, they examine its distributional properties in a sample of patients recently undergoing knee surgery. Postprocedure, each patient is asked to rate pain on the following scale: no pain, minimal pain, some pain, moderate pain, or severe pain. The investigators hypothesize that the distribution of responses will be approximately normal, on the order of 1 to 2 to 4 to 2 to 1 across the response categories. Use the following data to test the claim at a 5% level of significance:

	Pain				
	None	Minimal	Some	Moderate	Severe
Number of patients:	15	25	46	36	18

25. Suppose the measure described in Problem 24 is used to compare a newly developed pain medication against a standard medication with respect to self-reported pain. Using the following data, is there a difference in the pain levels of patients on the different medications? Run the appropriate test at a 5% level of significance.

	Pain				
	None	Minimal	Some	Moderate	Severe
New:	20	35	41	15	6
Standard:	15	25	46	36	18

26. In the application described in Problem 25, suppose instead of using the five-level pain measure, the investigators collapse the responses as follows: {None, Minimal, and Some = Low Pain} and {Moderate and

Severe = High Pain}. Is there a significant difference in the proportions of patients with High Pain between medication groups? Run the appropriate test at a 5% level of significance.

27. A study is conducted comparing three different prenatal care programs among women at high risk for preterm delivery. The programs differ in intensity of medical intervention. Women who meet the criteria for high risk of preterm delivery are asked to participate in the study and are randomly assigned to one of the three prenatal care programs. At the time of delivery, they are classified as preterm or term delivery. Based on the following data, is there a relationship between the prenatal care programs and preterm delivery? Run the appropriate test at $\alpha = 0.05$.

	Program 1: Minimal Intensity	Program 2: Moderate Intensity	Program 3: High Intensity
Preterm:	34	18	12
Term:	36	52	58

28. A national study reports that 28% of high school students smoke. We wish to test if the smoking rate is higher than the national rate among freshmen at a local university. To run the test, we take a random sample of 200 freshmen, and 32% report that they smoke. Run the appropriate test at a 5% level of significance.

SAS Problems

Use SAS to solve the following problems.

1. Recent studies have investigated the relationship between gender and career advancement. The following data represent a random sample of mathematicians classified by gender and academic rank:

		Academic Rank		
	Instructor	Assistant Professor	Associate Professor	Full Professor
Female:	12	15	18	7
Male:	21	25	30	22

Use SAS Proc Freq to generate a contingency table and run a chi-square test of independence. Use a 5% level of significance.

2. A study is conducted over 10 years to investigate long-term compli-cation rates in patients treated with two different therapies. The data are

Therapy	Complications	
	No	Yes
1	911	89
2	873	127

Use SAS Proc Freq to generate a contingency table and test if there is a significant difference in the proportions of patients with complications between therapies.

3. Prior to being randomized to one of two competing therapies, the severity of participants' migraines is clinically assessed. The following table displays the severity classifications for patients assigned to the medical and the nontraditional therapies:

Therapy	Severity Classification			
	Minimal	Moderate	Severe	Total
Medical:	90	60	50	200
Nontraditional:	50	60	90	200
Total:	140	120	140	400

Use SAS Proc Freq to generate a contingency table and run a chi-square test of independence. Use a 5% level of significance.

4. Use SAS to estimate the sample sizes required in each group in Problem 3 to test the hypothesis $H_0: p_1 = p_2$. Consider a two-sided test. Suppose that $p_1 = 0.4$, and consider the following values for p_2: 0.20, 0.25, 0.30. How many subjects would be required to detect the specified differences with a power of 80% at a 5% level of significance?

5. Suppose we wish to estimate what proportion of patients in an HMO spend more than $500 on prescription medications over 12 months. In a random sample of 150 patients, 34% spent more than $500.

   a. Use SAS to determine the number of subjects that would be required to estimate the true proportion who spend more than $500 on prescription medications per year with a margin of error no more than 2% with 95% confidence.

b. Consider scenarios where the margin of error is 1%, 3%, and 5%. What is the effect of changing the margin of error on the number of subjects required?

c. Suppose that the sample described was not available. What would the estimate be in (a) without that information?

8

Comparing Risks in Two Populations

In Chapter 7 we introduced estimation and statistical inference procedures for categorical variables. We presented statistical inference techniques for both one- and two-sample cases where the analytic variable was dichotomous. We also considered multinomial distributions and introduced chi-square tests.

In this chapter we extend our discussion of the two-sample case with a dichotomous analytic variable and consider the specific application of comparing risks in two populations. This situation is very common in biostatistical research. For example, consider a clinical trial of a proposed stroke-prevention medication. Participants are randomly assigned to one of two treatments and are followed over the course of a 5-year study period. The analytic outcome variable is dichotomous: The participant either had a stroke during the follow-up period or did not. Another example is a longitudinal study of two populations in which the outcome variable of interest is the development of cardiovascular disease. In both of these situations, the interest is in comparing the risks of the outcome, or the proportion who develop disease in the two populations.

In Section 8.1, we introduce several effect measures used to compare risks in two populations, and in Section 8.2, we present confidence intervals for these effect measures. In Section 8.3, we review the use of the chi-square test in comparing risks in two populations and present a computational formula for the test statistic. We describe in Section 8.4 a test to be used when the assumptions of the chi-square test are not met. In Section 8.5, we present a method for calculating an adjusted relative risk and performing an adjusted chi-square test. In Section 8.6, we review the power and sample size calculations presented in Chapter 7. We summarize key formulas and present statistical computing applications in Sections 8.7 and 8.8, respectively. In Section 8.9, we use data from the Framingham Heart Study to illustrate the applications presented here.

8.1 Effect Measures

Dichotomous outcome variables in biostatistical applications usually represent events such as the development of a disease, a change in disease severity, or mortality. The parameters of interest are the population proportions, or the conditional probabilities of the event in the two populations. For example, consider the example in which one group receives treatment 1 and the other receives treatment 2 and the event of interest is stroke. The two parameters are the probability of having a stroke during a 5-year follow-up period conditional on receiving treatment 1 (p_1) and the probability of having a stroke during the 5-year follow-up period conditional on receiving treatment 2 (p_2). The probability of having the outcome of interest is often called the *risk* of that outcome. As described in Chapter 7, we estimate these probabilities, or risks, using the sample proportions in each treatment group, $\hat{p}_1$ and $\hat{p}_2$.

EXAMPLE 8.1

Risk of Coronary Abnormalities on Gamma Globulin and Aspirin

A clinical trial of gamma globulin in the treatment of children with Kawasaki syndrome randomized approximately half of the patients to receive gamma globulin. The standard treatment for Kawasaki syndrome was a regimen of aspirin; however, about one-quarter of these patients developed coronary abnormalities even under the standard treatment. The outcome of interest was the development of coronary abnormalities (CA) over a 7-week follow-up period. The following 2×2 cross-tabulation table summarizes the results of the trial.

Treatment Group	Coronary Abnormalities, $CA = 1$	No Coronary Abnormalities, $CA = 0$	Total
Gamma Globulin, $GG = 1$:	5	78	83
Aspirin, $GG = 0$:	21	63	84
Total:	26	141	167

Overall, 26 of the 167 patients developed coronary abnormalities. The estimated conditional probability or risk of developing coronary abnormalities given the standard treatment (aspirin) is $\hat{p}_0 = 21/84 = 0.25$. The risk of CA given treatment with gamma globulin is $\hat{p}_1 = 5/83 = 0.06$. ▪

A number of statistics are used to compare conditional probabilities of outcomes between populations (or treatments). Measures of difference in risk are known as *effect* measures. Three of these measures are the risk difference, the relative risk, and the odds ratio.

The simple difference between risks is called the *risk difference* and is estimated as follows:

$$\text{Estimate of risk difference} = \hat{R}D = \hat{p}_1 - \hat{p}_0 \tag{8.1}$$

A risk difference of zero indicates no difference in risks, a positive RD indicates higher risk in group 1, and a negative RD indicates lower risk in group 1. In Example 8.1, the risk difference is estimated as $\hat{R}D = 0.06 - 0.25 = -0.19$. The risk of CA in patients treated with gamma globulin is 0.19 lower than the risk in patients on the standard treatment. Note that you can reverse the roles of the groups and calculate the risk difference as $RD = \hat{p}_0 - \hat{p}_1$. In Example 8.1, this would yield an estimate of 0.19 (instead of -0.19), indicating a higher risk in group 0. The convention is to estimate the risk difference using (8.1), where $\hat{p}_0$ is the estimate of risk in the control or standard treatment group.

The relative risk is the ratio of the risks and is estimated as follows:

$$\text{Estimate of relative risk} = \hat{R}R = \hat{p}_1/\hat{p}_0 \tag{8.2}$$

A relative risk of 1 indicates no difference in risks, a RR greater than 1 indicates a higher risk in group 1, and a RR less than 1 indicates a lower risk in group 1. In Example 8.1, the relative risk is estimated as $\hat{R}R = (0.06/0.25) = 0.24$. The risk of CA in patients treated with gamma globulin is 24% (less than a quarter) of the risk of CA in those on standard treatment. Again, we can reverse the groups and estimate the relative risk as $\hat{R}R = \hat{p}_0/\hat{p}_1$. However, in many cases, such as in clinical trials, it is easier to interpret a relative risk in which group 1 is compared to group 0. For example, in a clinical trial, the relative risk as defined in (8.2) compares the treated group to the control group. In Example 8.1, the estimated $\hat{R}R = 0.24$, which is the risk in the gamma globulin treatment group relative to the risk in the standard treatment group. Reversing the comparison groups would yield $\hat{R}R = (0.25/0.06) = 4.17$, which is interpreted (awkwardly) as lack of treatment with gamma globulin more than quadruples the risk of coronary abnormalities.

The third measure commonly used to compare risks in two populations is the odds ratio, based on a comparison of the odds of the outcome in the two groups. Suppose that $x =$ the number of outcome events in a trial of size n. We estimate the risk of the event as $\hat{p} = x/n$. The odds of the event are defined as $\hat{o} = x/(n - x)$, the ratio of events to nonevents.

In Example 8.1, the odds of CA in the standard treatment group (GG = 0) are estimated at $\hat{o}_0 = 21/63 = 0.333$. The odds of CA in the gamma globulin group are estimated at $\hat{o}_1 = 5/78 = 0.064$. The odds can also be estimated using the sample proportion, as follows:

$$\text{Estimate of odds} = \hat{o} = \frac{x}{(n - x)} = \frac{x/n}{(n - x)/n} = \frac{x/n}{(1 - x/n)} = \frac{\hat{p}}{(1 - \hat{p})}$$

The odds ratio is estimated by the ratio of the odds in group 1 to the odds in group 2:

$$\text{Estimate of odds ratio} = \hat{O}R = \frac{\hat{o}_1}{\hat{o}_0} = \frac{\hat{p}_1/(1 - \hat{p}_1)}{\hat{p}_0/(1 - \hat{p}_0)} \qquad (8.3)$$

In Example 8.1, the odds ratio is estimated as $\hat{O}R = (5/78)/(21/63) = 0.064/0.333 = 0.192$. The odds of CA in the gamma globulin group are less than a fifth the odds of CA in the standard treatment group.

The interpretation of the odds ratio is not as intuitive as is the relative risk. However, there are some research designs in which the relative risk cannot be estimated, and in those situations, the odds ratio can be used to estimate a relative risk. If the event is rare (i.e., p is small), the odds ratio is a very good estimate of relative risk, because when p is small, $(1 - p)$ is very close to 1, so the odds $o = p/(1 - p)$ are very close to p. For example, if $p = 0.1$, then $(1 - p) = 0.9$ and $o = (0.1/0.9) = 0.11$, which is close to $p = 0.1$. For more common events, the odds are not a good estimate of the probability of that event. For example, if $p = 0.5$, then $(1 - p) = 0.5$ and $o = (0.5/0.5) = 1.0$, which is not close to p.

When the prevalence is less than 0.10, the odds of an event generally provide a good estimate of the probability of the event. In Example 8.1, the risk of CA is low in the GG group (0.06) and the estimated odds $\hat{o}_1 = 0.064$, is very close to $\hat{p}_1 = 0.060$. In the standard treatment group, the risk is higher (0.250) and $\hat{o}_0 = 0.333$ is larger than $\hat{p}_0 = 0.250$. Overall, the risk of CA is 0.156. The estimate of the odds ratio, $\hat{OR} = 0.192$, is smaller than the estimate of the relative risk, $\hat{RR} = 0.240$. ■

8.2 Confidence Intervals for Effect Measures

In Chapter 7, we presented techniques for statistical inference concerning the difference in proportions and introduced the chi-square goodness-of-fit tests and tests of independence. In this section, we provide formulas for calculating confidence intervals around the three effect measures used to compare risks in two populations.

The general case involving two populations with a dichotomous outcome variable can be represented by the general 2×2 table in Table 8.1. This framework facilitates many of the calculations needed for statistical inference. In this framework, the letter a represents x_1, the number of successes in group 1, and $(a + b)$ represents n_1, the sample size in group 1. Likewise, the letter c represents x_0, the number of successes in group 0, and $(c + d)$ represents n_0, the sample size in group 0.

The convention is to label events as 1 if present and 0 if absent. Similarly, the active or experimental treatment is usually labeled 1 and the control (e.g., placebo) is usually labeled 0. The estimated risks and effect measures can be expressed as follows using the notation of Table 8.1:

$$\hat{p}_1 = \frac{a}{(a + b)}, \qquad \hat{o}_1 = a/b$$

$$\hat{p}_0 = \frac{c}{(c + d)}, \qquad \hat{o}_0 = c/d$$

Table 8.1 *General Form of a 2 × 2 Table*

Treatment or Comparison Group	Outcome		
	1	*0*	
1	a	b	$a + b$
0	c	d	$c + d$
	$a + c$	$b + d$	N

Table 8.2 *Confidence Intervals for RD, RR, and OR*

Risk Difference:	$\hat{RD} \pm Z_{1-(\alpha/2)} \sqrt{\left(\dfrac{\hat{p}_0(1-\hat{p}_0)}{n_0}\right) + \left(\dfrac{\hat{p}_1(1-\hat{p}_1)}{n_1}\right)}$
Relative Risk:	$\exp\left(\ln(\hat{RR}) \pm Z_{1-(\alpha/2)} \sqrt{\dfrac{(d/c)}{n_0} + \dfrac{(b/a)}{n_1}}\right)$
Odds Ratio:	$\exp\left(\ln(\hat{OR}) \pm Z_{1-(\alpha/2)} \sqrt{\left(\dfrac{1}{a} + \dfrac{1}{b} + \dfrac{1}{c} + \dfrac{1}{d}\right)}\right)$

$$\text{Estimate of risk difference} = \hat{RD} = (\hat{p}_1 - \hat{p}_0) = \frac{a}{a+b} - \frac{c}{c+d} \quad (8.4)$$

$$\text{Estimate of relative risk} = \hat{RR} = \hat{p}_1/\hat{p}_0 = \frac{a/(a+b)}{c/(c+d)} \quad (8.5)$$

$$\text{Estimate of odds ratio} = \hat{OR} = \frac{\hat{O}_1}{\hat{O}_0} = \frac{a/b}{c/d} \quad (8.6)$$

The risk difference defined in (8.1) and (8.4) is simply the point estimate for the difference in proportions $(p_1 - p_0)$ introduced in Chapter 7. The confidence interval estimate of the risk difference is given in Table 7.3 and again in Table 8.2. Confidence interval formulas for the other two effect measures are also given in Table 8.2. Notice that the formulas for the confidence intervals for RR and OR are given in terms of the notation in Table 8.1.

As in Table 7.3, the three confidence intervals in Table 8.2 all assume that $\min(n_0\hat{p}_0, n_0(1-\hat{p}_0)) \geq 5$ *and* $\min(n_1\hat{p}_1, n_1(1-\hat{p}_1)) \geq 5$. This assumption is satisfied if the cell frequencies a, b, c, and d are each at least 5.

Recall Example 8.1 in which we compared gamma globulin to standard treatment with respect to the development of coronary abnormalities. The results are summarized next using the notation of Table 8.1.

EXAMPLE 8.1

Estimating Difference in Risk of Coronary Abnormalities on Gamma Globulin and Aspirin (continued)

Treatment Group	Coronary Abnormalities, CA = 1	No Coronary Abnormalities, CA = 0	Total
Gamma Globulin, GG = 1:	$a = 5$	$b = 78$	83
Aspirin, GG = 0:	$c = 21$	$d = 63$	84
Total:	26	141	167

We now calculate 95% confidence intervals for the RD, RR, and OR using the formulas in Table 8.2. First we check the sample size assumption, and note that each of the cell frequencies is at least 5. Next, we substitute the following into the formulas in Table 8.2:

$$\hat{RD} = -0.19, \qquad \hat{RR} = 0.24, \qquad \hat{OR} = 0.19$$

$$\hat{p}_0 = 0.25, \qquad \hat{p}_1 = 0.06, \qquad n_0 = 84, \qquad n_1 = 83$$

$$a = 5, \qquad b = 78, \qquad c = 21, \qquad d = 63$$

A 95% confidence interval for the *risk difference* is given by

$$\hat{RD} \pm Z_{1-(\alpha/2)} \sqrt{\left(\frac{\hat{p}_0(1-\hat{p}_0)}{n_0}\right) + \left(\frac{\hat{p}_1(1-\hat{p}_1)}{n_1}\right)}$$

$$-0.19 \pm 1.96 \sqrt{\left(\frac{0.25(0.75)}{84}\right) + \left(\frac{0.06(0.94)}{83}\right)}$$

$$-0.19 \pm 1.96(.054)$$

$$-0.19 \pm 0.106$$

$$(-0.296, -0.084)$$

The risk of coronary abnormalities in patients treated with gamma globulin is *lower* than that in patients on the standard treatment by 19%. We are 95% confident that the true difference in risk of coronary abnormalities in patients treated with gamma globulin as compared to patients on the standard treatment is between −29.6% and −8.4% (or is from 8.4% to 29.6% lower).

A 95% confidence interval for the *relative risk* is given by

$$\exp\left(\ln(\hat{RR}) \pm Z_{1-(\alpha/2)} \sqrt{\frac{(d/c)}{n_0} + \frac{(b/a)}{n_1}}\right)$$

$$\exp\left(\ln(0.24) \pm 1.96 \sqrt{\frac{(63/21)}{84} + \frac{(78/5)}{83}}\right)$$

$$\exp(-1.423 \pm 1.96(0.473))$$

$$\exp(-1.423 \pm 0.927)$$

$$(0.095, 0.609)$$

The risk of coronary abnormalities in patients treated with gamma globulin i less than a quarter the risk in patients on the standard treatment ($RR = 0.24$). We are 95% confident that the true relative risk of coronary abnormalities in patients treated with gamma globulin as compared to patients on the stan dard treatment is between 0.095 and 0.609.

A 95% confidence interval for the *odds ratio* is given by

$$\exp\left(\ln(\hat{OR}) \pm Z_{1-(\alpha/2)}\sqrt{\left(\frac{1}{a} + \frac{1}{b} + \frac{1}{c} + \frac{1}{d}\right)}\right)$$

$$\exp\left(\ln(0.19) \pm 1.96\sqrt{\left(\frac{1}{5} + \frac{1}{78} + \frac{1}{21} + \frac{1}{63}\right)}\right)$$

$$\exp(-1.649 \pm 1.96(0.526))$$

$$\exp(-1.649 \pm 1.030)$$

$$(0.069, 0.539)$$

The odds of coronary abnormalities in patients treated with gamma glob ulin are less than one-fifth the odds in patients on the standard treatmen ($OR = 0.19$). We are 95% confident that the true relative risk of coronary ab normalities in patients treated with gamma globulin as compared to patient on the standard treatment is between 0.069 and 0.539.

SAS EXAMPLE 8.1 **Estimating Difference in Risk of Coronary Abnormalities on Gamma Globulin and Aspirin Using SAS**

The following output was generated for the data in Example 8.1 using SA Proc Freq, which produces a contingency table (or cross-tabulation) whe two variables are specified. Notice that the row percentages in the "CA column are 6.02% and 25% for those in the gamma globulin and standar treatment groups, respectively. These are the estimated risks we calculated a 0.06 and 0.25.

We requested that SAS provide the odds ratio and relative risk and 95% confidence intervals. It is important that the event of interest is reported in th first column, as SAS calculates the relative risk and odds ratios assuming tha is the case. The relative risks and odds ratios compare the row 1 group to th row 2 group. For that reason, we make sure that the GG = 1 group is i the first row so that the effect measures will compare the gamma globuli group to the standard treatment group. A brief interpretation appears afte the output.

SAS Output for Example 8.1

```
                     The FREQ Procedure
                  Table of group by event

   group       event

   Frequency|
   Percent  |
   Row Pct  |
   Col Pct  |CA        |noCA      |   Total
   ---------+--------+--------+
   GG       |       5 |      78 |      83
            |    2.99 |   46.71 |   49.70
            |    6.02 |   93.98 |
            |   19.23 |   55.32 |
   ---------+--------+--------+
   noGG     |      21 |      63 |      84
            |   12.57 |   37.72 |   50.30
            |   25.00 |   75.00 |
            |   80.77 |   44.68 |
   ---------+--------+--------+
   Total           26       141        167
                15.57     84.43     100.00

          Statistics for Table of group by event

        Estimates of the Relative Risk (Row1/Row2)
```

Type of Study	Value	95% Confidence Limits	
Case-Control (Odds Ratio)	0.1923	0.0686	0.5388
Cohort (Col1 Risk)	0.2410	0.0954	0.6089
Cohort (Col2 Risk)	1.2530	1.0948	1.4340

```
                  Sample Size = 167
```

Interpretation of SAS Output for Example 8.1

We requested that SAS provide the odds ratio and the relative risk. The *OR* is given in the first row and the *RR* is given in the next row, labeled Col1 Risk, as it is the relative risk of the event in the first column (CA) of the 2 × 2 table. Note that the values SAS provides for the *OR* and *RR* agree with those we calculated earlier. The 95% confidence limits are also given for the odds ratio and relative risk. ■

8.3 The Chi-Square Test of Homogeneity

The chi-square test was introduced in Chapter 7 as a technique to be used in tests for goodness of fit and independence. The chi-square test of homogeneity can be used to test hypotheses concerning risks in two populations. The null hypothesis is that the risks are the same in the two populations, or that the two populations are *homogeneous* with respect to risk.

$$H_0: p_0 = p_1$$
$$H_1: p_0 \neq p_1$$

Now consider the relationship between the effect measures and the risks. If the two risks are the same, then the risk difference must be equal to zero and both the relative risk and odds ratios must be equal to 1. Thus, the null hypothesis may equivalently be written in terms of the risk difference,

$$H_0: RD = 0$$
$$H_1: RD \neq 0$$

the relative risk,

$$H_0: RR = 1$$
$$H_1: RR \neq 1$$

or the odds ratio,

$$H_0: OR = 1$$
$$H_1: OR \neq 1$$

As stated in Chapter 7, χ^2 tests are based on the agreement between observed (sample) and expected (under H_0) frequencies. We therefore calculate expected frequencies using the fact that the risks in the two groups are equal under the null hypothesis.

| EXAMPLE 8.2 | **Testing Difference in Risk of Stroke Between Treatments** |

Consider again the example of a clinical trial of a proposed stroke prevention medication. Suppose that 250 participants are randomly assigned to receive either the new treatment ($n_1 = 120$) or a placebo ($n_0 = 130$) and are followed over the course of a 5-year follow-up period. During the 5-year follow-up period, 12 of the 120 subjects in the new treatment group (T = 1) and 28 of the 130 subjects in the placebo group (T = 0) had strokes. Thus, $\hat{p}_1 = 0.100$ and $\hat{p}_0 = 0.215$. These results are given in the following table:

Treatment Group	Stroke	Event No Stroke	Total
$T = 1$	12	108	120
$T = 0$	28	102	130
	40	210	250

Suppose we want to test the hypothesis that the risk of stroke is different between treatment groups.

1. Set up hypotheses.
$$H_0: p_0 = p_1$$
$$H_1: p_0 \neq p_1$$

Alternatively, the hypotheses can be phrased in terms of the relative risk of stroke in the new treatment group ($T = 1$) as compared to the placebo group ($T = 0$):
$$H_0: RR = 1$$
$$H_1: RR \neq 1$$

2a. Select the appropriate test statistic.

We test the null hypothesis of homogeneity using the χ^2 test of homogeneity:
$$\chi^2 = \sum \frac{(O - E)^2}{E} \tag{8.7}$$

where $\sum$ indicates summation over all four cells of the table
O = observed frequency
E = expected frequency

The test statistic χ^2 follows a χ^2 distribution with df $= 1$ as long as the expected frequencies in each cell are at least 5. The critical value (see Table B.5 in the Appendix) for a test with $\alpha = 0.05$ is $\chi^2 = 3.84$.

2b. Check that the test is valid.

We must calculate the expected frequencies and check that each is at least 5 so that we can be sure the test statistic follows the χ^2 distribution. Combining the two treatment groups, we see that 40 of the 250 subjects had strokes in the 5-year study period. The estimated 5-year risk of stroke is thus $\hat{p} = 40/250 = 0.16$. Assuming that the null hypothesis is true, the risk of stroke is the same in both treatment groups, and we would expect that 16% of the subjects in each group would have a stroke during the study period. Thus, among the

120 subjects in the new treatment group (T = 1), we expect that 16%, or (0.16)(120) = 19.2 subjects, would have a stroke. Similarly, we expect that 16% of the 130 subjects in the placebo group (T = 0), or (0.16)(130) = 20.8 subjects, would have a stroke. The following table contains the expected cell frequencies under the null hypothesis. The expected frequencies in the "No Stroke" column are obtained by subtraction (e.g., 120 − 19.2 = 100.8). Notice that we do not round the expected frequencies to integers.

	Event		
Treatment Group	*Stroke*	*No Stroke*	*Total*
T = 1	19.2	100.8	120
T = 0	20.8	109.2	130
	40	210	250

Each of the expected frequencies (19.2, 100.8, 20.8, and 109.2) is at least 5, so we can compare the test statistic to the critical value $\chi^2 = 3.84$.

3. Decision rule.

$$\text{Reject } H_0 \text{ if } \chi^2 \geq 3.84$$

$$\text{Do not reject } H_0 \text{ if } \chi^2 < 3.84$$

4. Test statistic.

   We now calculate the test statistic using equation (8.7) and the expected frequencies.

$$\chi^2 = \frac{(12 - 19.2)^2}{19.2} + \frac{(108 - 100.8)^2}{100.8} + \frac{(28 - 20.8)^2}{20.8}$$
$$+ \frac{(102 - 109.2)^2}{109.2} = 6.181$$

5. Conclusion.

   Reject H_0 since $6.181 \geq 3.84$. There is significant evidence of a difference in risk, or that the relative risk is not equal to 1.

A computational formula for the χ^2 statistic in the special situation of a 2×2 table is

$$\chi^2 = \frac{(ad - bc)^2(N)}{(a+b)(c+d)(a+c)(b+d)} \tag{8.8}$$

This formula does not require the calculation of expected frequencies in a separate step. However, it is still necessary to check that the cell sizes are sufficien (that each expected frequency is at least 5). We can use this formula to calculate the test statistic in Example 8.2.

$$\chi^2 = \frac{(ad - bc)^2(N)}{(a+b)(c+d)(a+c)(b+d)}$$

$$= \frac{\{(12)(102) - (108)(28)\}^2(250)}{(120)(130)(40)(210)}$$

$$= \frac{810,000,000}{131,040,000}$$

$$= 6.181$$

SAS EXAMPLE 8.2 Testing Difference in Risk of Stroke Between Treatments Using SAS

The following output was generated for the data in Example 8.2 using SAS Proc Freq. We requested that SAS provide the expected cell frequencies and the row percents and the odds ratio, relative risk, and 95% confidence intervals. We also requested the chi-square test of homogeneity. Again, we make sure that the event of interest (stroke) is reported in the first column and the treatment group is in the first row. A brief interpretation appears after the output.

SAS Output for Example 8.2

```
                    The FREQ Procedure
                  Table of group by stroke

    group           stroke


    Frequency |
    Expected  |
    Row Pct   |yes       |no        | Total
    ----------+----------+----------+
    Treatment |    12 |      108 |     120
              |    19.2 |   100.8 |
              |    10.00 |   90.00 |
    ----------+----------+----------+
    Placebo   |    28 |      102 |     130
              |    20.8 |   109.2 |
              |    21.54 |   78.46 |
    ----------+----------+----------+
    Total            40        210         250
```

```
                     Statistics for Table of group by stroke
          Statistic                      DF          Value          Prob
          -----------------------------------------------------------------

          Chi-Square                      1          6.1813         0.0129
          Likelihood Ratio Chi-Square     1          6.3540         0.0117
          Continuity Adj. Chi-Square      1          5.3526         0.0207
          Mantel-Haenszel Chi-Square      1          6.1566         0.0131
          Phi Coefficient                            -0.1572
          Contingency Coefficient                    0.1553
          Cramer's V                                 -0.1572


                           Fisher's Exact Test
                 ---------------------------------------------
                 Cell (1,1) Frequency (F)          12
                 Left-sided Pr <= F           0.0097
                 Right-sided Pr >= F          0.9965


                 Table Probability (P)        0.0062
                 Two-sided Pr <= P            0.0154


              Estimates of the Relative Risk (Row1/Row2)
        Type of Study                    Value      95% Confidence Limits
        ---------------------------------------------------------------------

        Case-Control (Odds Ratio)       0.4048      0.1954         0.8386
        Cohort (Col1 Risk)              0.4643      0.2475         0.8710
        Cohort (Col2 Risk)              1.1471      1.0296         1.2779


                         Sample Size = 250
```

Interpretation of SAS Output for Example 8.2

The first number in each cell is the observed frequency, the second is the expected frequency, and the final number is the row percent. For example, in the "Treatment"–"yes" cell (the "a" cell), the observed frequency is 12, the expected frequency is 10.2, and the row percent is 10%. The estimated relative risk is $\hat{R}R = 0.464$ with 95% confidence limits (0.248, 0.871). The risk of stroke in subjects on the new treatment is estimated to be less than half the risk of stroke in those in the placebo group. Notice that the confidence interval does not include the null value 1.

The requested chi-square procedure allows us to test the null hypothesis that the risk of stroke is the same in the two groups. Here we will phrase the hypotheses in terms of the relative risk, $H_0: RR = 1$ and $H_1: RR \neq 1$. The value of the chi-square statistic is 6.181, as we calculated earlier, and the associated p value is $p = 0.0129$. Assuming $\alpha = 0.05$, we reject H_0 since $p = 0.0129 < \alpha = 0.05$. There is significant evidence ($p = 0.0129$) that the relative risk of stroke in treated subjects as compared to those on placebo is not equal to 1. ▪

EXAMPLE 8.3

Testing Difference in Risk of Institutionalization Between Male and Female Stroke Survivors

A study of stroke patients who survived 6 months after the stroke found that 6/45 men and 22/63 women lived in an institution (such as an assisted living or nursing facility). Is there evidence of a difference in risk of living in an institution after stroke for men versus women?

The null hypothesis is that men and women stroke survivors are equally likely to live in an institution, or that the relative risk for men of living in an institution compared to women is equal to 1. First, we set up the 2×2 table.

	Institution		
Comparison Group: Gender	Yes	No	Total
Men:	6	39	45
Women:	22	41	63
	28	80	108

We estimate the probabilities of living in an institution for men and women separately: $\hat{p}_M = 0.133$ and $\hat{p}_W = 0.349$. The estimated relative risk comparing men to women is $\hat{RR} = 0.381$; among stroke survivors, men are only 38% as likely as women to live in an institution. Suppose that we want to test the hypothesis that the risk of living in an institution is different for men and women.

1. Set up hypotheses.

$$H_0: p_M = p_W$$
$$H_1: p_M \neq p_W$$

Again, the hypotheses can be phrased in terms of the relative risk of living in an institution for men as compared to women:

$$H_0: \ RR = 1$$
$$H_1: \ RR \neq 1$$

2a. Select the appropriate test statistic.

We test the null hypothesis of homogeneity using the χ^2 test of homogeneity.

$$\chi^2 = \sum \frac{(O - E)^2}{E}$$

where $\sum$ indicates summation over all four cells of the table
  O = observed frequency
  E = expected frequency

The test statistic χ^2 follows a χ^2 distribution with df = 1 as long as the expected frequencies in each cell are at least 5.

2b. Check that the test is valid.

Before we can use the chi-square test, we must check that each of the expected frequencies is at least 5. Under the null hypothesis we assume that the probability of living in an institution is the same for men and women ($p_M = p_W = p$). The best estimate of this probability is obtained by combining men and women and calculating the overall sample proportion. Based on this combined sample, the estimated probability of living in an institution is $\hat{p} = (28/108) = 0.259$. Thus, we expect about 25.9% of men and 25.9% of women to be living in an institution. Under the null hypothesis, in this sample of 45 men, we expect $(0.259)(45)$ or 11.67 men to be living in an institution, while the remaining 33.33 live at home. Similarly, among the women, we expect $(.259)(63) = 16.33$ to be living in an institution and 46.67 to be living at home. The expected frequencies are 11.67, 33.33, 16.33, and 46.67, and each is of sufficient size (i.e., each is at least 5), so we can use the chi-square test to test H_0.

3. Decision rule.

$$\text{Reject } H_0 \text{ if } \chi^2 \geq 3.84$$
$$\text{Do not reject } H_0 \text{ if } \chi^2 < 3.84$$

4. Test statistic.

We now calculate the test statistic using the computational formula (8.7).

$$\chi^2 = \frac{(ad - bc)^2(N)}{(a+b)(c+d)(a+c)(b+d)}$$

$$= \frac{\{(6)(41) - (39)(22)\}^2(108)}{(45)(63)(28)(80)}$$

$$= \frac{40,450,752}{6,350,400}$$

$$= 6.3698$$

5. Conclusion.

Reject H_0 since $\chi^2 = 6.37 > 3.84$. There is significant evidence that the probability of living in an institution is different for men and women stroke survivors. Another interpretation is that there is significant evidence that the relative risk of living in an institution comparing men and women is different from 1. ▪

8.4 Fisher's Exact Test

In Chapter 7 and in Section 8.3, we stressed that the chi-square tests are valid if each of the expected cell frequencies is at least 5. If one or more of the four expected cell frequencies in a 2×2 table is less than 5, the chi-square test is not valid and we must use another method. One such method is Fisher's Exact test. A discussion of the mechanics of this test is beyond the scope of this text, so we simply present examples using SAS.

SAS EXAMPLE 8.4 Testing Differences in Functional Ability Between Stroke Survivors and Controls

A substudy of the stroke study we have described involved a comparison of the functional ability of stroke patients to patients of the same age and gender who did not suffer stroke. As many as possible of the stroke survivors were matched to controls who were the same age and sex. Cases (stroke patients) and controls (persons who did not suffer stroke) were questioned with respect to various measures of disability. Among the 24 stroke cases, only 16 were able to walk unassisted, whereas 23 of the 24 controls were able to walk unassisted. Using the data shown in the SAS output, we test whether the stroke cases were more likely to need assistance walking as compared to age- and sex-matched controls. The analysis is conducted using SAS Proc Freq; a brief interpretation appears after the output.

SAS Output for Example 8.4

```
                    The FREQ Procedure
                  Table of group by walk

group            walk

Frequency     |
Expected      |
Row Pct       |Needs As|Able to |   Total
              |ssistanc|Walk    |
              |e       |        |
    ----------+--------+--------+
Stroke Cases  |      8 |     16 |    24
              |    4.5 |   19.5 |
              |  33.33 |  66.67 |
    ----------+--------+--------+
Controls      |      1 |     23 |    24
              |    4.5 |   19.5 |
              |   4.17 |  95.83 |
    ----------+--------+--------+
Total                9       39      48
```

Statistics for Table of group by walk

Statistic	DF	Value	Prob
Chi-Square	1	6.7009	0.0096
Likelihood Ratio Chi-Square	1	7.4609	0.0063
Continuity Adj. Chi-Square	1	4.9231	0.0265
Mantel-Haenszel Chi-Square	1	6.5613	0.0104
Phi Coefficient		0.3736	
Contingency Coefficient		0.3500	
Cramer's V		0.3736	

WARNING: 50% of the cells have expected counts less
         than 5. Chi-Square may not be a valid test.

Fisher's Exact Test

Cell (1,1) Frequency (F)	8
Left-sided Pr <= F	0.9992
Right-sided Pr >= F	0.0113
Table Probability (P)	0.0105
Two-sided Pr <= P	0.0226

Estimates of the Relative Risk (Row1/Row2)

Type of Study	Value	95% Confidence Limits	
Case-Control (Odds Ratio)	11.5000	1.3071	101.1816
Cohort (Col1 Risk)	8.0000	1.0823	59.1349
Cohort (Col2 Risk)	0.6957	0.5180	0.9343

Sample Size = 48

Interpretation of SAS Output for Example 8.4

The expected cell frequencies in the four cells are 4.5, 4.5, 19.5, and 19.5. Two of these are less than the required 5. Notice that SAS provides a "Warning" statement, indicating that 50% of the cells have expected counts less than 5 and that the chi-square test may not be valid. Below this, SAS provides results of the two-sided Fisher's Exact test, which is recommended when the expected counts are small (i.e., < 5).

One-third (33.3%) of the stroke cases need assistance to walk whereas only 4.2% of their age and sex-matched controls need assistance. The estimated RR is 8.0 (0.333/0.0417). The null hypothesis is H_0: $RR = 1$ and H_1: $RR \neq 1$. We use the two-sided Fisher's Exact test to test the hypothesis. Assuming $\alpha = 0.05$, we reject H_0 since $p = 0.0226 < \alpha = 0.05$. There is significant evidence ($p = 0.0226$) that stroke cases are more likely to need assistance walking as compared to age- and sex-matched controls. ■

8.5 Cochran–Mantel–Haenszel Method

The Cochran–Mantel–Haenszel method is an extension of the chi-square method and is applied when interest lies in comparing two groups in terms of a dichotomous outcome over several levels of a third variable. For example, suppose there are a series of 2×2 tables, one for each of several strata (maybe the strata reflect different levels of severity of the index condition or different clinical centers), and interest lies in combining the information to take into account the differences in the strata. In this section we will describe a method used to adjust the estimate of relative risk and the test statistic to account for a third variable in the analysis.

EXAMPLE 8.5

Testing Differences in Risk of Hypertension Between Drugs in Older and Younger Patients

Suppose we want to compare two medications, call them Drug A and Drug B, with respect to the development of or risk of hypertension (HTN). A total of 200 subjects are involved in the analysis, and half are randomized to receive Drug A and half are randomized to receive Drug B. The following table summarizes the results of the study:

| | HTN | | |
Medication	Yes	No	
Drug A	56	44	100
Drug B	32	68	100
Total	88	112	200

Overall, 88/200 subjects, or 44%, developed hypertension (HTN). The risk of HTN among subjects taking Drug A is $\hat{p}_A = 56/100 = 0.56$ and the risk of HTN among subjects taking Drug B is $\hat{p}_B = 32/100 = 0.32$, and the estimated relative risk comparing subjects on Drug A to those on Drug B is $\hat{R}R = (0.56/0.32) = 1.75$. A test of the hypothesis $H_0: RR = 1$ yields $\chi^2 = 11.688$ with $p < 0.001$. We reject H_0 and conclude that there is significant evidence that the relative risk of HTN comparing subjects taking Drug A to those taking Drug B is different from 1.

Half of the subjects were randomized to receive Drug A and the other half received Drug B. However, further inspection of the data revealed that this balance was not maintained within age groups. In fact, it turns out that 60% of the 100 older subjects (age 65 and older) received Drug A, and only 40% of the 100 younger subjects (age less than 65) received Drug A. We can repeat the analysis within the two age groups (i.e., two separate replications).

Age 65 + HTN				*Age < 65 HTN*		
	Yes	No			Yes	No
Drug A:	32	8	40	**Drug A:**	24	36	60
Drug B:	24	36	60	**Drug B:**	8	32	40
Total:	56	44	100	Total:	32	68	100

$$\hat{R}R = 0.8/0.4 = 2.0 \qquad\qquad \hat{R}R = 0.4/0.2 = 2.0$$

The overall risk of hypertension is 56% among those age 65 and older, and it is only 32% for those less than 65 years of age. However, the relative risk of HTN comparing those taking Drug A to those taking Drug B is the same in the two age groups. The baseline level of HTN is different, but the relative impact of the two drugs is the same.

This would appear to indicate that combining the two age groups and reporting results based on the combined data are fine. In fact, since the estimated relative risk is 2.0 in each age group, the relative risk based on the combined data should surely also be 2.0. However, recall that we actually obtained an estimate of $\hat{R}R = 1.75$. This is caused by the combination of different baseline risks in the age groups and the imbalance in the treatment group allocation in the age groups, which is called *confounding* by age group. ▪

In this section, we present the Cochran–Mantel–Haenszel method used to adjust the relative risk and the chi-square statistic to remove the effect of confounding. In Chapter 11, we introduce another method to adjust for confounding.

With a series of 2×2 tables, each table reflecting the relationship between group and event for a different strata (e.g., different level of a confounder), the Cochran–Mantel–Haenszel method can be used to calculate an *adjusted chi-square test statistic and an adjusted relative risk*. The procedure is as follows.

First, create a 2×2 table *within* each stratum of the stratification variable. As before, the basic notation we use for the 2×2 table is as follows:

Group	Stratum 1 Event 1	0	
1:	a	b	a + b
0:	c	d	c + d
	a + c	b + d	N

Next, calculate:

$$\chi^2_{CMH} = \frac{\left(\sum \frac{(ad - bc)}{N} \right)^2}{\sum \frac{(a+b)(c+d)(a+c)(b+d)}{(N-1)N^2}} \tag{8.9}$$

where the summations are over the strata. This test statistic has a χ^2 distribution with 1 df, so we compare the test statistic to the critical value of 3.84, assuming a 5% level of significance.

EXAMPLE 8.5

Testing Differences in Risk of Hypertension Between Drugs in Older and Younger Patients (continued)

Returning to Example 8.5, the adjusted test statistic is computed as follows:

$$\chi^2_{CMH} = \frac{\left(\sum \frac{(ad - bc)}{N} \right)^2}{\sum \frac{(a+b)(c+d)(a+c)(b+d)}{(N-1)N^2}}$$

$$= \frac{\left(\frac{(32)(36) - (8)(24)}{100} + \frac{(24)(32) - (36)(86)}{100} \right)^2}{\frac{(40)(60)(56)(44)}{(99)100^2} + \frac{(60)(40)(32)(68)}{(99)100^2}}$$

$$= \frac{207.36}{11.248} = 18.435$$

The null hypothesis is that the relative risk of hypertension comparing subjects on Drug A to subjects on Drug B, adjusted for age, is equal to 1. We reject H_0 since $\chi^2_{\text{MH}} = 18.435 > 3.84$ and conclude that, after adjusting for age, the risk of HTN in subjects taking Drugs A and B are not equal.

We can also calculate the adjusted estimate of the relative risk. The crude relative risk, $\hat{R}R_C$, is the relative risk obtained by combining all the data and estimating RR. In Example 8.5, $\hat{R}R_C = (0.56/0.32) = 1.75$. The Cochran–Mantel–Haenszel adjusted RR is estimated by the following:

$$\hat{R}R_{\text{CMH}} = \frac{\sum \dfrac{a(c+d)}{N}}{\sum \dfrac{c(a+b)}{N}} \tag{8.10}$$

where the summations are over the strata. In Example 8.5,

$$\hat{R}R_{\text{CMH}} = \frac{\dfrac{(32)(60)}{100} + \dfrac{(24)(40)}{100}}{\dfrac{(24)(40)}{100} + \dfrac{(8)(60)}{100}}$$

$$= \frac{28.8}{14.4}$$

$$= 2.0$$

The relative risk adjusted for age is $\hat{R}R_{\text{CMH}} = 2.0$, which is the same relative risk we obtained in each of the age groups. ■

SAS EXAMPLE 8.5 Testing Differences in Risk of Hypertension Between Drugs in Older and Younger Patients Using SAS

We can request that SAS perform the Cochran–Mantel–Haenszel adjusted chi-square test and produce a Cochran–Mantel–Haenszel adjusted relative risk. The analysis is conducted using SAS Proc Freq; a brief interpretation appears after the output.

SAS Output for Example 8.5

```
                    The FREQ Procedure

                Table 1 of group by htn
                Controlling for age=65+

  group        htn

  Frequency|
  Row Pct   |HTN     |noHTN   |  Total
  ---------+--------+--------+
  Drug A   |     32 |      8 |     40
           |  80.00 |  20.00 |
  ---------+--------+--------+
  Drug B   |     24 |     36 |     60
           |  40.00 |  60.00 |
  ---------+--------+--------+
  Total          56       44     100

  Table 2 of group by htn
  Controlling for age=<65

  group        htn

  Frequency|
  Row Pct   |HTN     |noHTN   |  Total
  ---------+--------+--------+
  Drug A   |     24 |     36 |     60
           |  40.00 |  60.00 |
  ---------+--------+--------+
  Drug B   |      8 |     32 |     40
           |  20.00 |  80.00 |
  ---------+--------+--------+
  Total          32       68     100

       Summary Statistics for group by htn
              Controlling for age
```

Cochran-Mantel-Haenszel Statistics (Based on Table Scores)

Statistic	Alternative Hypothesis	DF	Value	Prob
1	Nonzero Correlation	1	18.4345	<.0001
2	Row Mean Scores Differ	1	18.4345	<.0001
3	General Association	1	18.4345	<.0001

```
            Estimates of the Common Relative Risk (Row1/Row2)
Type of Study     Method              Value       95% Confidence Limits
-----------------------------------------------------------------------
Case-Control      Mantel-Haenszel     4.0000         2.0791        7.6955
   (Odds Ratio)   Logit               4.0000         2.0707        7.7268

Cohort            Mantel-Haenszel     2.0000         1.4427        2.7727
   (Col1 Risk)    Logit               2.0000         1.4670        2.7266

Cohort            Mantel-Haenszel     0.5714         0.4351        0.7505
   (Col2 Risk)    Logit               0.6722         0.5286        0.8546

                        Breslow-Day Test for
                   Homogeneity of the Odds Ratios
                   -----------------------------
                   Chi-Square                 1.4664
                   DF                              1
                   Pr > ChiSq                 0.2259
                    Total Sample Size = 200
```

Interpretation of SAS Output for Example 8.5

SAS produces individual 2×2 tables for each of the strata (age groups). The Cochran–Mantel–Haenszel adjusted chi-square statistic and its associated p value is given under "Cochran–Mantel–Haenszel Statistics (Based on Table Scores)"; in this situation, all three given statistics are identical. The Cochran–Mantel–Haenszel adjusted relative risk and the 95% confidence interval are given under "Estimates of the Common Relative Risk (Row1/ Row2)" in the row labeled "Type of Study = Cohort (Col 1 Risk)" and "Method = Mantel–Haenszel."

This method is only valid if the relative risks are homogeneous across strata. SAS provides the p value associated with the Breslow–Day test for the hypothesis of homogeneity. If this p value is > 0.05, we assume that the relative risks are homogeneous and that the Cochran–Mantel–Haenszel statistics are valid.

In this example, the p value for the Breslow–Day test is $p = 0.226 > 0.05$, so the Cochran–Mantel–Haenszel method is valid. From the output, we see that $\hat{R}R_{MH} = 2.0$, with 95% confidence interval $(1.44, 2.77)$. The $\chi^2_{CMH} = 18.435$, with $p =< 0.001$. ■

8.6 Precision, Power, and Sample Size Determination

The formulas given in Section 7.7 may be used to calculate the minimum number of subjects needed to ensure a specified level of power to detect a difference in proportions (or risks) between two groups. Equation (7.16) is given here using the terminology of this chapter.

$$n_i = \left(\frac{\sqrt{2\bar{p}\bar{q}}\, Z_{1-(\alpha/2)} + \sqrt{p_1 q_1 + p_0 q_0}\, Z_{1-\beta}}{\hat{R}D} \right)^2 \tag{8.11}$$

where $\bar{p} = (\hat{p}_1 + \hat{p}_0)/2$ and $\bar{q} = 1 - \bar{p}$

8.7 Key Formulas (using 2 × 2 table notation in Table 8.1)

Application	Notation/Formula	Description
Risk difference	$\hat{R}D = \hat{p}_1 - \hat{p}_0 = \dfrac{a}{(a+b)} - \dfrac{c}{(c+d)}$	
Relative risk	$\hat{R}R = \hat{p}_1/\hat{p}_0 = \dfrac{a/(a+b)}{c/(c+d)}$	
Odds ratio	$\hat{O}R = \dfrac{\hat{o}_1}{\hat{o}_0} = \dfrac{\hat{p}_1/(1-\hat{p}_1)}{\hat{p}_0/(1-\hat{p}_0)} = \dfrac{a/b}{c/d}$	
Confidence interval for risk difference	$\hat{R}D \pm Z_{1-(\alpha/2)}\sqrt{\left(\dfrac{\hat{p}_0(1-\hat{p}_0)}{n_0}\right) + \left(\dfrac{\hat{p}_1(1-\hat{p}_1)}{n_1}\right)}$	
Confidence interval for relative risk	$\exp\left(\ln(\hat{R}R) \pm Z_{1-(\alpha/2)}\sqrt{\dfrac{(d/c)}{n_0} + \dfrac{(b/a)}{n_1}} \right)$	
Confidence interval for odds ratio	$\exp\left(\ln(\hat{O}R) \pm Z_{1-(\alpha/2)}\sqrt{\left(\dfrac{1}{a} + \dfrac{1}{b} + \dfrac{1}{c} + \dfrac{1}{d}\right)} \right)$	
$H_0: RD = 0$ or $H_0: RR = 1$ or $H_0: OR = 1$	$\chi^2 = \sum \dfrac{(O-E)^2}{E}, \quad df = 1$	Chi-square test of homogeneity. Assumes all expected cell counts are ≥ 5
$H_0: RD = 0$ or $H_0: RR = 1$ or $H_0: OR = 1$	$\chi^2 = \dfrac{(ad-bc)^2(N)}{(a+b)(c+d)(a+c)(b+d)}$	Chi-square test of homogeneity: computational formula. Assumes all expected cell counts are ≥ 5
$H_0: RD = 0$ or $H_0: RR = 1$ or $H_0: OR = 1$ (each adjusted for confounder)	$\chi^2_{MH} = \dfrac{\left(\sum \dfrac{(ad-bc)}{N}\right)^2}{\sum \dfrac{(a+b)(c+d)(a+c)(b+d)}{(N-1)N^2}}$	Cochran–Mantel–Haenszel chi-square test of homogeneity, adjusted for confounder
Estimate of relative risk, adjusted for confounder	$RR_{MH} = \left(\sum \dfrac{a(c+d)}{N}\right) \Big/ \left(\sum \dfrac{c(a+b)}{N}\right)$	Cochran–Mantel–Haenszel estimate of relative risk, adjusted for confounder
Sample size required per group to test $H_0: RD = 0$ with power $1 - \beta$	$n_i = \left(\dfrac{\sqrt{2\bar{p}\bar{q}}\, Z_{1-(\alpha/2)} + \sqrt{p_1 q_1 + p_0 q_0}\, Z_{1-\beta}}{\hat{R}D} \right)^2$	

8.8 Statistical Computing

Following are the SAS programs used to generate the analyses presented in this chapter. The SAS procedures and brief descriptions of their use are noted in the header to each example. Notes are provided to the right of the SAS programs (in blue) for orientation purposes and are not part of the programs. In addition, there are blank lines in the programs that are solely to accommodate the notes. Blank lines and spaces can be used throughout SAS programs to enhance readability. A summary of the SAS procedures used in the examples is provided at the end of this section.

SAS EXAMPLE 8.1 **Estimate Relative Risk and Odds Ratio**

Compare Risk of Coronary Abnormalities on Gamma Globulin as Compared to Aspirin (Example 8.1)

A trial of gamma globulin in the treatment of children with Kawasaki syndrome randomized approximately half of the patients to receive gamma globulin plus aspirin; the other half received standard treatment of aspirin. The outcome of interest was the development of coronary abnormalities (CA) within seven weeks of treatment. The following 2 × 2 cross-tabulation table summarizes the results of the trial. Use SAS to estimate the relative risk (and odds ratio) of CA in patients treated with gamma globulin as compared to those on standard treatment.

Treatment Group	Coronary Abnormalities CA = 1	No Coronary Abnormalities CA = 0	Total
Gamma Globulin, GG = 1	5	78	83
Aspirin, GG = 0	21	63	84
Total	26	141	167

Program Code

```
options ps=62 ls=80;

data in;
  input group $ event $ f;
```

Formats the output page to 62 lines in length and 80 columns in width
Beginning of Data Step
Inputs three variables, **group** (noGG or GG), **event** (CA or noCA), and *f*, the cell frequency. **Group** and **event** are defined as character variables using the $.

```
cards;
noGG noCA 63
noGG CA 21
GG noCA 78
GG CA 5
run;
proc freq;


  tables group*event/relrisk;






  weight f;


run;
```

Beginning of Raw Data section.
Actual observations (values of
   group, event, and *f* on each line)

Procedure call. Proc freq generates
   a 2 × 2 table for two categorical
   variables.

Specifies the analytic variables to
   form the rows (**group**) and
   columns (**event**) of the table. The
   relrisk option requests that SAS
   generate estimates of the relative
   risk and odds ratio.

Specifies the variable that contains
   the cell counts, *f*.

End of procedure section. ■

SAS EXAMPLE 8.2 **Estimate Relative Risk and Test H_0: $RR = 1$ Versus H_1: $RR \neq 1$**
Estimate the Relative Risk of Stroke Comparing a Proposed Stroke
Medication to Placebo, and Test the Hypothesis That the Relative Risk Is
Equal to 1 (Example 8.2)

In a clinical trial 250 participants are randomly assigned to receive either a
proposed stroke prevention medication (T_1) or a placebo (T_0) and are followed over the course of a 5-year study period. These results are given in the
following table. Using SAS, estimate the relative risk of stroke comparing
those on the medication to those on placebo, and test the hypothesis that the
relative risk is not equal to 1.

	Event		
Treatment Group	Stroke	No Stroke	Total
$T = 1$	12	108	120
$T = 0$	28	102	130
	40	210	250

Program Code

```
options ps=62 ls=80;

proc format;

  value eventf 1='yes' 2='no';
  value grpf 1='Treatment' 2='Placebo';




run;

data in;
  input group stroke f;

  format stroke eventf. group grpf.;








cards;
1 1 12
1 2 108
2 1 28
2 2 102
run;

proc freq;

  tables group*stroke/nocol nopercent
         expected relrisk chisq;













  weight f;

run;
```

Formats the output page to 62 lines in length and 80 columns in width

Proc format defines formats to label the values of the variables.

Variables with values of 1 and 2 will be labeled as 'yes' and 'no,' respectively, if formatted with the **eventf** format. Variables with values of 1 and 2 will be labeled as 'Treatment' and 'Placebo,' respectively, if formatted with the **grpf** format.

End of format procedure.

Beginning of Data Step

Inputs three variables **group** (1 or 2), **stroke** (1 or 2), and *f* (the cell frequency).

The format statement assigns the format **eventf** to the variable **stroke,** and the format **grpf** to the variable **group.** Note that the format names are followed by a period to distinguish them from variable names.

Beginning of Raw Data section.

Actual observations (values of **group, stroke,** and *f* on each line).

Procedure call. Proc freq generates a 2 × 2 table for two categorical variables.

Specifies the analytic variables to form the rows (**group**) and columns (**stroke**) of the table. The nocol and nopercent options suppress the printing of the column and overall percents, respectively. The relrisk option requests that SAS generate estimates of the relative risk and odds ratio. The chisq option requests the Chi-Square test.

Specifies the variable that contains the cell counts, *f.*

End of procedure section. ▪

SAS EXAMPLE 8.4 **Estimate Relative Risk and Test H_0: $RR = 1$ Versus H_1: $RR \neq 1$**

Are Stroke Cases More Likely to Need Assistance Walking as Compared to Age- and Sex-Matched Controls? (Example 8.4)

As part of the stroke study described earlier, as many as possible of the stroke survivors were matched to controls who were the same age and sex. Cases and controls were questioned with respect to various measures of disability. Among the 24 stroke cases, only 16 were able to walk unassisted, whereas 23 of the 24 controls were able to walk unassisted. Use SAS to test whether stroke cases are more likely to need assistance walking as compared to age- and sex-matched controls.

Program Code

```
options ps=62 ls=80;
```
Formats the output page to 62 lines in length and 80 columns in width

```
proc format;
```
Proc format defines formats to label the values of the variables.

```
  value eventf 1='Needs Assistance'
               2='Able to Walk';
```
Variables with values of 1 and 2 will be labeled as 'Needs Assistance' and 'Able to Walk,' respectively, if formatted with the **eventf** format.

```
  value grpf 1='Stroke Cases'
             2='Controls';
```
Variables with values of 1 and 2 will be labeled as 'Stroke Cases' and 'Controls,' respectively, if formatted with the **grpf** format.

```
run;
```
End of format procedure.

```
data in;
  input group walk f;
```
Beginning of Data Step
Inputs three variables **group** (1 or 2), **walk** (1 or 2), and *f* (the cell frequency).

```
  format walk eventf. group grpf.;
```
The format statement assigns the format **eventf** to the variable **walk,** and the format **grpf** to the variable **group.** Note that the format names are followed by a period to distinguish them from variable names.

```
cards;
1 1 8
1 2 16
2 1 1
2 2 23
run;
```
Beginning of Raw Data section.
Actual observations (values of **group, walk,** and *f* on each line).

```
proc freq;
```
Procedure call. Proc freq generates a 2 × 2 table for two categorical variables.

```
tables group*walk/nocol nopercent
   expected relrisk chisq;
```

Specifies the analytic variables to form the rows (**group**) and columns (**walk**) of the table. The nocol and nopercent options suppress the printing of the column and overall percents, respectively. The relrisk option requests that SAS generate estimates of the relative risk and odds ratio. The chisq option requests the Chi-Square test.

```
   weight f;
```

Specifies the variable that contains the cell counts, f.

```
run;
```

End of procedure section. ■

SAS EXAMPLE 8.5 Estimate Cochran–Mantel–Haenszel Adjusted Relative Risk and

Perform Cochran–Mantel–Haenszel Chi-Square Test of Homogeneity (Example 8.5)

We want to compare the risk of hypertension (HTN) in two groups of subjects, those treated with Drug A and those treated with Drug B, adjusted for age (< 65 versus $65+$). The assignments to drug treatment and the outcome status (Hypertension yes/no) for each age group are summarized in the tables below. Use SAS to estimate a relative risk adjusted for age and perform the Cochran–Mantel–Haenszel test of homogeneity adjusting for age.

	Age 65 + HTN				Age < 65 HTN		
	Yes	*No*			*Yes*	*No*	
Drug A:	32	8	40	*Drug A:*	24	36	60
Drug B:	24	36	60	*Drug B:*	8	32	40
Total:	56	44	100	*Total:*	32	68	100

Program Code

```
options ps=62 ls=80;
```

Formats the output page to 62 lines in length and 80 columns in width

```
proc format;
```

Proc format defines formats to label the values of the variables.

```
 value eventf 1='HTN' 2='noHTN';
```

Variables with values of 1 and 2 will be labeled as 'HTN' and 'noHTN,' respectively, if formatted with the **eventf** format.

```
value grpf 1='Drug A' 2='Drug B';
```
Variables with values of 1 and 2 will be labeled as 'Drug A' and 'Drug B,' respectively, if formatted with the **grpf** format.

```
value agef 1='65+' 2='<65';
```
Variables with values of 1 and 2 will be labeled as '65+' and '<65,' respectively, if formatted with the **agef** format.

```
run;
```
End of format procedure.

```
data in;
```
Beginning of Data Step.

```
  input group htn age f;
```
Inputs four variables **group** (1 or 2), **htn** (1 or 2), age (1 or 2), and *f* (the cell frequency).

```
  format htn eventf. group grpf. age agef.;
```
The format statement assigns the format **eventf** to the variable **htn**, the format **grpf** to the variable **group,** and the format **agef** to the variable **age.** Note that the format names are followed by a period to distinguish them from variable names.

```
cards;
1 1 1 32
1 2 1 8
2 1 1 24
2 2 1 36
1 1 2 24
1 2 2 36
2 1 2 8
2 2 2 32
run;
```
Beginning of Raw Data section.

```
proc freq;
```
Procedure call. Proc freq generates a 2×2 table for two categorical variables.

```
  tables group*htn/nocol nopercent relrisk
    chisq;
```
Specifies the analytic variables to form the rows (**group**) and columns (**htn**) of the table. The nocol and nopercent options suppress the printing of the column and overall percents, respectively. The relrisk option requests that SAS generate estimates of the crude relative risk and odds ratio. The chisq option requests the Chi-Square test.

```
  weight f;
```
Specifies the variable that contains the cell counts, *f.*

```
run;
proc freq;
```
End of procedure section.

Procedure call. Proc freq generates a 2×2 table for two categorical variables.

```
tables age*group*htn/cmh nocol nopercent;
```
Specifies the analytic variables to form the rows (**group**) and columns (**htn**) of the table, stratified by the third variable (**age**). The cmh option requests an estimate of the Cochran-Mantel-Haenszel relative risk and requests the Mantel-Haenszel test of homogeneity. Again, the nocol and nopercent options suppress the printing of the column and overall percents, respectively.

```
weight f;
```
Specifies the variable that contains the cell counts, *f*.

```
run;
```
End of procedure section.   ■

8.8.1 Summary of SAS Procedures

The SAS Freq Procedure is used to generate $R \times C$ tables for categorical variables. Specific options can be requested to produce crude and adjusted estimates of relative risks and odds ratios and to run unadjusted and adjusted chi-square tests of homogeneity. The specific options are shown in italics in the following table. Users should refer to the examples in this section for complete descriptions of the procedure and specific options. A general description of the procedure and options is provided in the table.

Procedure	Sample Procedure Call	Description

proc freq	proc freq;
	    tables a*b;
	    weight f;
		Generates a 2 × 2 contingency table with row variable *a* (a dichotomous variable) and column variable *b* (a dichotomous variable). The weight option indicates that summary data are input, and the variable *f* contains the cell frequencies.

	proc freq; tables a*b/*relrisk chisq;*	Generates a 2 × 2 contingency table (*a* by *b*) and requests estimates of the crude or unadjusted relative risk and odds ratio and runs the unadjusted chi-square test of homogeneity.
	proc freq; tables strata*a*b/*cmh;*	Generates 2 × 2 contingency tables (*a* by *b*) stratified by the third variable strata. The cmh option requests estimates of the adjusted relative risk and odds ratio and runs the Cochran–Mantel–Haenszel adjusted chi-square test of homogeneity.

8.9 Analysis of Framingham Heart Study Data

The Framingham data set includes data collected from the original cohort. Participants contributed up to three examination cycles of data. Here we use data collected in the first examination cycle (called the period = 1 examination) to ascertain data on the comparison groups. In this analysis, we will compare participants with diabetes to those without diabetes at baseline in terms of their risk for development of cardiovascular disease over the 24-year follow-up period. We use SAS Proc Freq to generate 2×2 tables to assess the effect of diabetes status on the development of CVD for the total sample and then for men and women separately. We then conduct the Cochran–Mantel–Haenszel test to assess whether sex is a confounder. The SAS code to run these analyses is given next.

Framingham Data Analysis—SAS Code

```
data fhs;
  set in.frmgham;
  if period=1;
run;


proc freq data=fhs;
  tables diabetes*cvd/riskdiff relrisk chisq;
run;


proc sort data=fhs;
  by sex;
run;


proc freq data=fhs;
  tables diabetes*cvd/riskdiff relrisk chisq;
  by sex;
run;


proc freq data=fhs;
  tables sex*diabetes*cvd/cmh;
run;
```

Framingham Data Analysis—SAS Output

```
                      The FREQ Procedure
                   Table of DIABETES by CVD

DIABETES(Diabetic Y/N)
          CVD(Incident Hosp MI or Stroke, Fatal or Non)
Frequency|
Percent  |
Row Pct  |
Col Pct  |Yes      |No       |  Total
---------+--------+--------+
Yes      |      74 |      47 |    121
         |    1.67 |    1.06 |   2.73
         |   61.16 |   38.84 |
         |    6.40 |    1.43 |
---------+--------+--------+
No       |    1083 |    3230 |   4313
         |   24.42 |   72.85 |  97.27
         |   25.11 |   74.89 |
         |   93.60 |   98.57 |
---------+--------+--------+
Total        1157      3277     4434
            26.09     73.91 ·  100.00
```

Statistics for Table of DIABETES by CVD

Statistic	DF	Value	Prob
Chi-Square	1	79.3024	<.0001
Likelihood Ratio Chi-Square	1	67.7732	<.0001
Continuity Adj. Chi-Square	1	77.4443	<.0001
Mantel-Haenszel Chi-Square	1	79.2845	<.0001
Phi Coefficient		0.1337	
Contingency Coefficient		0.1326	
Cramer's V		0.1337	

Fisher's Exact Test

```
-----------------------------------------
     Cell (1,1) Frequency (F)         74
     Left-sided Pr <= F           1.0000
     Right-sided Pr >= F          1.848E-16

     Table Probability (P)        2.220E-16
     Two-sided Pr <= P            2.562E-16
```

The FREQ Procedure
Statistics for Table of DIABETES by CVD

Column 1 Risk Estimates

	Risk	ASE	(Asymptotic) 95% Confidence Limits		(Exact) 95% Confidence Limits	
Row 1	0.6116	0.0443	0.5247	0.6984	0.5187	0.6988
Row 2	0.2511	0.0066	0.2382	0.2640	0.2382	0.2643
Total	0.2609	0.0066	0.2480	0.2739	0.2481	0.2741
Difference	0.3605	0.0448	0.2727	0.4483		

Difference is (Row 1 - Row 2)

Column 2 Risk Estimates

	Risk	ASE	(Asymptotic) 95% Confidence Limits		(Exact) 95% Confidence Limits	
Row 1	0.3884	0.0443	0.3016	0.4753	0.3012	0.4813
Row 2	0.7489	0.0066	0.7360	0.7618	0.7357	0.7618
Total	0.7391	0.0066	0.7261	0.7520	0.7259	0.7519
Difference	-0.3605	0.0448	-0.4483	-0.2727		

Difference is (Row 1 - Row 2)

Estimates of the Relative Risk (Row1/Row2)

Type of Study	Value	95% Confidence Limits	
Case-Control (Odds Ratio)	4.6958	3.2371	6.8118
Cohort (Col1 Risk)	2.4356	2.0941	2.8327
Cohort (Col2 Risk)	0.5187	0.4145	0.6490

Sample Size = 4434

In the output, SAS first generates a 2 × 2 table showing the relationship between diabetes status and incident CVD. Of interest are the row percents: the risk of CVD for diabetics is 61.2% as compared to 25.1% for nondiabetics. The difference is highly significant at $p < 0.0001$ (chi-square test). The Fisher's Exact test gives a similar result, but because the cell sizes are sufficiently large, the chi-square test is appropriate here. We requested that SAS estimate the risk difference, which it does considering column1 as the outcome of interest and again considering column2 as the outcome of interest. Here, column 1 (CVD = yes) is the outcome of interest, so the estimate of the risk difference is 36.1%, with a 95% confidence interval of (27.3%, 44.8%). SAS estimates the relative risk at 2.44 (diabetics are 2.44 times more likely to develop CVD as compared to nondiabetics), with a 95% confidence interval of (2.09, 2.83).

In the following, we perform similar analyses but stratify by sex. Is the effect of diabetes similar for men and women?

----------------------- SEX=M -----------------------

The FREQ Procedure
Table of DIABETES by CVD

DIABETES(Diabetic Y/N)
            CVD(Incident Hosp MI or Stroke, Fatal or Non)
Frequency|
Percent |
Row Pct |
Col Pct |Yes |No | Total
---------+--------+--------+
Yes | 38 | 21 | 59
         | 1.95 | 1.08 | 3.03
         | 64.41 | 35.59 |
         | 5.54 | 1.67 |
---------+--------+--------+
No | 648 | 1237 | 1885
         | 33.33 | 63.63 | 96.97
         | 34.38 | 65.62 |
         | 94.46 | 98.33 |
---------+--------+--------+
Total   686   1258   1944
               35.29   64.71   100.00

Statistics for Table of DIABETES by CVD

Statistic	DF	Value	Prob
Chi-Square	1	22.5927	<.0001
Likelihood Ratio Chi-Square	1	21.3085	<.0001
Continuity Adj. Chi-Square	1	21.2968	<.0001
Mantel-Haenszel Chi-Square	1	22.5811	<.0001
Phi Coefficient		0.1078	
Contingency Coefficient		0.1072	
Cramer's V		0.1078	

Fisher's Exact Test

Cell (1,1) Frequency (F)	38
Left-sided Pr <= F	1.0000
Right-sided Pr >= F	3.588E-06
Table Probability (P)	2.603E-06
Two-sided Pr <= P	5.109E-06

The FREQ Procedure
Statistics for Table of DIABETES by CVD

Column 1 Risk Estimates

	Risk	ASE	(Asymptotic) 95% Confidence Limits		(Exact) 95% Confidence Limits	
Row 1	0.6441	0.0623	0.5219	0.7662	0.5087	0.7645
Row 2	0.3438	0.0109	0.3223	0.3652	0.3223	0.3657
Total	0.3529	0.0108	0.3316	0.3741	0.3316	0.3746
Difference	0.3003	0.0633	0.1763	0.4243		

Difference is (Row 1 - Row 2)

Column 2 Risk Estimates

	Risk	ASE	(Asymptotic) 95% Confidence Limits		(Exact) 95% Confidence Limits	
Row 1	0.3559	0.0623	0.2338	0.4781	0.2355	0.4913
Row 2	0.6562	0.0109	0.6348	0.6777	0.6343	0.6777
Total	0.6471	0.0108	0.6259	0.6684	0.6254	0.6684
Difference	-0.3003	0.0633	-0.4243	-0.1763		

Difference is (Row 1 - Row 2)

Estimates of the Relative Risk (Row1/Row2)

Type of Study	Value	95% Confidence Limits	
Case-Control (Odds Ratio)	3.4543	2.0103	5.9355
Cohort (Col1 Risk)	1.8736	1.5344	2.2876
Cohort (Col2 Risk)	0.5424	0.3842	0.7657

Sample Size = 1944

---------------------- SEX=F ------------------------

The FREQ Procedure
Table of DIABETES by CVD

DIABETES(Diabetic Y/N)
            CVD(Incident Hosp MI or Stroke, Fatal or Non)

Frequency Percent Row Pct Col Pct	Yes	No	Total
Yes	36 1.45 58.06 7.64	26 1.04 41.94 1.29	62 2.49
No	435 17.47 17.92 92.36	1993 80.04 82.08 98.71	2428 97.51
Total	471 18.92	2019 81.08	2490 100.00

Statistics for Table of DIABETES by CVD

Statistic	DF	Value	Prob
Chi-Square	1	63.5363	<.0001
Likelihood Ratio Chi-Square	1	48.0701	<.0001
Continuity Adj. Chi-Square	1	60.9456	<.0001
Mantel-Haenszel Chi-Square	1	63.5108	<.0001
Phi Coefficient		0.1597	
Contingency Coefficient		0.1577	
Cramer's V		0.1597	

Fisher's Exact Test

Cell (1,1) Frequency (F)	36
Left-sided Pr <= F	1.0000
Right-sided Pr >= F	4.543E-12
Table Probability (P)	3.854E-12
Two-sided Pr <= P	4.543E-12

The FREQ Procedure
Statistics for Table of DIABETES by CVD

Column 1 Risk Estimates

	Risk	ASE	(Asymptotic) 95% Confidence Limits		(Exact) 95% Confidence Limits	
Row 1	0.5806	0.0627	0.4578	0.7035	0.4485	0.7049
Row 2	0.1792	0.0078	0.1639	0.1944	0.1641	0.1950
Total	0.1892	0.0078	0.1738	0.2045	0.1739	0.2051
Difference	0.4015	0.0632	0.2777	0.5253		

Difference is (Row 1 - Row 2)

Column 2 Risk Estimates

	Risk	ASE	(Asymptotic) 95% Confidence Limits		(Exact) 95% Confidence Limits	
Row 1	0.4194	0.0627	0.2965	0.5422	0.2951	0.5515
Row 2	0.8208	0.0078	0.8056	0.8361	0.8050	0.8359
Total	0.8108	0.0078	0.7955	0.8262	0.7949	0.8261
Difference	-0.4015	0.0632	-0.5253	-0.2777		

Difference is (Row 1 - Row 2)

Estimates of the Relative Risk (Row1/Row2)

Type of Study	Value	95% Confidence Limits	
Case-Control (Odds Ratio)	6.3438	3.7904	10.6171
Cohort (Col1 Risk)	3.2409	2.5801	4.0710
Cohort (Col2 Risk)	0.5109	0.3809	0.6851

Sample Size = 2490

What is the relative risk of CVD for diabetic versus nondiabetic men? What is the relative risk of CVD for diabetic versus nondiabetic women? Are the relative risks similar? Is sex a confounding variable? In the next analysis, we generate an adjusted relative risk.

The FREQ Procedure
Table 1 of DIABETES by CVD
Controlling for SEX=M

DIABETES(Diabetic Y/N)
          CVD(Incident Hosp MI or Stroke, Fatal or Non)

Frequency Percent Row Pct Col Pct	Yes	No	Total
Yes	38 1.95 64.41 5.54	21 1.08 35.59 1.67	59 3.03
No	648 33.33 34.38 94.46	1237 63.63 65.62 98.33	1885 96.97
Total	686 35.29	1258 64.71	1944 100.00

Table 2 of DIABETES by CVD
Controlling for SEX=F

DIABETES(Diabetic Y/N)
          CVD(Incident Hosp MI or Stroke, Fatal or Non)

```
Frequency|
Percent  |
Row Pct  |
Col Pct  |Yes      |No       |  Total
---------+--------+--------+
Yes      |      36 |      26 |     62
         |    1.45 |    1.04 |   2.49
         |   58.06 |   41.94 |
         |    7.64 |    1.29 |
---------+--------+--------+
No       |     435 |    1993 |   2428
         |   17.47 |   80.04 |  97.51
         |   17.92 |   82.08 |
         |   92.36 |   98.71 |
---------+--------+--------+
Total          471      2019     2490
             18.92     81.08   100.00
```

The FREQ Procedure

Summary Statistics for DIABETES by CVD
Controlling for SEX

Cochran-Mantel-Haenszel Statistics (Based on Table Scores)

Statistic	Alternative Hypothesis	DF	Value	Prob
1	Nonzero Correlation	1	76.8912	<.0001
2	Row Mean Scores Differ	1	76.8912	<.0001
3	General Association	1	76.8912	<.0001

```
                Estimates of the Common Relative Risk  (Row1/Row2)

Type of Study       Method                    Value       95% Confidence Limits
--------------------------------------------------------------------------------
Case-Control        Mantel-Haenszel           4.5914       3.1470        6.6987
   (Odds Ratio)     Logit                     4.7526       3.2726        6.9021

Cohort              Mantel-Haenszel           2.3592       2.0328        2.7380
   (Col1 Risk)      Logit                     2.3766       2.0451        2.7619

Cohort              Mantel-Haenszel           0.5245       0.4194        0.6559
   (Col2 Risk)      Logit                     0.5239       0.4190        0.6551


                          Breslow-Day Test for
                       Homogeneity of the Odds Ratios
                       ------------------------------
                       Chi-Square                2.5936
                       DF                             1
                       Pr > ChiSq                0.1073


                     Total Sample Size = 4434
```

Is the method valid (i.e., are relative risks homogeneous across sexes)? What is the adjusted relative risk? How does it compare to the relative risk for the pooled or combined sample and to the relative risks in men and in women?

8.10 Problems

1. A study is conducted over 10 years to investigate long-term complication rates in patients treated with two different therapies. The data are

Therapy	Complications	
	Yes	*No*
1:	89	911
2:	127	873

a. Estimate the risk difference.

b. Estimate the relative risk.

c. Estimate the odds ratio.

d. Based on (a)–(c), how do the therapies compare?

2. A study is conducted comparing an experimental treatment to a control treatment with respect to effectiveness in reducing joint pain in patients with arthritis. One hundred patients are randomly assigned to one of the competing treatments and the following data are collected, representing the numbers of patients reporting improvement in joint pain after the assigned treatment is administered:

	Control	Experimental
Number Reporting Improvement:	21	28
Total Number of Subjects:	50	50

Is there a significant difference in the proportions of patients reporting improvement in joint pain among the treatments? Run the appropriate test at the 5% level of significance.

3. Using the data in Problem 2,

a. Construct a 95% confidence interval for the risk difference of patients reporting improvement in joint pain between the Control and Experimental treatments.

b. Based on (a), is there a significant difference in the proportions of patients reporting improvement in joint pain between the Control and Experimental treatments? Justify your answer (be brief but complete).

4. Patients were enrolled in a study from two clinical centers. The objective of the study was to assess medication adherence (i.e., taking medications as prescribed). Some investigators suggest that adherence exceeding 85% is sufficient to classify a patient as adherent, whereas medication adherence below 85% suggests that the patient is not adherent to the prescribed schedule. Based on the following data, is there a significant difference in the proportions of adherent patients among the clinical centers? Run the appropriate test at $\alpha = 0.05$.

	Enrollment Site	
	Center 1	*Center 2*
Adherent (> 85%):	28	30
Not Adherent (< 85%):	21	29

5. Suppose an observational study is conducted to investigate the smoking behaviors of male and female patients with a history of coronary heart disease. Among 220 men surveyed, 80 were smokers. Among 190 women surveyed, 95 were smokers.

   a. Estimate the odds ratio of smoking for male versus female patients with a history of coronary heart disease.

   b. Construct a 95% confidence interval for the odds ratio.

   c. Based on (a) and (b), would you reject H_0: $OR = 1$ in favor of H_1: $OR \neq 1$? Justify your answer briefly.

6. Suppose a cross-sectional study is conducted to investigate cardiovascular risk factors among a sample of patients seeking medical care at one of two local hospitals. A total of 200 patients are enrolled. Construct a 95% confidence interval for the difference in proportions of patients with a family history of cardiovascular disease (CVD) between hospitals.

	Enrollment Site	
Family History of CVD	Hospital 1	Hospital 2
Yes:	24	14
No:	76	86
Total:	100	100

7. A randomized trial is conducted to compare a newly developed pain medication against a standard medication with respect to self-reported pain. Pain is reported on a 5-point scale. Suppose we are interested in the proportions of patients reporting moderate or severe pain between medications. Organize the data given into a dichotomous outcome {moderate or severe pain} versus {none, minimal or some pain}. Estimate the relative risk of moderate or severe pain between treatment groups. Test the hypotheses H_0: $RR = 1$ versus H_1: $RR \neq 1$ at a 5% level of significance.

	Pain				
	None	Minimal	Some	Moderate	Severe
New:	20	35	41	15	6
Standard:	15	25	46	36	18

8. A randomized trial is conducted comparing two different prenatal care programs among women at high risk for preterm delivery. The programs differ in intensity of medical intervention. Women who meet the criteria for high risk of preterm delivery are asked to participate in the study and are randomly assigned to one of the prenatal care programs. At the time

of delivery, they are classified as preterm or term delivery. The results are summarized here.

	Preterm Delivery	Term Delivery
Intensive Prenatal Care:	12	43
Standard Prenatal Care:	18	47

a. Estimate the relative risk of preterm delivery for women in the intensive prenatal care program as compared to the standard.
b. Construct a 95% confidence interval for the relative risk.
c. Based on (a), would you reject H_0: $RR = 1$ in favor of H_1: $RR \neq 1$? Justify your answer briefly.

9. A clinical trial of a new treatment for migraine headaches was conducted using a sample of 300 young adults with documented history of migraine headache. Among the 120 subjects on the new treatment (coded as 1), 62 experienced at least one migraine headache episode ($MH = 1$) during the study period, and 86 of the 180 subjects on the standard treatment (coded as 0) experienced at least one migraine headache episode during the study period.

a. Complete the following table of results.
b. Estimate the RR and test H_0: $RR = 1$.

	Migraine Headache (MH)	
Treatment	Yes (1)	No (0)
New (1):	62	
Standard (0):	86	
Total:		300

One of the investigators suggested adjustment for age since the risk of MH was higher in older subjects. The following results are given by age (older versus younger):

	Age = Old Migraine				Age = Young Migraine		
Trt	1	0		Trt	1	0	
1:	30	30	60	1:	32	28	60
0:	35	5	40	0:	51	89	140
Total:	65	35	100	Total:	83	117	200

c. Estimate the RR adjusted for age, and test H_0: $RR = 1$.

SAS Problems

Use SAS to solve the following problems.

1. A study is conducted over 10 years to investigate long-term complication rates in patients treated with two different therapies. The data are

	Complications	
Therapy	Yes	No
1:	89	911
2:	127	873

Use SAS Proc Freq to generate a 2 × 2 contingency table, and estimate the relative risk and odds ratio of complications. Test whether the risk of complications is different between therapies, using the chi-square test of homogeneity.

2. A randomized trial is conducted comparing two different prenatal care programs among women at high risk for preterm delivery. The programs differ in intensity of medical intervention. Women who meet the criteria for high risk of preterm delivery are asked to participate in the study and are randomly assigned to one of the prenatal care programs. At the time of delivery, they are classified as preterm or term delivery. The results are summarized here.

	Preterm Delivery	Term Delivery
Intensive Prenatal Care:	12	43
Standard Prenatal Care:	18	47

Use SAS Proc Freq to generate a 2 × 2 contingency table, and estimate the relative risk and odds ratio of complications. Generate 95% confidence intervals for the relative risk and odds ratio. Test whether the risk of complications is different between therapies, using the chi-square test of homogeneity.

3. A clinical trial of a new treatment for migraine headaches was conducted using a sample of 300 young adults with documented history of migraine headache. Among the 150 subjects on the new treatment (coded as 1), 62 experienced at least one migraine headache episode (MH = 1) during the study period, and 86 of the 100 subjects on the standard treatment (coded as 0) experienced at least one migraine headache episode during the study period. One of the investigators suggested adjustment for age

since the risk of MH was higher in older subjects. The results are given here by age (older versus younger).

	Age = Old Migraine				Age = Young Migraine		
Trt	1	0		Trt	1	0	
1:	30	30	60	1:	32	28	60
0:	35	5	40	0:	51	89	140
Total:	65	35	100	Total:	83	117	200

Use SAS to estimate the RR of treatment on migraine and test H_0: $RR = 1$. Use SAS to estimate the RR adjusted for age and test H_0: $RR = 1$.

Descriptive Statistics
(Ch. 2)

Probability
(Ch. 3)

Sampling Distributions
(Ch. 4)

Statistical Inference
(Chapters 5–13)

OUTCOME VARIABLE	GROUPING VARIABLE(S)/ PREDICTOR(S)	ANALYSIS	CHAPTER(S)
Continuous	—	Estimate μ; Compare μ to Known, Historical Value	5/12
Continuous	Dichotomous (2 groups)	Compare Independent Means (Estimate/Test $(\mu_1 - \mu_2)$) or the Mean Difference (μ_d)	6/12
Continuous	Discrete (>2 groups)	Test the Equality of k Means Using Analysis of Variance $(\mu_1 = \mu_2 = \cdots = \mu_k)$	9/12
Continuous	Continuous	Estimate Correlation or Determine Regression Equation	10/12
Continuous	Several Continuous or Dichotomous	Multiple Linear Regression Analysis	10
Dichotomous	—	Estimate p; Compare p to Known, Historical Value	7
Dichotomous	Dichotomous (2 groups)	Compare Independent Proportions (Estimate/Test $(p_1 - p_2)$)	7/8
Dichotomous	Discrete (> 2 groups)	Test the Equality of k Proportions (Chi-Square Test)	7
Dichotomous	Several Continuous or Dichotomous	Multiple Logistic Regression Analysis	11
Discrete	Discrete	Compare Distributions Among k Populations (Chi-Square Test)	7
Time to Event	Several Continuous or Dichotomous	Survival Analysis	13

Analysis of Variance

9

Analysis of variance (ANOVA) is one of the most widely used statistical techniques for testing the equality of population means. ANOVA is used to test the equality of more than two treatment means (to test the equality of two treatment means, we use the techniques described in Chapter 6). Specifically the hypotheses are

$$H_0: \mu_1 = \mu_2 = \mu_3 = \cdots = \mu_k$$
$$H_1: \text{means not all equal}$$

where $k =$ the number of populations under consideration $(k > 2)$

NOTE: The alternative hypothesis is not written $H_1: \mu_1 \neq \mu_2 \neq \mu_3 \neq \cdots \neq \mu_k$, as we want to reject the null hypothesis (H_0) if *any* of the population means are not equal (i.e., if at least one pair of means is not equal).

The assumptions necessary for valid applications of ANOVA are

1. k independent populations
2. Random samples from each of k $(k > 2)$ populations under consideration
3. Large samples ($n_i \geq 30$, where $i = 1, 2, \ldots, k$) or normal populations
4. Equal population variances (i.e., $\sigma_1^2 = \sigma_2^2 = \cdots = \sigma_k^2 = \sigma^2$).

The logic of the analysis of variance technique is presented in Section 9.1. Notation and computations are illustrated through examples in Section 9.2. In Section 9.3, we define fixed and random effects models. In Section 9.4, we present a statistic to assess the magnitude of the treatment effect. We define multiple comparison procedures and illustrate the use of two specific procedures in Section 9.5. In Section 9.6, we outline simple analysis of variance procedures for dependent samples, called repeated measures analysis of variance. Key formulas are summarized in Section 9.7, statistical computing applications are presented in Section 9.8, and in Section 9.9 we use data from the Framingham Heart Study to illustrate the applications presented here.

9.1 Background Logic

Consistent with other tests of hypotheses, we take random samples from each population of interest and evaluate sample statistics as a means of assessing the likelihood that H_0 is true. Consider the following examples, which illustrate the logic of the analysis of variance procedure.

EXAMPLE 9.1

Variation in Time to Relief of Symptoms Between and Within Treatments

An experiment is conducted in which three treatments are compared with respect to their effectiveness. For the purposes of this example, effectiveness is evaluated in terms of time to relief of symptoms, reported in minutes. We assume that the distribution of times to relief are approximately normal, and the test of interest is as follows:

$$H_0: \mu_1 = \mu_2 = \mu_3$$
$$H_1: \text{means not all equal}$$

Fifteen subjects are randomly selected to participate in the investigation. Five subjects are randomly assigned to each treatment and each subject reports the time to relief of symptoms, in minutes, following their assigned treatment. The sample data, and summary statistics, are as follows:

Treatment 1	Treatment 2	Treatment 3
29.0	25.1	20.1
29.2	25.0	20.0
29.1	25.0	19.9
28.9	24.9	19.8
28.8	25.0	20.2

Summary Statistics by Treatment

$\overline{X}_1 = 29.0$	$\overline{X}_2 = 25.0$	$\overline{X}_3 = 20.0$
$s_1^2 = 0.025$	$s_2^2 = 0.005$	$s_3^2 = 0.025$
$s_1 = 0.158$	$s_2 = 0.071$	$s_3 = 0.158$

From the summary statistics we see that the sample means are numerically different (i.e., 29.0 versus 25.0 versus 20.0 minutes). In addition, the variability *within* each sample is small (i.e., the standard deviations are 0.158, 0.071, 0.158, respectively), which implies that observations within each sample are tightly clustered about their respective sample means.

Suppose that the population means are equal (i.e., $H_0: \mu_1 = \mu_2 = \mu_3$ is true). We can assume, then, that the three samples are drawn from the same population and can pool all of the observations together (i.e., $n = 15$). The overall sample mean is $\overline{X} = 24.67$ minutes, with a sample variance $s^2 = 14.54$ and standard deviation $s = 3.81$. The variability in the pooled sample is large. In ANOVA, we compare the variation *within* samples to the variation *between* samples to assess the equality of the population means. If the observations within a sample are similar in value (i.e., small within-sample variation) and the means are different across samples (large between-sample variation), then a real difference is said to exist in the population means. Figure 9.1 displays the sample means and ranges of observations within each sample in Example 9.1.

Figure 9.1 *Variation Between and Within Treatments in Example 9.1*

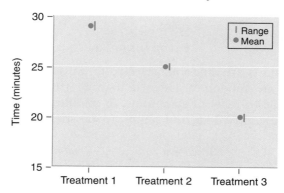

EXAMPLE 9.2

Variation in Time to Relief of Symptoms Between and Within Treatments

Consider the investigation described in Example 9.1. Suppose that the following sample data are observed in a similar investigation. Summary statistics for each sample are also shown.

Treatment 1	*Treatment 2*	*Treatment 3*
29.0	33.1	15.2
14.2	7.4	39.3
45.1	17.6	14.8
48.9	44.2	25.5
7.8	22.7	5.2

Summary Statistics by Treatment

$\overline{X}_1 = 29.0$	$\overline{X}_2 = 25.0$	$\overline{X}_3 = 20.0$
$s_1^2 = 330.87$	$s_2^2 = 201.07$	$s_3^2 = 167.96$
$s_1 = 18.19$	$s_2 = 14.18$	$s_3 = 12.96$

From the summary statistics we see that again the sample means are numerically different (i.e., 29.0 versus 25.0 versus 20.0 minutes). However, the variability within each sample is large (i.e., the standard deviations are 18.19, 14.18, 12.96, respectively), which implies that the observations within each sample are not tightly clustered about their respective sample means, but widely spread.

Suppose again we pool all of the observations together ($n = 15$) and compute summary statistics. The overall sample mean is $\overline{X} = 24.67$, the sample variance is $s^2 = 214.49$, and the standard deviation is $s = 14.65$. In

Figure 9.2 *Variation Between and Within Treatments in Example 9.2*

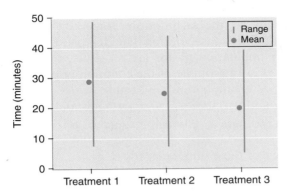

Example 9.2, the variation between sample means is the same as in Example 9.1; however, there is large variation within samples, which suggests that there is no real difference in the population means (see Figure 9.2). ■

In ANOVA, we wish to test the following: H_0: $\mu_1 = \mu_2 = \mu_3 = \cdots = \mu_k$ versus H_1: Means are not all equal (or at least one pair is not equal), where $k =$ the number of populations under consideration. To test H_0, we compute two estimates of the common population variance (σ^2). The first estimate is independent of H_0 (i.e., we do not assume that the population means are equal and we treat each sample separately). This estimate is called the estimate of the *within treatment variation*. The second estimate is based on the assumption that H_0 is true (i.e., population means are equal) and we pool all data together. This second estimate is called the estimate of the *between treatment variation*. The formulas for the estimates of the between and within variation follow for the case of equal sample sizes (i.e., $n_1 = n_2 = \cdots = n_k$). Sample sizes do not have to be equal in practice. The formulas presented in the next section illustrate the computations for both equal and unequal sample size applications.

Our first estimate is the estimate of the *within treatment variation*. To compute this estimate, we assume nothing about the population means. We do, however, assume that $\sigma_1^2 = \sigma_2^2 = \cdots = \sigma_k^2 = \sigma^2$. (This assumption is required for appropriate use of ANOVA.) It follows that each sample variance s_j^2 (where $j = 1, 2, \ldots, k$) is an estimate of σ^2 (the common population variance). Again, to simplify things, we assume that $n_1 = n_2 = \cdots = n_k$. An estimate of σ^2 is obtained by taking the mean of the sample variances (s_j^2) over the k treatments:

$$s_w^2 = \sum_{j=1}^{k} \frac{s_1^2}{k} = \frac{s_1^2 + s_2^2 + \cdots + s_k^2}{k} \tag{9.1}$$

where $s_w^2 =$ denotes the within treatment variance or within variation.

This estimate of σ^2 depends only on the assumptions for ANOVA, specifically on the assumption of equal population variances ($\sigma_1^2 = \sigma_2^2 = \cdots = \sigma_k^2 = \sigma^2$).

The second estimate of σ^2 is called the *between variation*. This second estimate depends on the assumptions for ANOVA (e.g., $\sigma_1^2 = \sigma_2^2 = \cdots = \sigma_k^2 = \sigma^2$) and also on the assumption that H_0 is true (i.e., $\mu_1 = \mu_2 = \mu_3 = \cdots = \mu_k = \mu$). If the population means are all equal, then each sample mean $\overline{X}_j$ ($j = 1, 2, \ldots, k$) is an estimate of the common population mean, μ. The $\overline{X}_j$'s can be viewed as a simple random sample of size k from a population with mean $\mu_{\overline{X}_j} = \mu$ and variance $\sigma_{\overline{X}_j}^2 = \sigma^2/n$. Our goal is to generate an estimate of σ^2. We can estimate $\sigma_{\overline{X}_j}^2$, which is equal to σ^2/n, and then use algebra to solve for σ^2.

The variance of the k sample means is

$$s_{\overline{X}_j}^2 = \sum_{j=1}^{k} \frac{(\overline{X}_j - \overline{X})^2}{k - 1} \tag{9.2}$$

where $\overline{X}$ is the overall mean (i.e., based on all observations pooled together)

$s_{\overline{X}_j}^2$ is an estimate of $\sigma_{\overline{X}_j}^2 = \sigma^2/n$. Therefore, $ns_{\overline{X}_j}^2$ is an estimate of σ^2:

$$s_b^2 = ns_{\overline{X}_j}^2 \tag{9.3}$$

where s_b^2 denotes the between treatment variance or between variation.

The test statistic in ANOVA is based on the ratio of these two estimates:

$$F = \frac{s_b^2}{s_w^2} \tag{9.4}$$

The test statistic follows an F distribution (see Figure 9.3). The F distribution is an asymmetric distribution that takes on values greater than or equal to zero.

If the two estimates of σ^2 are close in value (i.e., F is approximately equal to 1), then we have no reason to reject H_0. However, if the variation between samples (s_b^2) is large and the variation within samples (s_w^2) is small (i.e., F is large), then we reject H_0. To draw a conclusion regarding H_0, we need a critical

Figure 9.3 *The F Distribution*

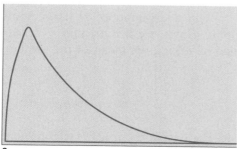

0

value from the F distribution. In order to select the appropriate value, we need 2 degrees of freedom: the numerator degrees of freedom, denoted $df_1 = k - 1$, and the denominator degrees of freedom, denoted $df_2 = k(n - 1)$, where $k =$ the number of populations or treatments under consideration and $n =$ the sample size per treatment. (*Note:* $k(n - 1) = kn - k$, where n is the common sample size or sample size in each group. We sometimes let $N = kn$, where $N =$ the total sample size (all groups combined).) Once the appropriate critical value is selected, we can construct our decision rule, which is of the form: Reject H_0 if $F \geq F_{k-1,N-k}$. Critical values of the F distribution are contained in Table B.4A in the Appendix for $\alpha = 0.05$ (and in Table B.4B for $\alpha = 0.025$).

The ANOVA technique is illustrated in the next section through examples. The computations are based on the logic presented here.

9.2 Notation and Examples

We now illustrate the computations using examples. In each example, the test of interest is a test of hypotheses involving more than two populations. Computations are illustrated for both equal and unequal sample size situations.

EXAMPLE 9.3

Testing Difference in Mean Time to Pain Relief Among 3 Treatments

An investigator wishes to compare the average time to relief of headache pain under three distinct medications, call them Drugs A, B, and C. Fifteen patients who suffer from chronic headaches are randomly selected for the investigation, and five subjects are randomly assigned to each treatment. The following data reflect times to relief (in minutes) after taking the assigned drug:

Drug A	Drug B	Drug C
30	25	15
35	20	20
40	30	25
25	25	20
35	30	20

Notation

X_{ij} denotes the *i*th observation in the *j*th treatment (e.g., $X_{11} = 30$, $X_{42} = 25$, $X_{53} = 20$)

A "." in place of a subscript (either *i* or *j*) denotes summation over that index: (e.g., $X_{.1} =$ sum over observations in treatment 1

$X_{.1} = 30 + 35 + 40 + 25 + 35 = 165$

$X_{1.} =$ sum first observations over treatments

$X_{1.} = 30 + 25 + 15 = 70$

$\overline{X}_{.1} =$ sample mean in treatment 1

$\overline{X}_{..} =$ overall sample mean (taken over all observations and treatments)

Using the notation, the summary statistics are:

Drug A	Drug B	Drug C
$\overline{X}_{.1} = 33.0$	$\overline{X}_{.2} = 26.0$	$\overline{X}_{.3} = 20.0$
$s_{.1} = 5.7$	$s_{.2} = 4.2$	$s_{.3} = 3.5$

To test whether the true mean times to relief under the three different drugs are equal, we use the same five-step procedure used in other tests of hypotheses.

1. Set up hypotheses.

$$H_0: \mu_1 = \mu_2 = \mu_3$$

$$H_1: \text{means not all equal,} \quad \alpha = 0.05$$

The assumptions for ANOVA are

1. Random samples from each of the three populations under consideration.
2. The times to relief are approximately normally distributed.
3. The three populations are independent.
4. The population variances are equal (i.e., $\sigma_1^2 = \sigma_2^2 = \sigma_3^2 = \sigma^2$).

2. Select the appropriate test statistic.

$$F = \frac{s_b^2}{s_w^2}$$

where $s_b^2 =$ denotes the between variation, which is also denoted MS_b (mean square between)

$s_w^2 =$ denotes the within variation, which is also denoted MS_w (mean square within) (see Table 9.1.)

Table 9.1 *Analysis of Variance Table*

Source of Variation	Sums of Squares (SS)	Degrees of Freedom (df)	Mean Squares (MS)	F
Between	$SS_b = \sum n_j (\overline{X}_{.j} - \overline{X}_{..})^2$	$k - 1$	$s_b^2 = MS_b = \dfrac{SS_b}{k-1}$	$F = \dfrac{MS_b}{MS_w}$
Within	$SS_w = \sum\sum (X_{ij} - \overline{X}_{.j})^2$	$N - k$	$s_w^2 = MS_w = \dfrac{SS_w}{N-k}$	
Total	$SS_{total} = \sum\sum (X_{ij} - \overline{X}_{..})^2$	$N - 1$		

where $X_{ij} = i$th observation in the jth treatment
$\overline{X}_{.j}$ = sample mean of jth treatment
$\overline{X}_{..}$ = overall sample mean
k = # treatments
$N = \sum n_j$ = total sample size

3. Decision rule.
   To select the appropriate critical value from the F distribution (Table B.4A), we first compute the numerator degrees of freedom (df_1) and the denominator degrees of freedom (df_2):

$$df_1 = k - 1 = 3 - 1 = 2$$
$$df_2 = N - k = 15 - 3 = 12$$

In ANOVA, we reject H_0 if the test statistic is larger than the critical value. The critical value of F with 2 and 12 degrees of freedom, relative to a 5% level of significance, is denoted $F_{2,12}$ and can be found in Table B.4A: $F_{2,12} = 3.89$. The decision rule is

Reject H_0 if $F \geq 3.89$

Do not reject H_0 if $F < 3.89$

4. Compute the test statistic.
   Generally, to organize the computations in ANOVA applications, an ANOVA table is constructed. The table contains all of the computations, the degrees of freedom used to select the appropriate critical value, and the test statistic. The general form of the ANOVA table is shown in Table 9.1.
   Now, using the data in Example 9.3, we construct an ANOVA table. We first compute the sums of squares. The between treatment sums of squares (also called the sums of square due to treatments) is computed by summing the squared differences between each treatment mean and the overall mean. We first compute the overall mean. In Example 9.3, the sample sizes are equal; therefore, the overall mean is the mean of the three treatment means:

$$\overline{X}_{..} = \frac{(33.0 + 26.0 + 20.0)}{3} = 26.3$$

The between treatment sums of squares is

$$SS_b = \sum n_j(\overline{X}_{.j} - \overline{X}_{..})^2 = 5(33 - 26.3)^2 + 5(26 - 26.3)^2$$
$$+ 5(20 - 26.3)^2 = 423.3$$

The within treatment sums of squares (also called the sums of square due to error) is computed by summing the squared differences between each observation and its treatment mean.

To compute the within sums of squares, $SS_w = \sum\sum(X_{ij} - \overline{X}_{.j})^2$, we construct the following table to organize our computations:

Drug A		Drug B		Drug C	
$(X_{i1} - \overline{X}_{.1})$	$(X_{i1} - \overline{X}_{.1})^2$	$(X_{i2} - \overline{X}_{.2})$	$(X_{i2} - \overline{X}_{.2})^2$	$(X_{i3} - \overline{X}_{.3})$	$(X_{i3} - \overline{X}_{.3})^2$
-3	9	-1	1	-5	25
2	4	-6	36	0	0
7	49	4	16	5	25
-8	64	-1	1	0	0
2	4	4	16	0	0
$\sum(X_{i1} - \overline{X}_{.1})$ $= 0$	$\sum(X_{i1} - \overline{X}_{.1})^2$ $= 130$	$\sum(X_{i2} - \overline{X}_{.2})$ $= 0$	$\sum(X_{i2} - \overline{X}_{.2})^2$ $= 70$	$\sum(X_{i3} - \overline{X}_{.3})$ $= 0$	$\sum(X_{i3} - \overline{X}_{.3})^2$ $= 50$

The within treatment sums of squares is

$$SS_w = \sum\sum(X_{ij} - \overline{X}_{.j})^2 = 130 + 70 + 50 = 250$$

The total sums of squares is computed by summing the squared differences between each observation and the overall mean:

$$SS_{total} = \sum\sum(X_{ij} - \overline{X}_{..})^2 = (30 - 26.3)^2 + \cdots + (20 - 26.3)^2 = 673.3$$

However, since $SS_{total} = SS_b + SS_w$, it is not necessary to compute SS_{total} directly: $SS_{total} = 423.3 + 250 = 673.3$.

We now construct the ANOVA table for Example 9.3.

Source of Variation	Sums of Squares (SS)	Degrees of Freedom (df)	Mean Squares (MS)	F
Between	423.3	2	211.67	10.16
Within	250.0	12	20.82	
Total	673.3	14		

5. Conclusion.

Reject H_0, since $10.16 > 3.89$. We have significant evidence, $\alpha = 0.05$, to show that the mean times to relief from headache pain under the three drugs A, B, and C are not all equal. Because we do not have more extensive tables for the F distribution here, we cannot compute a p value. However, when an ANOVA is run using SAS, an exact p value is generated. ■

SAS EXAMPLE 9.3 **Testing Difference in Mean Time to Pain Relief Among 3 Treatments Using SAS**

The following output was generated using SAS Proc ANOVA, which runs an analysis of variance test for equality of means. SAS produces the following. A brief interpretation appears after the output.

SAS Output for Example 9.3

```
                          The ANOVA Procedure
Dependent Variable: time

                                 Sum of
Source                  DF       Squares      Mean Square    F Value   Pr >

Model                    2     423.3333333    211.6666667     10.16    0.0026
Error                   12     250.0000000     20.8333333
Corrected Total         14     673.3333333


          R-Square     Coeff Var     Root MSE     time Mean
          0.628713     17.33299      4.564355     26.33333


Source                  DF      ANOVA SS     Mean Square    F Value   Pr > F
trt                      2     423.3333333    211.6666667     10.16    0.0026
```

Interpretation of SAS Output for Example 9.3

SAS has two procedures for analysis of variance applications. The first is the ANOVA procedure, which is used when the sample sizes are equal, and the second is the GLM (general linear models) procedure, which can be used when the sample sizes are unequal or equal. Since the sample sizes are equal in Example 9.3, we used the ANOVA procedure.

SAS produces an ANOVA table, similar to Table 9.1. SAS uses the term "Model" to refer to the between treatment variation and "Error" to refer to the within treatment variation. SAS also presents the degrees of freedom before the sums of squares; otherwise, the table is identical. In Example 9.3, the test statistic is $F = 10.16$ with $p = 0.0026$, which would lead to rejection of H_0 since $p = 0.0026 < \alpha = 0.05$. ▪

EXAMPLE 9.4 **Testing Difference in Mean Age at Completion of 8th Grade Among 3 School Districts**

The following data, collected from randomly selected students at rural, suburban, and urban schools, reflect ages of students at completion of eighth grade. Test if there is a significant difference in the mean age at completion of eighth grade for rural, suburban, and urban students using a 5% level of significance.

Sample Data:

Rural:	14	14	14	14	13	13	13	12	
Suburban:	14	14	14	13	13	13	13	13	12	12
Urban:	16	16	15	15	15	14	14	14	13	12

1. Set up hypotheses.

$$H_0: \mu_1 = \mu_2 = \mu_3$$
$$H_1: \text{means not all equal}, \quad \alpha = 0.05$$

2. Select the appropriate test statistic.

$$F = \frac{s_b^2}{s_w^2}$$

where s_b^2 = denotes the between variation, which is also denoted MS_b (mean square between)

s_w^2 = denotes the within variation, which is also denoted MS_w (mean square within) (see Table 9.1).

3. Decision rule.

To select the appropriate critical value from the F distribution (Table B.4), we first compute the numerator degrees of freedom (df_1) and the denominator degrees of freedom (df_2):

$$df_1 = k - 1 = 3 - 1 = 2$$
$$df_2 = N - k = 28 - 3 = 25$$

The critical value of F with 2 and 25 degrees of freedom, relative to a 5% level of significance, is found in Table B.4A: $F_{2, 25} = 3.39$. The decision rule is

$$\text{Reject } H_0 \text{ if } F \geq 3.39$$
$$\text{Do not reject } H_0 \text{ if } F < 3.39$$

4. Compute the test statistic.

Again, we will construct an ANOVA table to organize our computations. In this example, some of the formulas have been modified to accommodate the unequal sample sizes.

The following table contains summary statistics on the age data:

	Rural	Suburban	Urban
n_j	8	10	10
$\sum X_{ij}$	107	131	144
$\overline{X}_{\cdot j}$	13.4	13.1	14.4

The between sums of squares (also called the sums of squares due to treatments) is computed by summing the squared differences between each treatments) is computed by summing the squared differences between each treatment mean and the overall mean. In Example 9.4, the sample sizes are unequal; therefore, the overall mean is computed by summing all of the observations and dividing by N:

$$\overline{X}_{..} = \frac{(107 + 131 + 144)}{28} = 13.7$$

NOTE: When the sample sizes are equal, the overall mean can be computed by taking the mean of the sample means.

The between sums of squares is

$$SS_b = \sum n_j (\overline{X}_{.j} - \overline{X}_{..})^2 = 8(13.4 - 13.7)^2$$
$$+ 10(13.1 - 13.7)^2 + 10(14.4 - 13.7)^2 = 9.22$$

The within sums of squares (also called the sums of squares due to error) is computed by summing the squared differences between each observation and its treatment mean. To compute the within sums of squares, $SS_w = \sum\sum(X_{ij} - \overline{X}_{.j})^2$, we construct the following table:

Rural		Suburban		Urban	
$(X_{i1} - \overline{X}_{.1})$	$(X_{i1} - \overline{X}_{.1})^2$	$(X_{i2} - \overline{X}_{.2})$	$(X_{i2} - \overline{X}_{.2})^2$	$(X_{i3} - \overline{X}_{.3})$	$(X_{i3} - \overline{X}_{.3})^2$
0.6	0.36	0.9	0.81	1.6	2.56
0.6	0.36	0.9	0.81	1.6	2.56
0.6	0.36	0.9	0.81	0.6	0.36
0.6	0.36	−0.1	0.01	0.6	0.36
−0.4	0.16	−0.1	0.01	0.6	0.36
−0.4	0.16	−0.1	0.01	−0.4	0.16
−0.4	0.16	−0.1	0.01	−0.4	0.16
−1.4	1.96	−0.1	0.01	−0.4	0.16
		−1.1	1.21	−1.4	1.96
		−1.1	1.21	−2.4	5.76
$\sum(X_{i1} - \overline{X}_{.1})$ $= 0$	$\sum(X_{i1} - \overline{X}_{.1})^2$ $= 3.88$	$\sum(X_{i2} - \overline{X}_{.2})$ $= 0$	$\sum(X_{i2} - \overline{X}_{.2})^2$ $= 4.90$	$\sum(X_{i3} - \overline{X}_{.3})$ $= 0$	$\sum(X_{i3} - \overline{X}_{.3})^2$ $= 14.40$

The within sums of squares is

$$SS_w = \sum\sum(X_{ij} - \overline{X}_{.j})^2 = 3.88 + 4.90 + 14.40 = 23.18$$

The total sums of squares is computed by summing the squared differences between each observation and the overall mean:

$$SS_{total} = \sum\sum(X_{ij} - \overline{X}_{..})^2 = (14 - 13.7)^2 + \cdots + (12 - 13.7)^2 = 32.4$$

Again, since $SS_{total} = SS_b + SS_w$, it is not necessary to compute SS_{total} directly: $SS_{total} = 9.22 + 23.18 = 32.40$.

We now construct the ANOVA table for Example 9.4.

Source of Variation	Sums of Squares (SS)	Degrees of Freedom (df)	Mean Squares (MS)	F
Between	9.22	2	4.63	4.99
Within	23.18	25	0.93	
Total	32.40	27		

5. Conclusion.

Reject H_0, since $4.99 > 3.39$. We have significant evidence, $\alpha = 0.05$, to show that the mean ages at completion of eighth grade are not equal for rural, suburban, and urban students. ■

SAS EXAMPLE 9.4 Testing Difference in Mean Age at Completion of 8th Grade Among 3 School Districts Using SAS

The following output was generated using SAS Proc GLM, which runs an analysis of variance test for equality of means. GLM is used when the sample sizes are unequal. SAS produces the following. A brief interpretation appears after the output.

SAS Output for Example 9.4

The GLM Procedure

Dependent Variable: age

Source	DF	Sum of Squares	Mean Square	F Value	Pr > F
Model	2	9.25357143	4.62678571	4.99	0.0150
Error	25	23.17500000	0.92700000		
Corrected Total	27	32.42857143			

R-Square	Coeff Var	Root MSE	age Mean
0.285352	7.057234	0.962808	13.64286

Source	DF	Type I SS	Mean Square	F Value	Pr > F
school	2	9.25357143	4.62678571	4.99	0.0150

Source	DF	Type III SS	Mean Square	F Value	Pr > F
school	2	9.25357143	4.62678571	4.99	0.0150

Interpretation of SAS Output for Example 9.4

Here we used the GLM procedure to run the ANOVA because the sample sizes are unequal. SAS produces an ANOVA table similar to Table 9.1. Again, SAS uses the term "Model" to refer to the between treatment variation and "Error" to refer to the within treatment variation. SAS also presents the degrees of freedom before the sums of squares; otherwise, the table is identical. In Example 9.4, the test statistic is $F = 4.99$, with $p = 0.0150$, which would lead to rejection of H_0 since $p = 0.0150 < \alpha = 0.05$. ▪

EXAMPLE 9.5

Testing Difference in Mean Weight Gain Among 4 Different Diets

A study is developed to examine the effects of vitamin and milk supplements on infant weight gain. Four diet plans are considered: Diet A involves a regular diet plus the vitamin supplement, Diet B involves a regular diet plus the special milk formula, Diet C is our control diet (i.e., no restrictions or special considerations), and Diet D involves a regular diet plus the vitamin and the special milk formula. Twenty infants are selected for the investigation and each is randomized to one of the four competing diet programs. The following table displays weight gains, measured in pounds, after 1 month on the assigned diet.

Diet A	Diet B	Diet C	Diet D
2.0	1.6	1.5	2.1
1.5	1.9	2.0	2.4
2.4	2.1	1.8	1.9
1.9	1.1	1.3	1.8
2.6	1.7	1.2	2.2

1. Set up hypotheses.

$$H_0: \mu_1 = \mu_2 = \mu_3 = \mu_4$$
$$H_1: \text{means not all equal}, \quad \alpha = 0.05$$

2. Select the appropriate test statistic.

$$F = \frac{s_b^2}{s_w^2}$$

where s_b^2 = denotes the between variation, which is also denoted MS_b (mean square between)

s_w^2 = denotes the within variation, which is also denoted MS_w (mean square within) (see Table 9.1)

3. Decision rule.

    To select the appropriate critical value from the F distribution (Table B.4), we first compute the numerator degrees of freedom (df_1) and the denominator degrees of freedom (df_2):

$$df_1 = k - 1 = 4 - 1 = 3$$
$$df_2 = N - k = 20 - 4 = 16$$

The critical value of F with 3 and 16 degrees of freedom, relative to a 5% level of significance, is found in Table B.4a: $F_{3,16} = 3.24$. The decision rule is

$$\text{Reject } H_0 \text{ if } F \geq 3.24$$

$$\text{Do not reject } H_0 \text{ if } F < 3.24$$

4. Compute the test statistic.

    Again, we will construct an ANOVA table to organize our computations. The following table displays summary statistics on the infant weights:

	Diet A	Diet B	Diet C	Diet D
n_j	5	5	5	5
$\sum X_{ij}$	10.4	8.4	7.8	10.4
$\overline{X}_{.j}$	2.1	1.7	1.6	2.1

    The between sums of squares (also called the sums of squares due to treatments) is computed by summing the squared differences between each treatment mean and the overall mean. Since the sample sizes are equal, the overall mean can be found by computing the mean of the four treatment means:

$$\overline{X}_{..} = \frac{(2.1 + 1.7 + 1.6 + 2.1)}{4} = 1.88$$

The between sums of squares is

$$SS_b = \sum n_j (\overline{X}_{.j} - \overline{X}_{..})^2 = 5((2.1 - 1.88)^2 + (1.7 - 1.88)^2$$
$$+ (1.6 - 1.88)^2 + (2.1 - 1.88)^2) = 1.04$$

    The within sums of squares (also called the sums of squares due to error) is computed by summing the squared differences between each observation and its treatment mean. To compute the within sums of squares, $SS_w = \sum\sum(X_{ij} - \overline{X}_{.j})^2$, we construct a table similar to those presented in Examples 9.3 and 9.4. Here, we present only the results. The within sums of squares is

$$SS_w = \sum\sum(X_{ij} - \overline{X}_{.j})^2 = 0.75 + 0.57 + 0.46 + 0.23 = 2.01$$

The total sums of squares is computed by adding the between and within sums of squares:

$$SS_{total} = SS_b + SS_w = 1.04 + 2.01 = 3.05$$

We now construct the ANOVA table for Example 9.5.

Source of Variation	Sums of Squares (SS)	Degrees of Freedom (df)	Mean Squares (MS)	F
Between	1.04	3	0.35	2.69
Within	2.01	16	0.13	
Total	3.05	19		

5. Conclusion.
    Do not reject H_0, since $2.69 < 3.24$. We do not have significant evidence, $\alpha = 0.05$, to show that the mean weight gains under the four different diets are not equal. ■

SAS EXAMPLE 9.5 Testing Difference in Mean Weight Gain Among 4 Different Diets Using SAS

The following output was generated using SAS Proc GLM, which runs an analysis of variance test for equality of means. GLM can accommodate applications where the sample sizes are equal or unequal. SAS produces the following. A brief interpretation appears after the output.

SAS Output for Example 9.5

```
                          The GLM Procedure
Dependent Variable: gain
                                 Sum of
Source                   DF      Squares    Mean Square   F Value   Pr > F

Model                     3   1.09400000    0.36466667      2.92   0.0659
Error                    16   1.99600000    0.12475000
Corrected Total          19   3.09000000


           R-Square     Coeff Var     Root MSE     gain Mean
           0.354045      19.09187     0.353200      1.850000

Source                   DF    Type I SS    Mean Square   F Value   Pr > F
diet                      3   1.09400000    0.36466667      2.92   0.0659

Source                   DF  Type III SS    Mean Square   F Value   Pr > F
diet                      3   1.09400000    0.36466667      2.92   0.0659
```

Interpretation of SAS Output for Example 9.5

Here we used the GLM procedure to run the ANOVA. In Example 9.5, the test statistic is $F = 2.92$ with $p = 0.0659$. We do not reject H_0 since $p = 0.0659 > \alpha = 0.05$. In this example, the SAS calculations are slightly different from our hand calculations due to rounding. SAS carries many more decimal places in computations and produces a more exact solution. The conclusions of the tests (performed by hand and by SAS) are the same. It should be noted that the test is marginally significant. Although we did not reach the specified significance level of 0.05, these results should be evaluated carefully because $p = 0.0659$, suggesting that there are some differences among the diets. If we evaluate the mean weight gains, Diets A and D produce the largest gains; Diet B is not much different than the control diet, Diet C. ■

9.3 Fixed Versus Random Effects Models

There are two types of analysis of variance applications: fixed effects models and random effects models. In *fixed effects models*, the treatment groups under study—for example, the three headache medications (Drugs A, B, and C), the four infant diets (A, B, C, and D)—represent all treatments of interest. In our concluding statement we say there is (or is not) significant evidence of a difference in means among the treatments studied (e.g., there is a difference in the mean times to relief of headache pain under Drugs A, B, and C). In *random effects models*, we randomly select k treatments for the investigation from a larger pool of available treatments. For example, suppose there are 10 competing treatments for headache pain or 12 well-known infant diets and we randomly select 3 or 4 to study (e.g., Drugs A, B, and C or Diets A, B, C, and D). In our concluding statement we say there is (or is not) significant evidence of a difference in means among ALL treatments (e.g., there is a difference in weight gain among all 12 well-known infant diets), though we studied only a subset.

Basically, in random effects models we can generalize our results to the pool of all treatments since we randomly selected a subset for the investigation. In fixed effects models, our conclusions apply only to the treatments studied. The logic and the computations presented in the preceding sections are appropriate only for fixed effects models. Modifications beyond the scope of this book are necessary for random effects models (see Cobb, G.W. (1998). *Introduction to Design and Analysis of Experiments*, Springer-Verlag, Inc., New York).

9.4 Evaluating Treatment Effects

If an ANOVA is performed and it has been established that a difference in means exists (i.e., we reject H_0), we want to assess the magnitude of the effect *due* to the treatments. That is, we want to address the question, How much variation in the data is due to the treatments?

The following statistic, called "eta-squared," is the ratio of variation due to the treatments (SS_b) to the total variation:

$$\eta^2 = \frac{SS_b}{SS_{total}} \qquad (9.5)$$

where $0 \le \eta^2 \le 1$

Values of η^2 that are closer to 1 imply that more variation in the data is attributable to the treatments.

In Example 9.3, comparing the times to relief among the three headache medications,

$$\eta^2 = \frac{423.3}{673.3} = 0.629$$

Thus, 62.9% of the variation in the times to relief is due to the medications (i.e., Drug A, B, or C). In Example 9.4, comparing students' ages,

$$\eta^2 = \frac{9.25}{32.43} = 0.285$$

Thus, only 28.5% of the variation in the students' ages is due to the location of the school (i.e., rural, suburban, urban).

9.5 Multiple Comparisons Procedures

Once we reject $H_0: \mu_1 = \mu_2 = \cdots = \mu_k$ in an ANOVA application, we say there is a significant difference among all of the treatment means (or at least one pair of means are not equal). It is often of interest to then test specific hypotheses comparing certain treatments. For example, in Example 9.3 we concluded that the mean times to relief for the three headache medications were significantly different. Suppose we are particularly interested in comparing only the first two medications (i.e., $H_0: \mu_1 = \mu_2$) or the first and the third (i.e., $H_0: \mu_1 = \mu_3$). Tests of this type are called *pairwise comparisons,* since they involve pairs of treatment means. It is also possible to construct more complicated comparisons. For example, it may be of interest to compare the mean time to relief for patients assigned to either Drug A or B to the mean time to relief for patients assigned to Drug C. The hypotheses would be denoted as follows: $H_0: (\mu_1 + \mu_2)/2 = \mu_3$. Both pairwise (two-at-a-time) and more complicated comparisons are generally called *contrasts.*

There are a number of statistical procedures for handling these applications, which are called *multiple comparison procedures,* or MCPs. Different procedures are recommended for different applications. The procedures differ according to the types of comparisons of interest (e.g., pairwise comparisons), the number of comparisons, and the number of treatments in the ANOVA application. The procedures also differ with respect to their treatment of Type I errors (i.e., $P(\text{Reject } H_0 | H_0 \text{ true})$). Techniques such as the two independent samples t test can be used to test pairs of treatment means, but the Type I error rate over all comparisons of interest is not controlled. In applications involv ing k treatments, there are as many as $k(k-1)/2$ possible pairwise compar isons. In the worst possible case, the Type I error can be as large a $\alpha(k(k-1)/2)$. For example, if three pairwise comparisons are performed, th Type I error rate could be 15%, or as large as 50% if 10 pairwise comparison are performed. In most every application, these levels would be unacceptable Consider the following definitions:

$$\text{Error rate per comparison (ER\_PC)} = P(\text{Type I error}) \text{ on any one} \\ \text{test or comparison} \qquad (9.6$$

In general, the error rate per comparison is 0.05.

$$\text{Error rate per experiment (ER\_PE)} = \text{the number of Type I errors} \\ \text{we expect to make in any} \\ \text{experiment under } H_0 \qquad (9.7$$

For example, suppose we collect data on 100 different variables (e.g., systoli blood pressure, diastolic blood pressure, total cholesterol, age) from a randon sample of females and from a random sample of males and wish to test fo mean differences between males and females on each variable. The experimen involves 100 two independent samples t tests, each performed at the $\alpha = 0.0$ level. The error rate over the entire experiment (ER_PE) is $100(0.05) = 5$. Tha is, we expect 5 tests to be significant (i.e., we reject H_0 in 5 tests) solely b chance (i.e., we expect to make five Type I errors in the experiment). Notic that the error rate per experiment is a frequency and not a probability.

$$\text{Familywise error rate (FW\_ER)} = P(\text{at least 1 Type I error}) \\ \text{in experiment} \qquad (9.8$$

The FW_ER is computed by: $1 - (1 - \alpha_i)^c$, where α_i is the error rate per com parison (ER_PC) and c represents the number of contrasts, or comparisons, i the experiment. The formula is illustrated in Example 9.6.

EXAMPLE 9.6   **Error Rates with Multiple Comparisons**

Suppose we test the equality of five treatment means using ANOVA and th null hypothesis is rejected at $\alpha = 0.05$. Suppose that it is of interest to perform a pairwise comparisons. There are $k(k-1)/2 = 5(5-1)/2 = 10$ distinct pai wise comparisons (e.g., $H_0: \mu_1 = \mu_2$ versus $H_1: \mu_1 \neq \mu_2$, $H_0: \mu_1 = \mu_3$ versu $H_1: \mu_1 \neq \mu_3$, $H_0: \mu_1 = \mu_4$ versus $H_1: \mu_1 \neq \mu_4, \ldots, H_0: \mu_4 = \mu_5$ versus H $\mu_4 \neq \mu_5$). Suppose we wish to conduct each comparison at a 5% level o significance. It should be noted that one should perform only tests that are of substantive interest and not just all possible tests.

The error rate per comparison, ER_PC = 0.05.
The error rate per experiment, ER_PE = 10(0.05) = 0.5.
The familywise error rate, FW_ER = $1 - (1 - 0.05)^{10} = 0.401$.

In this example, we expect to make 0.5 Type I errors solely by chance, and the probability of at least one Type I error is large (40.1% chance). ■

Again, there are a number of multiple comparison procedures that differ according to their treatment of the error rates per experiment and familywise error rates. Other MCPs (not discussed here) include the Duncan procedure (also called the multiple range test), Fisher's Least Significant Difference, the Newman–Keuls test, and Dunnett's test (used to compare a control to several active treatments). For further details, see D'Agostino, R. B., Massaro, J., Kwan, H., Cabral, H. (1993). Strategies for dealing with multiple treatment comparisons in confirmatory clinical trials. *Drug Information Journal*, 27, 625–641. We now illustrate the use of two popular multiple comparison procedures, the Scheffe and Tukey procedures.

9.5.1 The Scheffe Procedure

The Scheffe procedure is a MCP that controls the familywise error rate. That is, the *P*(Type I error) is controlled (and equal to α) over the family of all comparisons. For example, if 6 or 8 or 20 comparisons are performed within a particular experiment, the familywise error rate is 5%. The Scheffe procedure is most desirable in applications involving more than a few contrasts; however, it is a conservative procedure (i.e., has lower statistical power) compared to competing procedures.

The Scheffe procedure is outlined next, for the case of pairwise comparisons in Example 9.7. More complicated contrasts are considered in Example 9.8.

1. Set up hypotheses.

$$H_0: \mu_i = \mu_j$$
$$H_1: \mu_i \neq \mu_j$$

where μ_i and μ_j are two of k treatment means that were found to be significantly different based on ANOVA

2. Select the appropriate test statistic.
    The test statistic for pairwise comparisons takes the following form:

$$F = \frac{(\overline{X}_{.i} - \overline{X}_{.j})^2}{s_w^2 \left(\frac{1}{n_i} + \frac{1}{n_j} \right)} = \frac{(\overline{X}_{.i} - \overline{X}_{.j})^2}{MS_{\text{error}} \left(\frac{1}{n_i} + \frac{1}{n_j} \right)}$$

where s_w^2 is the estimate of the within variation and equal to the mean square within or mean square error (from ANOVA table)

3. Decision rule.

The test statistic follows an F distribution; therefore a critical value is selected from the F distribution table (Table B.4). The critical value for the Scheffe procedure (pairwise as well as other contrasts) is the product of $(k - 1)$ and the critical value from the ANOVA:

$$\text{Reject } H_0 \text{ if } F \geq (k - 1) F_{k-1, N-k}$$

$$\text{Do not reject } H_0 \text{ if } F < (k - 1) F_{k-1, N-k}$$

EXAMPLE 9.7

Scheffe Pairwise Comparisons for Differences in Means Between Drugs

Consider Example 9.3 in which we compared the mean times to relief from headache pain under three competing medications. An ANOVA was performed at the 5% level of significance and we rejected $H_0: \mu_1 = \mu_2 = \mu_3$. Suppose we now wish to compare the medications taken two-at-a-time (i.e., pairwise comparisons). The summary statistics are

Drug A	Drug B	Drug C
$\overline{X}_1 = 33.0$	$\overline{X}_2 = 26.0$	$\overline{X}_3 = 20.0$
$s_1 = 5.7$	$s_2 = 4.2$	$s_3 = 3.5$

Drug A Versus Drug B

1. Set up hypotheses.

$$H_0: \mu_1 = \mu_2$$
$$H_1: \mu_1 \neq \mu_2, \quad \alpha = 0.05$$

2. Select the appropriate test statistic.

$$F = \frac{(\overline{X}_1 - \overline{X}_2)^2}{s_w^2 \left(\dfrac{1}{n_1} + \dfrac{1}{n_2} \right)} = \frac{(\overline{X}_1 - \overline{X}_2)^2}{MS_{error} \left(\dfrac{1}{n_1} + \dfrac{1}{n_2} \right)}$$

3. Decision rule.

Reject H_0 if $F \geq (k - 1) F_{2,12} = 2(3.89) = 7.78$ (where $F_{2,12} = 3.89$ was used in Example 9.3 in the ANOVA)

4. Compute the test statistic.

$$F = \frac{(33.0 - 26.0)^2}{20.82 \left(\dfrac{1}{5} + \dfrac{1}{5} \right)} = 5.88$$

5. Conclusion.

Do not reject H_0 since $5.88 < 7.78$. We do not have significant evidence, $\alpha = 0.05$, to show that $\mu_1 \neq \mu_2$.

Drug A Versus Drug C

1. Set up hypotheses.

$$H_0:\ \mu_1 = \mu_3$$
$$H_1:\ \mu_1 \neq \mu_3, \quad \alpha = 0.05$$

2. Select the appropriate test statistic.

$$F = \frac{(\overline{X}_{.1} - \overline{X}_{.3})^2}{s_w^2 \left(\dfrac{1}{n_1} + \dfrac{1}{n_3}\right)} = \frac{(\overline{X}_{.1} - \overline{X}_{.3})^2}{MS_{error} \left(\dfrac{1}{n_1} + \dfrac{1}{n_3}\right)}$$

3. Decision rule.

   Reject H_0 if $F \geq (k-1)F_{2,\,12} = 2(3.89) = 7.78$

4. Compute the test statistic.

$$F = \frac{(33.0 - 20.0)^2}{20.82 \left(\dfrac{1}{5} + \dfrac{1}{5}\right)} = 20.28$$

5. Conclusion.

   Reject H_0 since $20.28 \geq 7.78$. We have significant evidence, $\alpha = 0.05$, to show that $\mu_1 \neq \mu_3$.

Drug B Versus Drug C

1. Set up hypotheses.

$$H_0:\ \mu_2 = \mu_3$$
$$H_1:\ \mu_2 \neq \mu_3, \quad \alpha = 0.05$$

2. Select the appropriate test statistic.

$$F = \frac{(\overline{X}_{.2} - \overline{X}_{.3})^2}{s_w^2 \left(\dfrac{1}{n_2} + \dfrac{1}{n_3}\right)} = \frac{(\overline{X}_{.2} - \overline{X}_{.3})^2}{MS_{error} \left(\dfrac{1}{n_2} + \dfrac{1}{n_3}\right)}$$

3. Decision rule.

   Reject H_0 if $F \geq (k-1)F_{2,\,12} = 2(3.89) = 7.78$

4. Compute the test statistic.

$$F = \frac{(26.0 - 20.0)^2}{20.82 \left(\dfrac{1}{5} + \dfrac{1}{5}\right)} = 4.32$$

5. Conclusion.

   Do not reject H_0 since $4.32 < 7.78$. We do not have significant evidence, $\alpha = 0.05$, to show that $\mu_2 \neq \mu_3$. ■

SAS EXAMPLE 9.7 **Scheffe Pairwise Comparisons for Differences in Means Between Drugs Using SAS**

The following output was generated using SAS Proc ANOVA. We specified an option to conduct all pairwise comparisons using the Scheffe MCP. SAS produces the following. A brief interpretation appears after the output.

SAS Output for Example 9.7

The ANOVA Procedure

Dependent Variable: time

Source	DF	Sum of Squares	Mean Square	F Value	Pr > F
Model	2	423.3333333	211.6666667	10.16	0.0026
Error	12	250.0000000	20.8333333		
Corrected Total	14	673.3333333			

R-Square	Coeff Var	Root MSE	time Mean
0.628713	17.33299	4.564355	26.33333

Source	DF	ANOVA SS	Mean Square	F Value	Pr > F
trt	2	423.3333333	211.6666667	10.16	0.0026

Scheffe's Test for time

NOTE: This test controls the Type I experimentwise error rate.

Alpha	0.05
Error Degrees of Freedom	12
Error Mean Square	20.83333
Critical Value of F	3.88529
Minimum Significant Difference	8.047

Means with the same letter are not significantly different.

Scheffe Grouping		Mean	N	trt
	A	33.000	5	A
B	A	26.000	5	B
B		20.000	5	C

Interpretation of SAS Output for Example 9.7

Again, SAS produces an ANOVA table, similar to Table 9.1. In Example 9.3, we had a test statistic of $F = 10.16$ with $p = 0.0026$, which would lead to rejection of H_0 since $p = 0.0026 < \alpha = 0.05$.

The next section of the output displays the results of the Scheffe procedure for pairwise comparisons. Along with the results of the Scheffe pairwise comparisons, SAS prints a note that the Scheffe procedure is one that controls the

Type I error rate. This procedure also has a higher Type II error rate than alternative procedures. SAS also copies the mean square error (MS_{error}) from the preceding ANOVA table, which is used in the test statistics. The pairwise comparisons are performed internally and SAS indicates which means are significantly different from others by assigning letters ("Scheffe Grouping") to each treatment. If the same letters are assigned to different treatments, the treatment means are not significantly different. However, if different letters are assigned to the treatments, the treatment means are significantly different. In the output, the treatments (or drugs) A and B are assigned the letter "A," indicating that the means of Drugs A and B are not significantly different. Drug C is assigned the letter "B." Therefore, the means of Drugs A and C are significantly different. Drug B is also assigned the letter "B," indicating that the means of Drugs B and C are not significantly different. ■

EXAMPLE 9.8

Comparison Between Mean Age at Time to Completion of 8th Grade Between Urban versus Rural and Suburban Districts

Consider Example 9.4, comparing the ages of students at the completion of eighth grade from rural, suburban, and urban schools. A one-way ANOVA was performed in which $H_0: \mu_1 = \mu_2 = \mu_3$ was rejected at $\alpha = 0.05$. Suppose we wish to compare the urban students to the rural and suburban students combined. The summary statistics on the students' ages are

	Rural	Suburban	Urban
n_j	8	10	10
$\sum X_{ij}$	107	131	144
$\overline{X}_{.j}$	13.4	13.1	14.4

1. Set up hypotheses.

$$H_0: \tfrac{1}{2}(\mu_1 + \mu_2) = \mu_3$$

$$H_1: \tfrac{1}{2}(\mu_1 + \mu_2) \neq \mu_3, \quad \alpha = 0.05$$

NOTE: In the null hypothesis we state that the mean age for rural and suburban students combined is equal to the mean age for urban students. The null hypothesis is equivalent to $H_0: 1/2(\mu_1 + \mu_2) - \mu_3 = 0$; therefore, the weights for the sample means are $1/2, 1/2,$ and -1 (see step 2).

2. Select the appropriate test statistic.

$$F = \frac{\left(\dfrac{\overline{X}_{.1} + \overline{X}_{.2}}{2} - \overline{X}_{.3} \right)^2}{MS_{error} \left[\dfrac{1}{2^2}\left(\dfrac{1}{n_1}\right) + \dfrac{1}{2^2}\left(\dfrac{1}{n_2}\right) + \dfrac{1}{n_3} \right]}$$

In this example, we consider a more complicated contrast. Notice that the test statistic is modified accordingly. The numerator of the test statistic compares point estimates, and the denominator involves the reciprocal of each sample size, weighted by the coefficient associated with that population mean squared. For example, in H_0 we weight both μ_1 and μ_2 by 1/2, which is squared in the denominator of the statistic.

3. Decision rule.

Reject H_0 if $F \geq (k-1)F_{2,25} = 2(3.39) = 6.78$ (where $F_{2,25} = 3.39$ was used in Example 9.4 in the ANOVA)

4. Compute the test statistic.

$$F = \frac{\left(\dfrac{(13.4 + 13.1)}{2} - 14.4\right)^2}{0.927\left[\dfrac{1}{4}\left(\dfrac{1}{8}\right) + \dfrac{1}{4}\left(\dfrac{1}{10}\right) + \dfrac{1}{10}\right]} = 9.13$$

5. Conclusion.

Reject H_0 since $9.13 > 6.78$. We have significant evidence, $\alpha = 0.05$, to show that the mean age for rural and suburban students combined is not equal to the mean age of urban students. ■

9.5.2 The Tukey Procedure

The Tukey procedure, also called the Studentized Range test, is a popular, widely applied MCP that also controls the familywise error rate. The Tukey procedure is appropriate for pairwise comparisons. It does not handle general contrasts. It is a less conservative procedure (i.e., has better statistical power) than the Scheffe procedure when there are a large number of pairwise comparisons.

The Tukey procedure is outlined here and illustrated in Example 9.9. The procedure involves several steps. In the first step, treatments are ordered according to the magnitude of their respective sample means. Let $\overline{X}_{1'}$ denote the largest sample mean, $\overline{X}_{2'}$ denote the second largest sample mean, and so on, to $\overline{X}_{k'}$, which denotes the smallest sample mean. In the Tukey test, pairwise comparisons are made in a specific order. The first comparison involves a comparison of the treatments with the largest and smallest sample means. If this test is significant, then a test comparing the treatment with the largest sample mean to the treatment with the next-to-smallest sample mean is performed. If this test is significant, then one proceeds to compare the treatment with the largest sample mean to the treatment with the third-to-smallest sample mean, and so on. The specifics of each test are outlined here. The example refers to the first test in the sequence of tests that involves the treatments with the largest and smallest sample means.

1. Set up hypotheses.

$$H_0: \mu_{1'} = \mu_{k'}$$
$$H_1: \mu_{1'} \neq \mu_{k'}$$

where $\mu_{1'}$ and $\mu_{k'}$ are the means of the treatments with the largest and smallest sample means, respectively

2. Select the appropriate test statistic.

$$q_k = \frac{(\overline{X}_{1'} - \overline{X}_{k'})}{\sqrt{\dfrac{s_w^2}{n}}} = \frac{(\overline{X}_{1'} - \overline{X}_{k'})}{\sqrt{\dfrac{MS_{error}}{n}}}$$

where s_w^2 is the estimate of the within variation, and equal to the mean square within or mean square error (from the ANOVA table)

3. Decision rule.

The critical value for the Tukey test can be found in Table B.6: Critical Values of the Studentized Range Distribution. The critical value depends upon the level of significance, α, the number of treatments involved in the analysis, k, and the error degrees of freedom from the ANOVA table. Table B.6 contains critical values for $\alpha = 0.05$. The same critical value is used for all pairwise comparisons, and the decision rule is of the form:

$$\text{Reject } H_0 \text{ if } q_k \geq q_\alpha(k, \text{ df}_{error})$$
$$\text{Do not reject } H_0 \text{ if } q_k < q_\alpha(k, \text{ df}_{error})$$

EXAMPLE 9.9

Tukey Pairwise Comparisons for Differences in Means Between Drugs

Consider Example 9.3 in which we compared the mean times to relief from headache pain under three competing medications. An ANOVA was performed at the 5% level of significance and we rejected $H_0: \mu_1 = \mu_2 = \mu_3$. Suppose we now wish to compare the medications taken two-at-a-time (i.e., pairwise comparisons) using the Tukey procedure. The summary statistics are

Drug A	Drug B	Drug C
$\overline{X}_{.1} = 33.0$	$\overline{X}_{.2} = 26.0$	$\overline{X}_{.3} = 20.0$
$s_{.1} = 5.7$	$s_{.2} = 4.2$	$s_{.3} = 3.5$

The first step is to order the treatments according to the magnitude of their respective sample means: $\overline{X}_{1'} = 33.0$, $\overline{X}_{2'} = 26.0$, and $\overline{X}_{3'} = 20.0$. (*Note:* Only coincidentally do the sample means array from largest to smallest as presented.) The first test in the Tukey procedure involves a comparison of Drugs A and C (largest versus smallest sample means).

Drug A Versus Drug C

1. Set up hypotheses.

$$H_0: \mu_1 = \mu_3$$

$$H_1: \mu_1 \neq \mu_3, \quad \alpha = 0.05$$

2. Select the appropriate test statistic.

$$q_k = \frac{(\overline{X}_{.1} - \overline{X}_{.3})}{\sqrt{\dfrac{MS_{error}}{n}}}$$

where MS_{error} is the mean square error (or mean square within from the ANOVA table)

3. Decision rule.
   The appropriate critical value from Table B.6 for $k = 3$ and $df_{error} = 12$ is 3.77.

$$\text{Reject } H_0 \text{ if } q_k \geq 3.77$$

$$\text{Do not reject } H_0 \text{ if } q_k < 3.77$$

4. Compute the test statistic.

$$q_3 = \frac{(33.0 - 20.0)}{\sqrt{\dfrac{20.82}{5}}} = 6.37$$

5. Conclusion.
   Reject H_0 since $6.37 > 3.77$. We have significant evidence, $\alpha = 0.05$, to show that $\mu_1 \neq \mu_3$.
   Because the first test was significant, we proceed to test the equality of treatments whose sample means reflect the next-largest difference.

Drug A Versus Drug B

1. Set up hypotheses.

$$H_0: \mu_1 = \mu_2$$

$$H_1: \mu_1 \neq \mu_2, \quad \alpha = 0.05$$

2. Select the appropriate test statistic.

$$q_k = \frac{(\overline{X}_{.1} - \overline{X}_{.2})}{\sqrt{\dfrac{MS_{error}}{n}}}$$

where MS_{error} is the mean square error (or mean square within from the ANOVA table)

3. Decision rule.

$$\text{Reject } H_0 \text{ if } q_k \geq 3.77$$
$$\text{Do not reject } H_0 \text{ if } q_k < 3.77$$

4. Compute the test statistic.

$$q_3 = \frac{(33.0 - 26.0)}{\sqrt{\dfrac{20.82}{5}}} = 3.43$$

5. Conclusion.

Do not reject H_0 since $3.43 < 3.77$. We do not have significant evidence, $\alpha = 0.05$, to show that $\mu_1 \neq \mu_2$. Because this test is not significant, we do not go on to test H_0: $\mu_2 = \mu_3$ versus H_1: $\mu_2 \neq \mu_3$. ■

SAS EXAMPLE 9.9 **Tukey Pairwise Comparisons for Differences in Means Between Drugs Using SAS**

The following output was generated using SAS Proc ANOVA. We specified an option to conduct all pairwise comparisons using the Tukey MCP. A brief interpretation appears after the output.

SAS Output for Example 9.9

```
Analysis of Variance Procedure
Dependent Variable: TIME
                            Sum of              Mean
Source              DF      Squares             Square       F Value   Pr > F
Model                2      423.33333333   211.66666667      10.16     0.0026
Error               12      250.00000000    20.83333333
Corrected Total     14      673.33333333
```

	R-Square	C.V.	Root MSE	TIME Mean
	0.628713	17.33299	4.5643546	26.333333

Source	DF	ANOVA SS	Mean Square	F Value	Pr > F
TRT	2	423.33333333	211.66666667	10.16	0.0026

Tukey's Studentized Range (HSD) Test for time

NOTE: This test controls the Type I experimentwise error rate, but it generally has a higher Type II error rate than REGWQ.

```
Alpha                                          0.05
Error  Degrees of Freedom                        12
Error Mean Square                         20.83333
Critical Value of Studentized Range        3.77278
Minimum Significant Difference             7.7012
```

```
Means with the same letter are not significantly different.
    Tukey Grouping            Mean      N    trt
                 A          33.000      5    A
          B      A          26.000      5    B
          B                 20.000      5    C
```

Interpretation of SAS Output for Example 9.9

In the second section of the output, along with the results of the Tukey pair
wise comparisons, SAS prints a note that the Tukey procedure is one that controls the Type I error rate but has a higher Type II error rate than alternative
procedures. SAS also prints the level of significance, $\alpha = 0.05$, the error
degrees of freedom, df $= 12$, and the mean square error (MS_{error}) from the
ANOVA table ($MS_{error} = 20.83333$) used in the test statistics. The treatments
are ordered according to the magnitude of their respective sample means
(largest to smallest). The pairwise comparisons are performed internally and
SAS indicates which means are significantly different from others by assigning
letters ("Tukey Grouping") to each treatment. If the same letters are assigned
to different treatments, the treatment means are not significantly different.
However, if different letters are assigned to the treatments, the treatment
means are significantly different. Recall, in the Tukey procedure, one first compares the treatments with the largest and smallest sample means. In this appli
cation, Drug A has the largest mean and Drug C has the smallest. Drug A is
assigned the letter "A" and Drug C is assigned the letter "B." Since the Tukey
groupings (assigned letters) are different, the means of Drugs A and C are sig
nificantly different. The next test is the test comparing the means of Drugs A
and B. In the output, Drugs A and B are assigned the letter "A," indicating that
the means of Drugs A and B are not significantly different. Although SAS
allows for the test comparing Drugs B and C, the Tukey procedure should be
terminated following the nonsignificant result in the second test. ■

9.6 Repeated Measures Analysis of Variance

In some applications, it is of interest to assess changes in a particular measure
over time. For example, suppose an intervention is designed to improve
patients' medication adherence, which is a particularly important issue in the

management of many chronic diseases. The intervention is administered at a point in time and measurements are taken at predetermined intervals to assess adherence. A hypothesis might be that the intervention has a decreasing effect over time. The data layout is as follows:

Subject	Time 1	Time 2	. . .	Time k
1	X_{11}	X_{12}		X_{1k}
2	X_{21}	X_{22}		X_{2k}
.				
.				
.				
n	X_{n1}	X_{n2}		X_{nk}

where X_{sj} represents the measurement (X) on the sth subject $(s = 1, 2, \ldots, n)$ on the jth occasion $(j = 1, 2, \ldots, k)$

In these applications we have one sample of n subjects and take multiple, or repeated, measurements on each subject (k measurements in total). Without the subject column, the data layout is identical to the layout for analysis of variance procedures described in previous sections (assuming equal sample sizes). It is important to note that in these applications, there is one sample of subjects and repeated measures are taken on these subjects, introducing a dependency among the measurements. Because of this dependency, the test statistic needs modification.

For reference, recall the two independent and two dependent sample applications described in Chapter 6. In the two dependent samples applications, we focused on difference scores. Because there are now more than two measurements $(k > 2)$, the appropriate analysis is analysis of variance. The test is outlined next.

1. Set up hypotheses.

$$H_0: \mu_1 = \mu_2 = \cdots = \mu_k$$
$$H_1: \text{means not all equal}$$

2. Select the appropriate test statistic.

$$F = \frac{s_b^2}{s_w^2}$$

where s_b^2 = denotes the between variation, which is also denoted MS_b (mean square between)

s_w^2 = denotes the within variation, which is also denoted MS_w (mean square within)

This test statistic is identical in form to the test statistic used earlier. The analysis of variance table is different, however, and includes an additional

Table 9.2 *Repeated Measures Analysis of Variance Table*

Source of Variation	Sums of Squares (SS)	Degrees of Freedom (df)	Mean Squares (MS)	F
Between Subjects	$SS_{subj} = \sum k(\overline{X}_{s.} - \overline{X}_{..})^2$	$n - 1$		
Between Treatments	$SS_b = \sum n(\overline{X}_{.j} - \overline{X}_{..})^2$	$k - 1$	$S_b^2 = MS_b = \dfrac{SS_b}{k-1}$	$F = \dfrac{MS_b}{MS_w}$
Within	$SS_w = SS_{total} - SS_{subj} - SS_b$	$(n-1)(k-1)$	$S_w^2 = MS_w = \dfrac{SS_w}{(n-1)(k-1)}$	
Total	$SS_{total} = \sum\sum(X_{sj} - \overline{X}_{..})^2$	$nk - 1$		

where X_{sj} = measurement on the sth subject in the jth treatment (or at the jth time point)

$\overline{X}_{s.}$ = sample mean of sth subject

$\overline{X}_{.j}$ = sample mean of jth treatment (or jth time point)

$\overline{X}_{..}$ = overall sample mean

k = # measurements per subject

n = number of subjects

source of variation—variation due to the subjects. Because there are now multiple measurements taken on each subject, we can measure variation within given subjects (in the applications described in previous sections we had only a single measurement on each subject and could not measure variation within a given subject). The analysis of variable table for repeated measures analysis of variance procedures is given in Table 9.2.

3. Decision rule.

To select the appropriate critical value from the F distribution (Table B.4), we use the appropriate numerator and denominator degrees of freedom, df_1 and df_2, respectively ($df_1 = k - 1$ and $df_2 = (n-1)(k-1)$). Again, in ANOVA, we reject H_0 if the test statistic is larger than the critical value. We now illustrate the use of these formulas with an example.

EXAMPLE 9.10

Repeated Measures ANOVA to Test Difference in Mean Completion Times Among 3 Training Courses

An investigator is interested in comparing the cardiovascular fitness of elite runners on three different training courses, each of which covers 10 miles. The courses differ in terms of terrain, Course 1 is flat, Course 2 has graded inclines, and Course 3 includes steep inclines. Each runner's heart rate is monitored at mile 5 of the run on each course. Ten runners are involved, and their heart rates measured on each course are shown next.

Runner Number	Course 1	Course 2	Course 3
1	132	135	138
2	143	148	148
3	135	138	141
4	128	131	139
5	141	141	150
6	150	156	161
7	131	134	138
8	150	156	162
9	142	145	151
10	139	165	160

Is there a significant difference in the mean heart rates of runners on the three courses? Run the appropriate test at a 5% level of significance.

Because we have a single sample of 10 subjects, and three measures taken on each, the appropriate analysis is a repeated measures analysis of variance. The test is carried out next.

1. Set up hypotheses.

$$H_0: \mu_1 = \mu_2 = \mu_3$$

$$H_1: \text{means not all equal}, \quad \alpha = 0.05$$

2. Select the appropriate test statistic.

$$F = \frac{s_b^2}{s_w^2}$$

3. Decision rule.

To select the appropriate critical value from the F distribution (Table B.4), we first compute the numerator degrees of freedom (df_1) and the denominator degrees of freedom (df_2):

$$df_1 = k - 1 = 3 - 1 = 2 \qquad df_2 = (n-1)(k-1) = 9(2) = 18$$

The critical value of F with 2 and 18 degrees of freedom, relative to a 5% level of significance, is found in Table B.4A: $F_{2,18} = 3.55$. The decision rule is

$$\text{Reject } H_0 \text{ if } F \geq 3.55$$

$$\text{Do not reject } H_0 \text{ if } F < 3.55$$

4. Compute the test statistic.

Again, we will construct an ANOVA table to organize our computations. We will first compute the *between subjects* sums of squares (necessary to account for the repeated measurements taken on each subject). The between subjects sums of squares is computed by summing the squared differences between each subject's mean heart rate and the overall mean heart rate. The overall mean is computed by summing all of the measurements and dividing by the total number of measurements ($N = nk = 10(3) = 30$):

$$\overline{X}.. = \frac{4328}{30} = 144.3$$

Runner Number	Course 1	Course 2	Course 3	Subject Mean $\overline{X}_s.$	$(\overline{X}_s. - \overline{X}..)^2$
1	132	135	138	135.0	86.5
2	143	148	148	146.3	4.0
3	135	138	141	138.0	39.7
4	128	131	139	132.7	134.6
5	141	141	150	144.0	0.1
6	150	156	161	155.7	130.0
7	131	134	138	134.3	100.0
8	150	156	162	156.0	136.9
9	142	145	151	146.0	2.9
10	139	165	160	154.7	108.2
Course Means $\overline{X}._j$	139.1	144.9	148.8	$\overline{X}.. = 144.3$	742.9

The between subjects sums of squares is

$$SS_{\text{subj}} = \sum k(\overline{X}_s. - \overline{X}..)^2 = 3(742.9) = 2228.7$$

The *between treatments* sums of squares is computed by summing the squared differences between each treatment mean and the overall mean. The treatment (or course) means are shown along the bottom of the preceding table. The between treatments sums of squares is

$$SS_{\text{b}} = \sum n(\overline{X}._j - \overline{X}..)^2 = 10[(139.1 - 144.3)^2 + (144.9 - 144.3)^2 + (148.8 - 144.3)^2] = 477$$

The total sums of squares is computed by summing the squared differences between each observation and the overall mean. This is equivalent to the numerator of the sample variance. Recall from Chapter 2 the shortcut formula for the sample variance and the following alternative formula for the total sums of squares:

$$SS_{\text{total}} = \sum \sum (\overline{X}_{sj} - \overline{X}..)^2 = \sum X_{sj}^2 - \frac{(\sum X_{sj})^2}{N}$$

It is tedious to compute the sum of each observation squared, but for this example, $\sum X_{sj}^2 = 627{,}362$. The sum of the observations is $\sum X_{sj} = 4328$, and the total sums of squares is

$$SS_{total} = \sum X_{sj}^2 - \frac{(\sum X_{sj})^2}{N} = 627{,}362 - \frac{(4328)^2}{30} = 2975.9$$

The within sums of squares is computed by subtraction: $SS_{within} = SS_{total} - SS_{subj} - SS_b$.

$$SS_{within} = 2975.9 - 2228.7 - 477 = 270.2$$

We now construct the ANOVA table for Example 9.10.

Source of Variation	Sums of Squares (SS)	Degrees of Freedom (df)	Mean Squares (MS)	F
Between Subjects	2228.7	9		
Between Treatments	477	2	238.5	15.9
Within	270.2	18	15.0	
Total	2975.9	29		

5. Conclusion.

   Reject H_0, since $15.9 > 3.55$. We have significant evidence, $\alpha = 0.05$, to show that there is a difference in mean heart rates of runners on the three courses. ■

SAS EXAMPLE 9.10 Repeated Measures ANOVA to Test Difference in Mean Completion Times Among 3 Training Courses Using SAS

The following output was generated using SAS Proc GLM, which runs a repeated measures analysis of variance test for equality of means. The repeated option (see SAS program code in Section 9.9 for the details) is used to indicate that the measurements are dependent. A brief interpretation appears after the output.

SAS Output for Example 9.10

```
                    The GLM Procedure
            Repeated Measures Analysis of Variance
               Repeated Measures Level Information
        Dependent Variable    course1   course2   course3
            Level of course       1         2         3
```

The GLM Procedure
Repeated Measures Analysis of Variance
Univariate Tests of Hypotheses for Within Subject Effects

Source	DF	Type III SS	Mean Square	F Value	Pr > F
course	2	476.4666667	238.2333333	15.60	0.0001
Error(course)	18	274.8666667	15.2703704		

Interpretation of SAS Output for Example 9.10

The GLM procedure generates more output than is shown here for a repeated measures analysis of variance. The section shown is the most relevant for performing the test of interest. SAS generates an abbreviated ANOVA table, similar to Table 9.2. Again, SAS presents the degrees of freedom before the sums of squares. For the repeated measures applications, only the between treatment variation (labeled "course" in the output) and the within treatment variation (labeled "error(course)" in the output) rows of the ANOVA table are shown. These are the most relevant for computing the test statistic, which is $F = 15.60$ with $p = 0.0001$. We computed $F = 15.9$ by hand; the difference is due to rounding. With $p = 0.0001$, we would reject H_0 and conclude that the mean heart rates are different on the three courses. ■

9.7 Key Formulas

Application	Notation/Formula	Description
Test $H_0: \mu_1 = \mu_2 = \cdots = \mu_k$	$F = \dfrac{s_b^2}{s_w^2}$	see Table 9.1 for ANOVA computations (Table 9.2 for repeated measures ANOVA)
Variation explained by treatments	$\eta^2 = \dfrac{SS_b}{SS_{total}}$	see (9.5)
Test $H_0: \mu_i = \mu_j$ using Scheffe MCP*	$F = \dfrac{(\overline{X}_{.i} - \overline{X}_{.j})^2}{MS_{error}\left(\frac{1}{n_i} + \frac{1}{n_j}\right)}$	MCP that controls familywise error rate
Test $H_0: \mu_i = \mu_j$ using Tukey MCP*	$q_k = \dfrac{(\overline{X}_{1'} - \overline{X}_{k'})}{\sqrt{\frac{MS_{error}}{n}}}$	MCP that controls familywise error rate

* These tests should only be performed if $H_0: \mu_1 = \mu_2 = \mu_3 = \cdots = \mu_k$ is rejected.

9.8 Statistical Computing

Following are the SAS programs that were used to conduct tests of equality of k means ($k > 2$) using ANOVA. Also shown are programs to run Scheffe and Tukey multiple comparisons (pairwise comparisons). The SAS procedures and brief descriptions of their use are noted in the header to each example. Notes are provided to the right of the SAS programs (in blue) for orientation purposes and are not part of the programs. In addition, there are blank lines in the programs that are solely to accommodate the notes. Blank lines and spaces can be used throughout SAS programs to enhance readability. A summary of the SAS procedures used in the examples is provided at the end of this section.

SAS EXAMPLE 9.3

Analysis of Variance (ANOVA): Equal Sample Sizes

Compare Mean Times to Relief Among Three Treatments (Example 9.3)

An investigator wishes to compare the average time to relief of headache pain under three distinct medications—call them Drugs A, B, and C. Fifteen patients who suffer from chronic headaches are randomly selected for the investigation, and five subjects are randomly assigned to each treatment. The following data reflect times to relief (in minutes) after taking the assigned drug. Run an ANOVA using SAS.

Drug A	Drug B	Drug C
30	25	15
35	20	20
40	30	25
25	25	20
35	30	20

Program Code

```
options ps=62 ls=80;
```
Formats the output page to 62 lines in length and 80 columns in width

```
data in;
   input trt $ time;
```
Beginning of Data Step
Inputs two variables **trt** and **time**, where **trt** is a character variable (A, B, or C).

```
cards;
A 30
A 35
A 40
A 25
A 35
B 25
B 20
B 30
```
Beginning of Raw Data section.
actual observations (value of **trt** and **time** on each line)

```
B 25
B 30
C 15
C 20
C 25
C 20
C 20
run;

proc anova;


  class trt;


  model time=trt;




run;
```

proc anova;	Procedure call. Proc ANOVA tests the equality of *k* treatment means when sample sizes are equal.
class trt;	Specification of grouping variable (i.e., variable that defines *k* comparison groups).
model time=trt;	Specification of outcome variable (**time**). SAS requires a model statement relating the outcome to the grouping variable (**trt**).
run;	End of procedure section. ■

SAS EXAMPLE 9.4   Analysis of Variance (ANOVA): Unequal Sample Sizes

Compare Mean Ages Among Three Groups of Students (Example 9.4)

The following data reflect ages of students at completion of eighth grade. Test if there is a significant difference in the mean age at completion of eighth grade for rural, suburban, and urban students using SAS and a 5% level of significance. The following data were collected from randomly selected students at rural, suburban, and urban schools.

Rural:	14	14	14	14	13	13	13	12		
Suburban:	14	14	14	13	13	13	13	13	12	12
Urban:	16	16	15	15	15	14	14	14	13	12

Program Code

```
options ps=62 ls=80;


data in;
 input school $ age;
```

options ps=62 ls=80;	Formats the output page to 62 lines in length and 80 columns in width
data in;	Beginning of Data Step
input school $ age;	Inputs two variables **school** and **age**, where **school** = Rural, Suburban, or Urban.

```
cards;
rural 14
rural 14
rural 14
rural 14
rural 13
rural 13
rural 13
rural 12
suburban 14
suburban 14
suburban 14
suburban 13
suburban 13
suburban 13
suburban 13
suburban 13
suburban 12
suburban 12
urban 16
urban 16
urban 15
urban 15
urban 15
urban 14
urban 14
urban 14
urban 13
urban 12
run;


proc glm;



  class school;



  model age=school;



 run;
```

Beginning of Raw Data section.
actual observations (value of **school**
and **age** on each line)

Procedure call. Proc Glm tests the
  equality of *k* treatment means
  when sample sizes are equal or
  unequal.
Specification of grouping variable
  (i.e., variable that defines k
  comparison groups).
Specification of outcome variable
  (**age**). SAS requires a model
  statement relating the outcome to
  the grouping variable (**school**).
End of procedure section.   ■

SAS EXAMPLE 9.5 **Analysis of Variance (ANOVA)**

Compare Mean Weight Gains Among Four Diets (Example 9.5)

A study is developed to examine the effects of vitamin and milk supplement on infant weight gain. Four diet plans are considered: Diet A involves a regular diet plus the vitamin supplement, Diet B involves a regular diet plus the special milk formula, Diet C is our control diet (i.e., no restrictions or special considerations), and Diet D involves a regular diet plus the vitamin and the special milk formula. Twenty infants are selected for the investigation and each is randomized to one of the four competing diet programs. The table displays weight gains, measured in pounds, after 1 month on the respective diet. Run an ANOVA using SAS.

Diet A	*Diet B*	*Diet C*	*Diet D*
2.0	1.6	1.5	2.1
1.5	1.9	2.0	2.4
2.4	2.1	1.8	1.9
1.9	1.1	1.3	1.8
2.6	1.7	1.2	2.2

Program Code

`options ps=62 ls=80;`	Formats the output page to 62 lines in length and 80 columns in width
`data in;`	Beginning of Data Step
` input diet $ gain;`	Inputs two variables **diet** and **gain**, where **diet** = A, B, C, or D.
`cards;`	Beginning of Raw Data section.
`A 2.0`	actual observations (value of **diet** and
`A 1.5`	**gain** on each line)
`A 2.4`	
`A 1.9`	
`A 2.6`	
`B 1.6`	
`B 1.9`	
`B 2.1`	
`B 1.1`	
`B 1.7`	
`C 1.5`	
`C 2.0`	
`C 1.8`	

```
C 1.3
C 1.2
D 2.1
D 2.4
D 1.9
D 1.8
D 2.2
run;
```

```
proc glm;
```
Procedure call. Proc Glm tests the equality of *k* treatment means when sample sizes are equal or unequal.

```
  class diet;
```
Specification of grouping variable (i.e., variable that defines *k* comparison groups).

```
  model gain=diet;
```
Specification of outcome variable (**gain**). SAS requires a model statement relating the outcome to the grouping variable (**diet**).

```
run;
```
End of procedure section. ■

SAS EXAMPLE 9.7 **Analysis of Variance (ANOVA): Pairwise Comparisons Using Scheffe and Tukey**

Pairwise Multiple Comparisons (Examples 9.7 and 9.9)

In SAS EXAMPLE 9.3 we ran an ANOVA and rejected H_0. Run pairwise comparisons using the Scheffe and Tukey procedures to determine which means are different.

Program Code

```
options ps=62 ls=80;
```
Formats the output page to 62 lines in length and 80 columns in width

```
data in;
  input trt $ time;
```
Beginning of Data Step

Inputs two variables **trt** and **time**, where **trt** = A, B, or C.

```
cards;
A 30
A 35
A 40
A 25
A 35
```
Beginning of Raw Data section.

actual observations (value of **trt** and **time** on each line)

```
B 25
B 20
B 30
B 25
B 30
C 15
C 20
C 25
C 20
C 20
run;
```

```
proc anova;
```
Procedure call. Proc ANOVA tests the equality of *k* treatment means when sample sizes are equal.

```
  class trt;
```
Specification of grouping variable (i.e., variable that defines *k* comparison groups).

```
  model time=trt;
```
Specification of outcome variable (**time**). SAS requires a model statement relating the outcome to the grouping variable (**trt**).

```
  means trt/scheffe;
```
Means option requires a comparison of means among the comparison groups defined by **trt**, using the Scheffe MCP. (SAS Example 9.7)

```
  means trt/tukey;
```
Means option requires a comparison of means among the comparison groups defined by **trt**, using the Tukey MCP. (SAS Example 9.9)

```
run;
```
End of procedure section.

SAS Example 9.10 Repeated Measures Analysis of Variance (ANOVA)

Compare Mean Heart Rates on Three Training Courses (Example 9.10)

An investigator is interested in comparing the cardiovascular fitness of elite runners on three different training courses, each of which covers 10 miles. The courses differ in terms of terrain: One includes steep inclines, the other more graded inclines, and the third is flat. Each runner's heart rate is monitored at mile 5 of the run on each course. Ten runners are involved and their heart rates as measured on each course are shown here. Run a repeated measures ANOVA using SAS.

Runner Number	Course 1	Course 2	Course 3
1	132	135	138
2	143	148	148
3	135	138	141
4	128	131	139
5	141	141	150
6	150	156	161
7	131	134	138
8	150	156	162
9	142	145	151
10	139	165	160

Program Code

```
options ps=62 ls=80;

data in;
  input runnerid course1 course2 course3;



  subjmean=mean(course1,course2,course3);


cards;
1     132     135     138
2     143     148     148
3     135     138     141
4     128     131     139
5     141     141     150
6     150     156     161
7     131     134     138
8     150     156     162
9     142     145     151
10    139     165     160
run;
proc print;


  var course1 course2 course3 subjmean;
run;
```

Formats the output page to 62 lines in length and 80 columns in width

Beginning of Data Step

Inputs four variables **runnerid** (subject identifier) and 3 measurements on each subject— **course1, course2**, and **course3**.

Computes a new variable, **subjmean**, which is the mean heart rate for each subject.

Beginning of Raw Data section.

actual observations (value of **runnerid, course1, course2** and **course3** on each line)

Procedure call. Proc Print lists the values of the specified variables.

Specification of variables for listing.

```proc means;```	Procedure call. Proc Means generates summary statistics on specified variables.
``` var course1 course2 course3 subjmean;```	Specification of variables (we are most interested in the means for each course. The mean of **subjmean** is the overall mean).
```run;```	
```proc glm;```	Procedure call. Proc Glm is used for analysis of variance applications.
``` model course1 course2 course3=/nouni;```	Specification of variables for analysis In repeated measures analysis, the variables listed after the model statement are those measured on each subject. The nouni option indicates that we do not want univariate tests (which test if the mean for each variable is zero or not).
``` repeated course;```	The repeated option indicates a repeated measures ANOVA. After the repeated statement, the user specifies a label for the repeated measurements, which appears on the output (**course**).
```run;```	

9.8.1 Summary of SAS Procedures

The SAS Anova procedure is used to run an ANOVA when the sample sizes are equal in all comparison groups. The SAS Glm procedure is used to run an ANOVA when the sample sizes are either equal or unequal. Specific options can be requested in these procedures to run pairwise multiple comparisons (e.g., Scheffe or Tukey). The options are shown in italics. Users should refer to the examples in this section for complete descriptions of the procedure and specific options. A general description of the procedure and options is provided in the table.

Procedure	*Sample Procedure Call*	*Description*
proc anova	proc anova; class group; model outcome=group;	Runs an ANOVA comparing the mean outcome scores among groups, when sample sizes are equal in all comparison groups.
proc glm	proc glm; class group; model outcome=group;	Runs an ANOVA comparing the mean outcome scores among groups.

proc anova; class group; model outcome=group; means group/*scheffe*;	Runs an ANOVA comparing the mean outcome scores among groups and generates pairwise comparisons using the Scheffe procedure. Here we assume equal sample sizes.
proc glm; class group; model outcome=group; means group/*tukey*;	Runs an ANOVA comparing the mean outcome scores among groups and generates pairwise comparisons using the Tukey procedure.
proc glm; model outcome1 outcome2 ... outcomek=/nouni; repeated label;	Runs a repeated measures ANOVA comparing the mean outcome scores over time. The nouni option suppresses univariate tests, and the user specifies a label describing the nature of the repeated assessments.

9.9 Analysis of Framingham Heart Study Data

The Framingham data set includes data collected from the original cohort. Participants contributed up to three examination cycles of data. Here we analyze data collected in the first examination cycle (called the period = 1 examination) and use SAS Proc GLM to compare mean systolic blood pressure levels for participants with different body mass indices. We organized BMI into categories as follows: BMI < 18.5 (underweight), 18.5–24.9 (normal weight), 25.0–29.9 (overweight), and ≥ 30.0 (obese). We then performed Scheffe multiple comparisons to assess differences in systolic blood pressure between BMI groups taken two-at-a-time. The SAS code to create this variable and to attach a format for better interpretability is given here along with the procedure calls.

Framingham Data Analysis—SAS Code

```
proc format;
 value bmifmt 1='<18.5      ' 2='18.5-24.9' 3='25.0-29.9' 4='30.0+';
run;

data fhs;
 set in.frmgham;
 if period=1;

if ole bmi lt 18.5 then bmi_grp=1;
else if 18.5 le bmi lt 25.0 then bmi_grp=2;
```

```
else if 25.0 le bmi lt 30.0 then bmi_grp=3;
else if bmi ge 30.0 then bmi_grp=4;
format bmi_grp bmifmt.;
run;

proc glm data=fhs;
  class bmi_grp;
  model sysbp=bmi_grp;
  means bmi_grp;
run;
proc glm data=fhs;
  class bmi_grp;
  model sysbp=bmi_grp;
  means bmi_grp/scheffe cldiff;
run;
```

Framingham Data Analysis—SAS Output

The GLM Procedure

Class Level Information

Class	Levels	Values
bmi_grp	4	18.5-24.9 25.0-29.9 30.0+ <18.5

Number of observations   4434

The GLM Procedure

Dependent Variable: SYSBP   Systolic BP mmHg

Source	DF	Sum of Squares	Mean Square	F Value	Pr > F
Model	3	181059.901	60353.300	130.58	<.0001
Error	4430	2047533.372	462.197		
Corrected Total	4433	2228593.273			

R-Square	Coeff Var	Root MSE	SYSBP Mean
0.081244	16.17571	21.49877	132.9078

Source	DF	Type I SS	Mean Square	F Value	Pr > F
bmi_grp	3	181059.9012	60353.3004	130.58	<.0001

Source	DF	Type III SS	Mean Square	F Value	Pr > F
bmi_grp	3	181059.9012	60353.3004	130.58	<.0001

The SAS System   3

The GLM Procedure

Level of bmi_grp	N	-----------SYSBP----------- Mean	Std Dev
<18.5	76	123.927632	23.9394659
18.5-24.9	1936	126.790289	20.3968744
25.0-29.9	1845	135.873171	21.4538212
30.0+	577	145.134315	24.6783770

There is a highly significant difference in mean systolic blood pressure across the BMI groups. The means option produces the mean and standard deviation in systolic blood pressure for each BMI level. These statistics are very useful in understanding the nature of the difference (or trend, in this case) across comparison groups.

In the following output, we generate Scheffe comparisons to test for differences in mean systolic blood pressures between BMI groups taken two-at-a-time. Here we asked SAS to produce confidence intervals for each pair of comparison groups using the cldiff option. SAS indicates which BMI groups are significantly different in terms of systolic blood pressure.

The GLM Procedure
Class Level Information

Class	Levels	Values
bmi_grp	4	18.5-24.9 25.0-29.9 30.0+ <18.5

Number of observations   4434

The GLM Procedure

Dependent Variable: SYSBP   Systolic BP mmHg

Source	DF	Sum of Squares	Mean Square	F Value	Pr > F
Model	3	181059.901	60353.300	130.58	<.0001
Error	4430	2047533.372	462.197		
Corrected Total	4433	2228593.273			

R-Square	Coeff Var	Root MSE	SYSBP Mean
0.081244	16.17571	21.49877	132.9078

Source	DF	Type I SS	Mean Square	F Value	Pr > F
bmi_grp	3	181059.9012	60353.3004	130.58	<.0001

Source	DF	Type III SS	Mean Square	F Value	Pr > F
bmi_grp	3	181059.9012	60353.3004	130.58	<.0001

```
                          Scheffe's Test for SYSBP
NOTE: This test controls the Type I experimentwise error rate, but it generally
   has a higher Type II error rate than Tukey's for all pairwise comparisons.

                     Alpha                        0.05
                     Error Degrees of Freedom     4430
                     Error Mean Square         462.1971
                     Critical Value of F         2.60691

      Comparisons significant at the 0.05 level are indicated by ***.

                                   Difference
                    bmi_grp          Between         Simultaneous 95%
                  Comparison          Means        Confidence Limits

       30.0+      - 25.0-29.9         9.2611          6.3934   12.1289   ***
       30.0+      - 18.5-24.9        18.3440         15.4924   21.1957   ***
       30.0+      - <18.5           21.2067         13.8700   28.5434   ***
       25.0-29.9  - 30.0+           -9.2611        -12.1289   -6.3934   ***
       25.0-29.9  - 18.5-24.9         9.0829          7.1268   11.0390   ***
       25.0-29.9  - <18.5           11.9455          4.9084   18.9827   ***
       18.5-24.9  - 30.0+          -18.3440        -21.1957  -15.4924   ***
       18.5-24.9  - 25.0-29.9        -9.0829        -11.0390   -7.1268   ***
       18.5-24.9  - <18.5            2.8627         -4.1679    9.8933
       <18.5      - 30.0+          -21.2067        -28.5434  -13.8700   ***
       <18.5      - 25.0-29.9       -11.9455        -18.9827   -4.9084   ***
       <18.5      - 18.5-24.9        -2.8627         -9.8933    4.1679
```

9.10 Problems

1. A pharmaceutical company is interested in the effectiveness of a new preparation designed to relieve arthritis pain. Three variations of the compound have been prepared for investigation, which differ according to the proportion of the active ingredients: T15 contains 15% active ingredients, T40 contains 40% active ingredients, and T50 contains 50% active ingredients. A sample of 20 patients is selected to participate in a study comparing the three variations of the compound. A control compound, which is currently available over the counter, is also included in the investigation. Patients are randomly assigned to one of the four treatments (control, T15, T40, T50) and the time (in minutes) until pain relief is recorded on each subject. The data are

Control:	12	15	18	16	20
T15:	20	21	22	19	20
T40:	17	16	19	15	19
T50:	14	13	12	14	11

a. Test if there is a difference in the mean time to relief among the four treatments. Use a 5% level of significance.

b. Using Scheffe multiple comparisons, test if there is a significant difference in the mean time to relief between the control and each of the experimental treatments (i.e., T15, T40, and T50), considered separately.

2. A study is performed to compare mean numbers of primary-care visits over 3 years among four different health maintenance organizations (HMOs). Fifty patients are randomly sampled from each HMO.

a. Write the hypotheses to be tested.

b. Complete the following ANOVA table:

Source of Variation	Sums of Squares	Degrees of Freedom	Mean Squares	F
Between	574.3			
Within				
Total	2759.8			

c. Is there a significant difference in mean numbers of primary-care visits among the four HMOs? Use a 5% level of significance.

3. Six different doses of a particular drug are compared in an effectiveness study. The study involves 30 subjects, and equal numbers of subjects are randomly assigned to each dose group.

a. What are the null and alternative hypotheses in the comparison?

b. Complete the following ANOVA table:

Source of Variation	Sums of Squares	Degrees of Freedom	Mean Squares	F
Between	189.85			
Within				
Total	352.57			

c. Is there a significant difference in the effectiveness among the doses? Use $\alpha = 0.05$.

d. Suppose we wish to compare dose groups 1 and 2 and the following are available: $\overline{X}_1 = 21.4$, $\overline{X}_2 = 27.6$. Run the appropriate test to assess whether there is a significant difference in effectiveness between dose groups 1 and 2 at the 5% level of significance.

4. The following data were collected as part of a study comparing a control treatment to an active treatment. Three doses of the active

treatment were considered in the study. The following table displays summary statistics on the ages of participants enrolled in the study classified by treatment group:

Treatment	# Participants	Mean Age	SD
Control	8	29.5	3.74
Low dose	8	34.5	2.88
Moderate dose	8	15.9	3.72
High dose	8	44.0	6.65

a. Test if there is a significant difference in the mean ages of participants across treatment groups. Complete the following table and show all parts of the test. Use $\alpha = 0.05$.

Source	Sums of Squares	Degrees of Freedom	Mean Squares	F
Between				
Within				
Total	3860.97			

b. Is there a significant difference in the mean ages of participants in the control and low dose groups? Run the appropriate test at $\alpha = 0.05$.

5. An investigation is performed to evaluate two new experimental treatments for allergies. Eighteen subjects who suffer from allergies are enrolled in the study and randomly assigned to one of three treatments: control treatment, experimental treatment 1, or experimental treatment 2. Each subject is instructed to take the assigned treatment, and symptoms of allergies are recorded on a scale of 1 to 20, with higher scores indicating worse symptoms. The data are

Control Treatment	Experimental Treatment 1	Experimental Treatment 2
19	12	5
18	14	6
16	13	3
15	10	2
12	9	3
17	10	4
$\overline{X}_1 = 16.2$	$\overline{X}_2 = 11.3$	$\overline{X}_3 = 3.8$

a. Test if there is a significant difference in mean symptom scores among the three treatments under investigation. Use a 5% level of significance. (*Hint:* $SS_{total} = 524.4$.)

b. Which treatment is the "best" of those investigated? (Justify your answer briefly.)

6. A randomized trial is conducted to compare four treatment regimens for HIV. Each regimen is based on a combination of medications. Twenty patients are involved in the investigation and are randomly assigned to one of four treatments: A, B, C, or D (5 subjects per treatment group). An overall symptom score, ranging from 0 to 20, is computed for each individual by aggregating their reports of the frequency and severity of an array of symptoms. Higher symptom scores indicate more frequent and/or severe symptoms. The summary statistics are

Treatment Regimen	Symptom Score
A	7.9
B	5.4
C	12.4
D	5.9

Test whether the mean symptom scores are equal among treatment regimens. Run the appropriate test at the 5% level of significance. (*Hint:* $SS_{within} = SS_{error} = 135.4$.)

7. A study is conducted among college students who smoke to assess whether there is a relationship between the number of cigarettes they smoke per day and the smoking status of their parents. For the purposes of the study, smoking status is defined as follows: never smoked, former smokers, or current smokers. The number of cigarettes smoked per day by each student is recorded and the data are

Parent's Smoking Status	Number of Students	Mean Number of Cigarettes Smoked/Day	SD
Never smoked	30	12.6	3.1
Former smokers	34	14.1	3.7
Current smokers	53	18.3	4.3
ALL	117	15.6	6.5

Based on the data, is there a significant difference in the mean numbers of cigarettes smoked per day according to the parent's smoking status? Run the appropriate test at $\alpha = 0.05$. (*Hint:* $SS_{total} = 3428.4$.)

8. A study is conducted comparing birthweights (in pounds) of infants born to mothers of various ages. The data are

Mother's Age		
<20 Years	20–29 Years	30+ Years
8.4	7.5	6.9
7.3	6.3	7.1
9.1	6.9	5.7
7.8	5.4	6.5
8.4	7.1	6.6

Is there a significant difference in the mean birthweights for mothers of different ages? Run the appropriate test at $\alpha = 0.05$.

9. Consider a continuous measure of medication adherence (scores from 0 to 100), and use the following data to test if there is a significant difference in the mean medication adherence scores in patients of different age groups. Use the following data to run the appropriate test at $\alpha = 0.05$. (*Hint:* $\sum \sum (X_{ij} - \overline{X})^2 = 29{,}159.26$.)

	Age Group			
	20–29	30–39	40–49	50–59
Number of patients:	48	53	37	12
Mean medication adherence:	69.2	83.3	82.1	83.4
Standard deviation:	11.9	13.2	12.8	11.3

10. A clinical trial is performed comparing a test (newly developed) drug to an active control (a drug already proven effective) and to a placebo. Persons with diagnosed hypertension who are at least 18 years of age are eligible for the trial. Persons agreeing to participate are randomly assigned to one of the competing drugs. The outcome measure is systolic blood pressure (SBP), which is measured 4 weeks postrandomization. Summary statistics are

Drug	*n*	Mean (SD) SBP
Test	15	125 (25)
Control	15	135 (21)
Placebo	15	160 (22)

a. Is there a significant difference in mean SBPs 4 weeks postrandomization? Run the appropriate test at a 5% level of significance. (*Hint:* $SS_{total} = 31,450$.)

b. Is there a significant difference in mean SBPs 4 weeks postrandomization between the test drug and placebo? Run the appropriate test at a 5% level of significance.

c. Is there a significant difference in mean SBPs 4 weeks postrandomization between the test and control drugs? Run the appropriate test at a 5% level of significance.

11. The following output was generated from SAS:

```
            Analysis of Variance Procedure
                Class Level Information
            Class      Levels     Values
            GROUP         3       a b c
        Number of observations in data set = 24
```

Dependent Variable: SCORE

Source	DF	Sum of Squares	Mean Square	F Value	Pr > F
Model	2	839.58333333	419.79166667	43.16	0.0001
Error	21	204.25000000	9.72619048		
Corrected Total	23	1043.83333333			

a. Test if there is a significant difference in mean scores between treatments. Write the hypotheses and justify your conclusion (use the SAS output).

b. How much of the variation in scores is explained by the groups?

12. The following table summarizes data collected in a multicenter study. The variable summarized is body mass index (BMI) computed as the ratio of weight in kilograms to height in meters squared.

BMI	Overall	Enrollment Site Hospital 1	Hospital 2	Hospital 3
n:	300	100	100	100
Mean:	24.8	21.6	24.8	27.9
SD:	2.5	2.1	1.8	1.3

Test if there is a significant difference in the mean BMI scores among hospitals. Show all parts of the test and use a 5% level of significance. (*Hint:* $MS_{within} = MS_{error} = 3.1$.)

13. A research group wishes to conduct a randomized trial to compare a newly approved medication, an experimental medication (one not yet available on market), and a medication they consider standard care. One hundred and fifty patients with hypertension are enrolled and randomized to one of the three comparison treatments. After taking the assigned medication for 6 weeks, each patient's systolic blood pressure (SBP) is measured. Summary statistics are given here. Use the data to test if there is a significant difference in systolic blood pressures among medication groups. Run the appropriate test at a 5% level of significance.

Treatment	Number of Patients	Mean SBP	SD
New	50	130	12
Standard	50	135	10
Experimental	50	115	17

Is there a difference in systolic blood pressures among the treatments? Run the appropriate test using a 5% level of significance. (*Hint:* $SS_{within} = SS_{error} = 26,117$, and $SS_{total} = 36,951$.)

14. The following data represent birthweights of siblings born to six different mothers:

| Mother | Birthweights | | | |
	Child 1	Child 2	Child 3	Child 4
1	6.4	6.9	6.7	7.1
2	8.5	7.8	7.8	8.3
3	7.6	8.7	9.9	8.2
4	5.3	6.7	7.5	6.4
5	6.2	5.6	6.4	5.5
6	7.0	7.8	8.6	6.6

Is there a significant difference in birthweights of siblings? Run the appropriate test at $\alpha = 0.05$.

15. Suppose in a clinical trial that systolic blood pressures are measured at 4, 8, and 12 weeks postrandomization in a subgroup of patients receiving a test drug. We wish to test if there are significant differences in systolic blood pressures over time.

	Systolic Blood Pressure		
Subject	4 weeks	8 weeks	12 weeks
1	120	125	130
2	110	115	118
3	105	110	100
4	140	130	140
5	150	145	140

Test if there is a significant difference in mean systolic blood pressures over time using a 5% level of significance.

16. Suppose the data in the previous problem were collected from three independent random samples of subjects (i.e., $n_1 = 5, n_2 = 5, n_3 = 5$, total sample size $= 15$). Test if there is a significant difference in mean systolic blood pressures over time using a 5% level of significance. (*Hint:* You do not need to recalculate the sums of squares—compare formulas first!)

SAS Problems

Use SAS to solve the following problems.

1. A pharmaceutical company is interested in the effectiveness of a new preparation designed to relieve arthritis pain. Three variations of the compound have been prepared for investigation, which differ according to the proportion of the active ingredients: T15 contains 15% active ingredients, T40 contains 40% active ingredients, and T50 contains 50% active ingredients. A sample of 20 patients is selected to participate in a study comparing the three variations of the compound. A control compound, which is currently available over the counter, is also included in the investigation. Patients are randomly assigned to one of the four treatments (control, T15, T40, T50) and the time (in minutes) until pain relief is recorded on each subject. The data are

Control:	12	15	18	16	20
T15:	20	21	22	19	20
T40:	17	16	19	15	19
T50:	14	13	12	14	11

Use SAS Proc Anova to test the equality of means. In addition, run all pairwise comparisons using the Scheffe procedure. Use a 5% level of significance.

2. An investigation is performed to evaluate two new experimental treatments for allergies. Eighteen subjects who suffer from allergies are enrolled in the study and randomly assigned to one of three treatments: control treatment, experimental treatment 1, or experimental treatment 2. Each subject is instructed to take the assigned treatment, and symptoms of allergies are recorded on a scale of 1 to 20, with higher scores indicating worse symptoms. The data are

Control Treatment	Experimental Treatment 1	Experimental Treatment 2
19	12	5
18	14	6
16	13	3
15	10	2
12	9	3
17	10	4

Use SAS Proc Anova to test the equality of means. In addition, run all pairwise comparisons using the Tukey procedure. Use a 5% level of significance.

3. A study is conducted comparing birthweights (in pounds) of infants born to mothers of various ages. The data are

Mother's Age		
<20 Years	20–29 Years	30+ Years
8.4	7.5	6.9
7.3	6.3	7.1
9.1	6.9	5.7
7.8	5.4	6.5
8.4	7.1	6.6

Use SAS Proc Glm to test if there is a significant difference in the mean birthweights for mothers of different ages. Run the appropriate test at $\alpha = 0.05$.

4. The following data represent birthweights of siblings born to six different mothers:

		Birthweights		
Mother	Child 1	Child 2	Child 3	Child 4
1	6.4	6.9	6.7	7.1
2	8.5	7.8	7.8	8.3
3	7.6	8.7	9.9	8.2
4	5.3	6.7	7.5	6.4
5	6.2	5.6	6.4	5.5
6	7.0	7.8	8.6	6.6

Use SAS Proc Glm (with a repeated option) to test if there is a significant difference in birthweights of siblings. Run the appropriate test at $\alpha = 0.05$.

5. Suppose in a clinical trial that systolic blood pressures are measured at 4, 8, and 12 weeks postrandomization in a subgroup of patients receiving a test drug. We wish to test if there are significant differences in systolic blood pressures over time. The following data were collected at 4 weeks, 8 weeks, and 12 weeks postrandomization in a sample of five patients receiving the test drug.

	Systolic Blood Pressure		
Subject	4 weeks	8 weeks	12 weeks
1	120	125	130
2	110	115	118
3	105	110	100
4	140	130	140
5	150	145	140

Use SAS Proc Glm (with a repeated option) to test if there is a significant difference in birthweights of siblings. Run the appropriate test at $\alpha = 0.05$.

Descriptive Statistics
(Ch. 2)

Probability
(Ch. 3)

Sampling Distributions
(Ch. 4)

Statistical Inference
(Chapters 5–12)

OUTCOME VARIABLE	GROUPING VARIABLE(S)/ PREDICTOR(S)	ANALYSIS	CHAPTER(S)
Continuous	—	Estimate μ; Compare μ to Known, Historical Value	5/12
Continuous	Dichotomous (2 groups)	Compare Independent Means (Estimate/Test $(\mu_1 - \mu_2)$) or the Mean Difference (μ_d)	6/12
Continuous	Discrete (>2 groups)	Test the Equality of k Means using Analysis of Variance $(\mu_1 = \mu_2 \cdots = \mu_k)$	9/12
Continuous	Continuous	Estimate Correlation or Determine Regression Equation	10/12
Continuous	Several Continuous or Dichotomous	Multiple Linear Regression Analysis	10
Dichotomous	—	Estimate p; Compare p to Known, Historical Value	7
Dichotomous	Dichotomous (2 groups)	Compare Independent Proportions (Estimate/Test $(p_1 - p_2)$)	7/8
Dichotomous	Discrete (>2 groups)	Test the Equality of k Proportions (Chi-Square Test)	7
Dichotomous	Several Continuous or Dichotomous	Multiple Logistic Regression Analysis	11
Discrete	Discrete	Compare Distributions Among k Populations (Chi-Square Test)	7
Time to Event	Several Continuous or Dichotomous	Survival Analysis	13

Correlation
and Regression

IO

In correlation and regression applications, we consider the relationship between two continuous (or measurement) variables. For example, we might be interested in the relationship between age and systolic blood pressure, or the relationship between the number of hours of aerobic exercise per week and percent body fat. In correlation and regression applications, we measure both variables on each of n randomly selected subjects. We denote the variables X and Y. (In prior applications, we used the variable name X to denote the single characteristic of interest.) The variable name X is used to represent the *independent, or predictor, variable,* and the variable name Y is used to represent the *dependent, outcome or response, variable.* In many applications, it will be clear which is the independent or predictor variable and which is the dependent or outcome variable. In some applications, the investigator must specify explicitly which variable should be considered the independent and which should be considered the dependent variable.

In Section 10.1 we discuss correlation analysis. We present and illustrate the computation of the sample correlation coefficient and then present techniques for statistical inference concerning the correlation coefficient. In Section 10.2 we present and illustrate simple linear regression analysis. In Section 10.3 we provide an introduction to multiple regression analysis, and in Section 10.4 we introduce logistic regression analysis. In Section 10.5 we summarize key formulas, and in Section 10.6 we display the statistical computing programs used to generate correlation and regression analyses presented in this chapter. In Section 10.7 we use data from the Framingham Heart Study to illustrate the applications presented here.

10.1 Correlation Analysis

The goal of correlation analysis is to understand the nature and strength of the association between the two measurement variables, denoted X and Y. A first step in understanding the relationship between two variables is through a *scatter diagram*. A scatter diagram is a plot of the (X,Y) pairs recorded on each of the n subjects. The X (independent or predictor) variable is plotted on the horizontal axis and the Y (dependent or outcome) variable is plotted on the vertical axis. The scatter diagram shown in Figure 10.1 indicates a positive or direct linear relationship between X and Y.

Figure 10.2 displays an negative or inverse linear association between two variables X and Y.

The population correlation coefficient, ρ (rho), quantifies the nature and strength of the linear relationship between X and Y. The population correlation coefficient takes on values in the range of -1 to 1 ($-1 \leq \rho \leq +1$). The sign of the correlation coefficient indicates the nature of the relationship between X and Y (i.e., positive or direct, negative or inverse), and the magnitude of the correlation coefficient indicates the strength of the linear association

Figure 10.1 *Direct Linear Relationship Between X and Y*

Figure 10.2 *Inverse Linear Relationship Between X and Y*

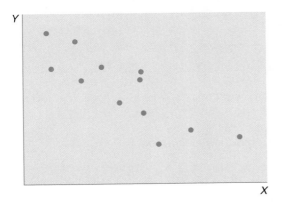

between the two variables. Figures 10.3a–d display scatter diagrams corresponding to the following values of the correlation coefficient: $\rho = -1$, $\rho = -0.5$, $\rho = 0.5$, and $\rho = 1$. These values represent, respectively, a perfect inverse relationship between X and Y ($\rho = -1.0$), a moderate inverse relationship between X and Y ($\rho = -0.5$), a moderate direct relationship between X and Y ($\rho = 0.5$), and a perfect direct relationship between X and Y ($\rho = 1.0$). A correlation of zero indicates that there is no linear association between X and Y.

The correlation coefficient is a measure of the *linear* association between X and Y. One must be cautious in interpreting the value of the correlation coefficient. It is always useful to generate a scatter diagram to assist in the interpretation. For example, the data displayed in both Figures 10.4a and 10.4b

Figure 10.3 *The Correlation Coefficient*

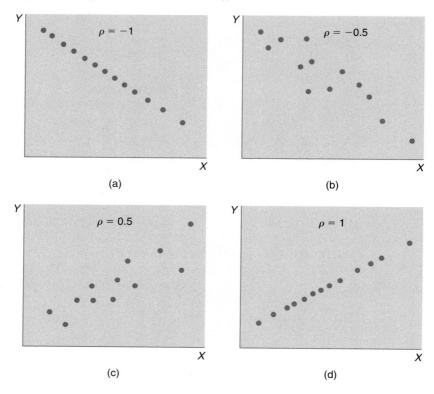

(a)
(b)
(c)
(d)

Figure 10.4 *Correlation Coefficient = 0*

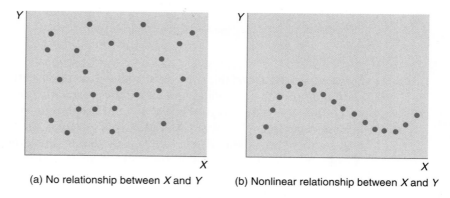

(a) No relationship between *X* and *Y*   (b) Nonlinear relationship between *X* and *Y*

produce correlation coefficients of zero. In Figure 10.4a, there is no association between *X* and *Y*. However, in Figure 10.4b there is an association between *X* and *Y*, though not a linear one.

The correlation coefficient can be affected by truncation. For example, suppose we analyze the relationship between SAT scores measured during the senior year of high school and grade point averages (GPAs) measured at the completion of the freshman year in college. Because individuals who do poorly on the SAT are less likely to attend college, the correlations might be distorted due to the fact that these individuals are not included.

In other situations, a correlation between two variables, X and Y, may turn out to be zero due to a confounding variable (i.e., a variable that affects either X or Y or both). For example, suppose we investigate the relationship between the size of a home and its selling price. Selling prices might be different each year depending on the market and the economy, but if we pool data from several years, there may appear to be no linear association. In other applications, a correlation may be large due to a confounding variable. For example, say we investigate the association between age of first job and starting salary. Observed salaries may be higher for individuals who start working later. This might be due to the fact that these individuals completed a college education, thus delaying their entry into the workforce.

10.1.1 The Sample Correlation Coefficient r

As with other applications, we will have data measured on a sample of subjects. The sample correlation coefficient, denoted r, is computed as follows:

$$r = \frac{\text{Cov}(X, Y)}{\sqrt{\text{Var}(X)\,\text{Var}(Y)}} \tag{10.1}$$

where $\text{Cov}(X, Y)$ is the covariance of X and Y (defined next), and $\text{Var}(X)$ and $\text{Var}(Y)$ are the sample variances of X and Y, respectively. Recall $\text{Var}(X) = \sum(X - \overline{X})^2/(n - 1)$, and $\text{Var}(Y) = \sum(Y - \overline{Y})^2/(n - 1)$.

$$\text{Cov}(X, Y) = \frac{\sum(X - \overline{X})(Y - \overline{Y})}{n - 1} \tag{10.2}$$

We now use examples to illustrate the computation of the sample correlation coefficient.

EXAMPLE 10.1

Correlation Between Body Mass Index and Systolic Blood Pressure

Suppose we are interested in the relationship between body mass index (computed as the ratio of weight in kilograms to height in meters squared) and systolic blood pressure in males 50 years of age. A random sample of 10 males 50 years of age is selected and their weights, heights, and systolic blood pressures are measured. Their weights and heights are transformed into body mass index scores and are given in the following table. In this analysis, the independent (or predictor) variable is body mass index and the dependent (or outcome) variable is systolic blood pressure.

X = Body Mass Index	Y = Systolic Blood Pressure
18.4	120
20.1	110
22.4	120
25.9	135
26.5	140
28.9	115
30.1	150
32.9	165
33.0	160
34.7	180

The first step in assessing the relationship between body mass index an systolic blood pressure is through a scatter diagram (Figure 10.5). Notice tha the independent variable (body mass index) is displayed on the horizonta axis and the dependent variable (systolic blood pressure) is displayed on th vertical axis. From the scatter diagram, it appears that there is a positiv (direct) association between body mass index and systolic blood pressure. W now compute the sample correlation coefficient, r, to quantify the degree o linear association between body mass index and systolic blood pressure. I order to compute r, we must first compute the variances of X and Y as well a the covariance between X and Y.

Figure 10.5 *Scatter Diagram Relating Body Mass Index and Systolic Blood Pressure*

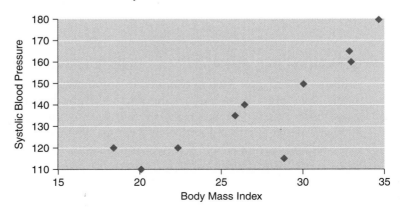

We first compute the variance of X: $\text{Var}(X) = \sum(X - \overline{X})^2/(n-1)$. The following table summarizes the computations:

X = Body Mass Index	$(X - \overline{X})$	$(X - \overline{X})^2$
18.4	−8.89	79.032
20.1	−7.19	51.696
22.4	−4.89	23.912
25.9	−1.39	1.932
26.5	−0.79	0.624
28.9	1.61	2.592
30.1	2.81	7.896
32.9	5.61	31.472
33.0	5.71	32.604
34.7	7.41	54.908
$\sum X = 272.9, \overline{X} = 27.29$	0	286.669

So, $\text{Var}(X) = \sum(X - \overline{X})^2/(n-1) = 286.669/9 = 31.852$.

We now compute the variance of Y: $\text{Var}(Y) = \sum(Y - \overline{Y})^2/(n-1)$. The following table summarizes the computations:

Y = Systolic Blood Pressure	$(Y - \overline{Y})$	$(Y - \overline{Y})^2$
120	−19.5	380.25
110	−29.5	870.25
120	−19.5	380.25
135	−4.5	20.25
140	0.5	0.25
115	−24.5	600.25
150	10.5	110.25
165	25.5	650.25
160	20.5	420.25
180	40.5	1640.25
$\sum Y = 1395.0, \overline{Y} = 139.5$	0	5072.50

So, $\text{Var}(Y) = \sum(Y - \overline{Y})^2/(n-1) = 5072.50/9 = 563.611$.

Finally, we compute the covariance of X and Y: $\text{Cov}(X, Y) = \sum(X - \overline{X})(Y - \overline{Y})/(n - 1)$. The following table summarizes the computations:

$(X - \overline{X})$	$(Y - \overline{Y})$	$(X - \overline{X})(Y - \overline{Y})$
−8.89	−19.5	173.355
−7.19	−29.5	212.105
−4.89	−19.5	95.355
−1.39	−4.5	6.255
−0.79	0.5	−0.395
1.61	−24.5	−39.455
2.81	10.5	29.505
5.61	25.5	143.055
5.71	20.5	117.055
7.41	40.5	300.105
		1036.95

So, $\text{Cov}(X, Y) = \sum(X - \overline{X})(Y - \overline{Y})/(n - 1) = 1036.95/9 = 115.22$. Substituting into (10.1), the sample correlation coefficient is

$$r = \frac{115.22}{\sqrt{(31.852)(563.611)}} = 0.859$$

Based on the sign and the magnitude of r, there is a strong, positive association between body mass index and systolic blood pressure. In fact, this correlation is artificially large (the data are hypothetical). In practice, correlations on the order of 0.3 or larger in absolute value are usually indicative of meaningful or important relationships. ■

10.1.2 Statistical Inference Concerning ρ

It is often of interest to draw inferences about the correlation between two variables in the population through a formal test of hypothesis. The sample correlation coefficient, r, is a point estimate for the population correlation coefficient, ρ. In general, tests of hypothesis concerning ρ address whether there is a linear association in the population ($\rho \neq 0$) or not ($\rho = 0$). The hypotheses are of the form:

$$H_0\colon \rho = 0 \quad \text{(no linear association)}$$
$$H_1\colon \rho \neq 0 \quad \text{(linear association)}$$

The test statistic follows a t distribution with $n - 2$ degrees of freedom:

$$t = r\sqrt{\frac{n-2}{1-r^2}}, \quad df = n - 2 \tag{10.3}$$

NOTE: The t statistic can be used regardless of the sample size (even when n is large), as the critical value of t (Table B.3) reflects the exact sample size. For example, when n is large, the two-sided critical value of t for $\alpha = 0.05$ is 1.96.

We now illustrate the test using the data from Example 10.1. The issue at hand is whether there is a significant correlation between systolic blood pressure and body mass index among all males 50 years of age. In a random sample of 10 males 50 years of age we observed a sample correlation coefficient of 0.859.

1. Set up hypotheses.

$$H_0: \rho = 0$$
$$H_1: \rho \neq 0, \quad \alpha = 0.05$$

2. Select the appropriate test statistic.

$$t = r\sqrt{\frac{n-2}{1-r^2}}$$

3. Decision rule (two-sided test, $\alpha = 0.05$).
   To determine the appropriate value from the t distribution table, we first compute the degrees of freedom. For Example 10.1, df $= n - 2 = 10 - 2 = 8$. The critical value is $t = 2.306$. The decision rule is

$$\text{Reject } H_0 \text{ if } t \geq 2.306 \text{ or if } t \leq -2.306$$
$$\text{Do not reject } H_0 \text{ if } -2.306 < t < 2.306$$

4. Test statistic.

$$t = r\sqrt{\frac{n-2}{1-r^2}} = 0.859\sqrt{\frac{10-2}{1-0.859^2}} = 4.75$$

5. Conclusion.
   Reject H_0 since $4.75 \geq 2.306$. We have significant evidence, $\alpha = 0.05$, to show that $\rho \neq 0$. For this example, $p < 0.01$ (see Table B.3). Therefore, there is evidence of a significant linear association between systolic blood pressure and body mass index among all males 50 years of age.

EXAMPLE 10.2

Correlation Between Number of Hours of Exercise and Systolic Blood Pressure

Consider the application described in Example 10.1. Suppose for the same sample, we also recorded the number of hours of vigorous exercise in a typical week. We wish to investigate the relationship between the number of hours of exercise per week and systolic blood pressure in males 50 years of age. In this analysis, the independent (or predictor) variable is number of hours of exercise per week and the dependent (or outcome) variable is systolic blood pressure. A scatter diagram is shown in Figure 10.6.

$X = $ Number of Hours of Exercise per Week	$Y = $ Systolic Blood Pressure
4	120
10	110
2	120
3	135
3	140
5	115
1	150
2	165
2	160
0	180

In order to compute r, we must first compute the variances of X and Y as well as the covariance between X and Y. We first compute the variance

Figure 10.6 *Scatter Diagram Relating Hours of Exercise and Systolic Blood Pressure*

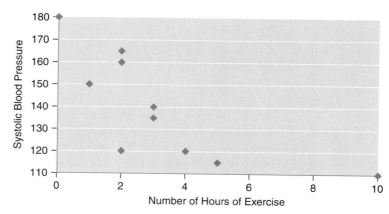

of X: $\text{Var}(X) = \sum(X - \overline{X})^2/(n - 1)$. The following table summarizes the computations:

X = Number of Hours of Exercise per Week	$(X - \overline{X})$	$(X - \overline{X})^2$
4	0.8	0.64
10	6.8	46.24
2	−1.2	1.44
3	−0.2	0.04
3	−0.2	0.04
5	1.8	3.24
1	−2.2	4.84
2	−1.2	1.44
2	−1.2	1.44
0	−3.2	10.24
$\sum X = 32, \overline{X} = 3.2$	0	69.60

So, $\text{Var}(X) = \sum(X - \overline{X})^2/(n - 1) = 69.60/9 = 7.73$.

We computed the variance of Y in Example 10.1, $\text{Var}(Y) = \sum(Y - \overline{Y})^2/(n - 1) = 5072.50/9 = 563.611$. We now need to compute the covariance of X and Y: $\text{Cov}(X, Y) = \sum(X - \overline{X})(Y - \overline{Y})/(n - 1)$. The following table summarizes the computations:

$(X - \overline{X})$	$(Y - \overline{Y})$	$(X - \overline{X})(Y - \overline{Y})$
0.8	−19.5	−15.6
6.8	−29.5	−200.6
−1.2	−19.5	23.4
−0.2	−4.5	0.9
−0.2	0.5	−0.1
1.8	−24.5	−44.1
−2.2	10.5	−23.1
−1.2	25.5	−30.6
−1.2	20.5	−24.6
−3.2	40.5	−129.6
		−444.0

So, $\text{Cov}(X, Y) = \sum(X - \overline{X})(Y - \overline{Y})/(n - 1) = -444.0/9 = -49.33$.

Substituting into (10.1), the sample correlation coefficient is

$$r = \frac{-49.33}{\sqrt{(7.73)(563.611)}} = -0.75$$

Based on the magnitude and sign of r, there is a strong, negative association between the number of hours of exercise per week and systolic blood pressure (i.e., more hours of exercise per week are associated with lower systolic blood pressures).

Using the same data (Example 10.2), we now test whether there is a significant correlation between systolic blood pressure and the number of hours of exercise per week among all males 50 years of age. In a random sample of 10 males 50 years of age we observed a sample correlation coefficient of -0.75.

1. Set up hypotheses.

$$H_0: \rho = 0$$
$$H_1: \rho \neq 0, \quad \alpha = 0.05$$

2. Select the appropriate test statistic.

$$t = r\sqrt{\frac{n-2}{1-r^2}}$$

3. Decision rule (two-sided test, $\alpha = 0.05$).

To determine the appropriate value from the t distribution table, we first compute the degrees of freedom. For Example 10.1, df $= n - 2 = 10 - 2 = 8$. The critical value is $t = 2.306$. The decision rule is

Reject H_0 if $t \geq 2.306$ or if $t \leq -2.306$

Do not reject H_0 if $-2.306 < t < 2.306$

4. Test statistic.

$$t = r\sqrt{\frac{n-2}{1-r^2}} = -0.75\sqrt{\frac{10-2}{1-(-0.75)^2}} = -3.18$$

5. Conclusion.

Reject H_0 since $-3.18 \leq -2.306$. We have significant evidence, $\alpha = 0.05$, that $\rho \neq 0$. For this example, $p < 0.02$ (see Table B.3). Therefore, there is evidence of a significant linear association between systolic blood pressure and the number of hours of exercise per week among all males 50 years of age. ■

10.2 Simple Linear Regression

In regression analysis, we develop the mathematical equation that best describes the relationship between two variables, X and Y. In correlation analysis, it is actually not necessary to specify which of the two variables is the independent and which is the dependent variable. In contrast, with regression analysis the independent and dependent variables must be specified. In regression analysis we address the following issues:

1. What mathematical equation best describes the relationship between X and Y (e.g., a line or a curve of some form)?
2. How do we estimate the equation that describes the relationship between X and Y?
3. Is the form specified in (1) appropriate?

We begin with the simplest situation, the one in which the relationship between X and Y is linear. The equation of the line relating Y to X is called the *simple linear regression equation* and is given here:

$$Y = \beta_0 + \beta_1 X + \varepsilon \qquad (10.4)$$

where Y is the dependent variable
$\quad$ X is the independent variable
$\quad$ β_0 is the Y-intercept (i.e., the value of Y when $X = 0$)
$\quad$ β_1 is the slope (i.e., the expected change in Y relative to one unit change in X)
$\quad$ ε is the random error

The estimates of β_0 and β_1, denoted $\hat{\beta}_0$ and $\hat{\beta}_1$, respectively, are determined using the following equations:

$$\hat{\beta}_1 = r\sqrt{\frac{\text{Var}(Y)}{\text{Var}(X)}} \qquad (10.5)$$

$$\hat{\beta}_0 = \overline{Y} - \hat{\beta}_1 \overline{X}$$

These estimates (10.5) are called the *least squares estimates* of the slope and intercept. The formulas shown are those that minimize the squared errors (i.e., minimize $\sum \varepsilon^2$); the derivations of the formulas will not be shown.

The estimate of the simple linear regression equation is given by substituting the least squares estimates (10.5) into equation (10.4):

$$\hat{Y} = \hat{\beta}_0 + \hat{\beta}_1 X \qquad (10.6)$$

where $\hat{Y}$ is the expected value of Y for a given value of X

EXAMPLE 10.1   **Regression Analysis of Body Mass Index on Systolic Blood Pressure (continued)**

We now estimate the simple linear regression equation for the data given in Example 10.1. The dependent variable (Y) is systolic blood pressure, the independent variable, X, is body mass index, and the correlation was estimated at 0.859. We first estimate the slope by substituting the appropriate statistics into (10.5):

$$\hat{\beta}_1 = r\sqrt{\frac{\text{Var}(Y)}{\text{Var}(X)}} = 0.859\sqrt{\frac{563.611}{31.852}} = 3.61$$

Now, substituting again, we compute the Y-intercept:

$$\hat{\beta}_0 = \overline{Y} - \hat{\beta}_1\overline{X} = 139.5 - (3.61)(27.29) = 40.98$$

The simple linear regression equation for Example 10.1 is

$$\hat{Y} = 40.98 + 3.61X$$

The Y-intercept is 40.98, which is the expected systolic blood pressure (Y) when body mass index (X) is zero. In this example, the Y-intercept is not meaningful since it is not possible to observe a body mass index equal to zero. However, the estimated slope, $\hat{\beta}_1 = 3.61$, indicates that a 1-unit increase in body mass index is associated with an expected increase of 3.61 units in systolic blood pressure. If we compare two males 50 years of age, the first with a body mass index 10 units higher than the second, we would expect the first subject's systolic blood pressure to be $10(3.61) = 36.1$ units higher than the second subject's.

We can also can use the equation to generate an estimate of systolic blood pressure (Y) for a person with a specific body mass index (X). For example, suppose we wish to estimate the systolic blood pressure of a male aged 50 whose body mass index is 20. Using the simple linear regression equation:

$$\hat{Y} = 40.98 + 3.61X = 40.98 + 3.61(20) = 113.81$$

This can be interpreted in two ways. It is the expected systolic blood pressure of *a* male age 50 whose body mass index is 20. It is also the expected systolic blood pressure for *all* males age 50 with body mass index of 20.   ■

SAS EXAMPLE 10.1 **Correlation and Regression Analysis of Body Mass Index on Systolic Blood Pressure Using SAS**

The following output was generated using SAS Proc Plot, SAS Proc Corr, and SAS Proc Reg, which generate, respectively, a scatter diagram and perform correlation and regression analyses. A brief interpretation appears after the output.

SAS Output for Example 10.1

```
Plot of sbp*bmi. Legend: A = 1 obs, B = 2 obs, etc.
```

```
                              The CORR Procedure
                      2   Variables:   bmi   sbp

                          Covariance Matrix, DF = 9
                                  bmi                sbp
                  bmi         31.8521111        115.2166667
                  sbp        115.2166667        563.6111111

                              Simple Statistics
Variable    N        Mean      Std Dev         Sum     Minimum        Maximum
bmi        10     27.29000     5.64377    272.90000    18.40000      34.70000
sbp        10    139.50000    23.74050         1395   110.00000     180.00000

                 Pearson Correlation Coefficients, N = 10
                      Prob > |r| under H0: Rho = 0

                                  bmi                sbp
                  bmi          1.00000            0.85992
                                                 0.0014
                  sbp          0.85992            1.00000
                               0.0014
```

```
                          The REG Procedure
                           Model: MODEL1
                      Dependent Variable: sbp

                          Analysis of Variance
                              Sum of          Mean
Source                 DF    Squares        Square     F Value    Pr > F
Model                   1    3750.89494    3750.89494    22.71     0.0014
Error                   8    1321.60506     165.20063
Corrected Total         9    5072.50000

            Root MSE              12.85304   R-Square   0.7395
            Dependent Mean       139.50000   Adj R-Sq   0.7069
            Coeff Var              9.21365

                          Parameter Estimates
                       Parameter      Standard
Variable        DF      Estimate        Error      t Value    Pr > |t|
Intercept        1      40.78558       21.11158      1.93       0.0895
bmi              1       3.61724        0.75913      4.76       0.0014
```

Interpretation of SAS Output for Example 10.1

SAS can produce high-level graphical displays; however, these require some programming to implement. The Plot procedure is easy to use and generates a scatter diagram for two continuous variables. SAS displays points in the scatter diagram with letters of the alphabet. The letter "A" appears when there is a single point in a particular location, "B" indicates that two points fall in the same location, and so on. Although the scatter diagram is somewhat crude, it clearly conveys the nature of the relationship between the two variables under investigation. In Example 10.1 there is a strong positive association between BMI and SBP.

The SAS Corr procedure generates a correlation analysis. In this example, we requested that SAS produce a Covariance Matrix, which appears at the top of the correlation output. The Covariance Matrix contains covariances between the variables in the rows and columns of the matrix. The covariance between a variable and itself is identical to the variance of that variable. For example, the Cov(SBP,SBP) = Var(SBP) = 563.61, the Cov(SBP,BMI) = Cov(BMI,SBP) = 115.22, and Cov(BMI,BMI) = Var(BMI) = 31.85. By default, the Corr procedure also generates summary statistics for each variable. The last section of the output contains the Correlation Matrix. The Correlation Matrix contains sample correlations (r) between variables in the rows and columns of the matrix. Underneath each sample correlation is a two-sided p value for testing H_0: $\rho = 0$ against H_1: $\rho \neq 0$. The correlation between a variable and itself is always 1.00 (and no test is performed). Of interest are the correlations between distinct variables. Specifically, Corr(SBP, BMI) = Corr(BMI,SBP) = 0.85992, and the correlation between SBP and BMI is significant at $p = 0.0014 < 0.05$.

The SAS Reg procedure generates an ANOVA table used to test whether the regression is significant or not, and then provides estimates of the parameters of the regression equation (e.g., estimates of the intercept and slope). The ANOVA table is set up exactly like the ANOVA tables we used in analysis of variance applications to test the equality of k treatment means. In regression analysis, the total sum of squares represents the variation in the dependent variable Y. The total variation is partitioned into two components, labeled Model and Error. The Model sum of squares is also referred to as the regression sums of squares and reflects the variation in Y accounted for by the regression equation. The Error sum of squares is also referred to as the residual sum of squares and reflects the variation in Y not accounted for by the regression. The p value (0.0014) is used to test whether the regression is significant. When there is a single independent variable (i.e., simple linear regression), this p value is identical to the p value in the correlation analysis and also identical to the p value used to test if the slope is significant. The next part of the regression output includes estimates of the regression parameters. The estimate of the intercept is 40.79 and the estimate of the slope is 3.62. SAS produces two-sided p values to test if the intercept and slope are significantly different from zero. It is usually not of interest to test if the intercept is significantly different from zero, but it is of interest to test if the slope is different from zero. Here, $p = 0.0014$, indicating that the slope (reflecting the change in SBP associated with a 1-unit change in BMI) is significant. ▪

If a regression is run and it has been established that the regression is significant, we often want to quantify how much variation in the dependent variable is "explained" by the independent variable (or set of independent variables, in the case of multiple regression analysis, described in Section 10.3).

The *coefficient of determination*, denoted R^2, "R-squared," is the ratio of the regression (or Model) sums of squares to the total sums of squares (from the ANOVA table).

$$R^2 = \frac{SS_{model}}{SS_{total}} = \frac{SS_{regression}}{SS_{total}} \tag{10.7}$$

where $0 \leq R^2 \leq 1$

Higher values of R^2 imply that more variation in the dependent variable is "explained" by the independent variable(s).

In Example 10.1:

$$R^2 = \frac{3750.89}{5072.50} = 0.7395$$

Thus, 73.9% of the variation in systolic blood pressures is explained by body mass index. Because this example is artificial, the value of R^2 is very high. In practice, values of $R^2 > 0.1$ can be clinically significant.

EXAMPLE 10.2

Regression Analysis of Number of Hours of Exercise on Systolic Blood Pressure (continued)

We now estimate the simple linear regression equation for the data given in Example 10.2. The dependent variable (Y) is systolic blood pressure, the independent variable (X) is the number of hours of exercise per week, and the correlation was estimated at -0.75.

We first estimate the slope by substituting the appropriate statistics into (10.5):

$$\hat{\beta}_1 = r\sqrt{\frac{Var(Y)}{Var(X)}} = -0.75\sqrt{\frac{563.611}{7.73}} = -6.38$$

Now, substituting, we compute the Y-intercept:

$$\hat{\beta}_0 = \overline{Y} - \hat{\beta}_1\overline{X} = 139.5 - (-6.38)(3.2) = 159.9$$

The simple linear regression equation for Example 10.2 is

$$\hat{Y} = 159.9 - 6.38X$$

The Y-intercept is 159.9, which is the expected systolic blood pressure (Y) when the number of hours of exercise (X) is zero. In this example, the Y-intercept is meaningful because it is possible to observe $X = 0$ (i.e., no exercise). The estimated slope, $\hat{\beta}_1 = -6.38$, indicates that each additional hour of exercise per week (a 1-unit increase) is associated with a decrease of 6.38 units in systolic blood pressure. If we compare two males 50 years of age, the first exercising 5 hours in a typical week and the second exercising 4 hours in a typical week, we would expect the first subject's systolic blood pressure to be 6.38 units lower than the second subject's.

We can also use the equation to generate estimates of values of systolic blood pressure (Y) for a person who exercises a specific number of hours per week (X). For example, suppose we wish to estimate the systolic blood pressure of a male aged 50 who exercises 3 hours per week. Using the simple linear regression equation:

$$\hat{Y} = 159.9 - 6.38(3) = 159.9 - 19.14 = 140.76$$ ▪

SAS EXAMPLE 10.2 Correlation and Regression Analysis of Number of Hours of Exercise on Systolic Blood Pressure Using SAS

The following output was generated using SAS Proc Corr and SAS Proc Reg, which perform, respectively, correlation and regression analyses. A brief interpretation appears after the output.

SAS Output for Example 10.2

```
                    The CORR Procedure
                2 Variables: exercise sbp

                        Simple Statistics
Variable    N      Mean     Std Dev      Sum     Minimum     Maximum
exercise   10    3.20000    2.78089   32.00000         0    10.00000
sbp        10  139.50000   23.74050       1395  110.00000  180.00000

           Pearson Correlation Coefficients, N = 10
                 Prob > |r| under H0: Rho=0

                        exercise          sbp
            exercise    1.00000      -0.74725
                                      0.0130

            sbp        -0.74725       1.00000
                        0.0130

                    The REG Procedure
                    Model: MODEL1
                Dependent Variable: sbp

                    Analysis of Variance
                        Sum of           Mean
Source            DF    Squares         Square    F Value    Pr > F
Model              1  2832.41379    2832.41379      10.12    0.0130
Error              8  2240.08621     280.01078
Corrected Total    9  5072.50000
```

```
Root MSE              16.73352   R-Square   0.5584
Dependent Mean       139.50000   Adj R-Sq   0.5032
Coeff Var             11.99536
```

		Parameter Estimates			
		Parameter	Standard		
Variable	DF	Estimate	Error	t Value	Pr > |t|
Intercept	1	159.91379	8.31854	19.22	<.0001
exercise	1	-6.37931	2.00578	-3.18	0.0130

Interpretation of SAS Output for Example 10.2

The SAS Corr procedure generates a correlation analysis. In this example, we did not request that SAS produce a Covariance Matrix (as we had requested in Example 10.1). The first part of the output contains summary statistics for each variable. The next section of the output includes the Correlation Matrix. The Correlation Matrix contains sample correlations (r) between variables showing in the rows and columns of the matrix. Underneath each sample correlation is a two-sided p value for testing $H_0: \rho = 0$ against $H_1: \rho \neq 0$. The correlation between a variable and itself is always 1.00. Of interest are the correlations between distinct variables. Specifically, Corr(SBP,EXERCISE) = Corr(EXERCISE,SBP) = -0.74725, and this correlation between SBP and EXERCISE is significant at $p = 0.0130 < 0.05$.

The SAS Reg procedure generates an ANOVA table used to test whether the regression is significant or not and then provides estimates of the parameters of the regression equation (e.g., estimates of the intercept and slope). In regression analysis, the total sums of squares represents the variation in the dependent variable Y. The total variation is partitioned into two components, labeled Model and Error. The Model sums of squares is also referred to as the regression sums of squares and reflects the variation in Y accounted for by the regression equation. The Error sums of squares is also referred to as the residual sums of squares and reflects the variation in Y that is not accounted for by the regression. The p value (0.0130) is used to test whether the regression is significant. When there is a single independent variable (i.e., simple linear regression), this p value is identical to the p value in the correlation analysis and also identical to the p value used to test if the slope is significant. The next part of the regression output includes estimates of the regression parameters. The estimate of the intercept is 159.91 and the estimate of the slope is -6.38. SAS produces two-sided p values to test if the intercept and slope are significantly different from zero. It is usually not of interest to test if the intercept is significantly different from zero, but it is of interest to test if the slope is different from zero. Here, $p = 0.0130$, indicating that the slope (reflecting the change in SBP associated with a 1-unit change in the number of hours of exercise per week) is significant. In this example, $R^2 = 0.56$, suggesting that 56% of the variation in systolic blood pressures is explained by the number of hours of exercise per week. ▪

10.3 Multiple Regression Analysis

In Examples 10.1 and 10.2, we found that body mass index and the number of hours of exercise per week were significantly associated with systolic blood pressure (when considered separately). There are many characteristics that might be related to systolic blood pressure, such as age, gender, diet, family history of hypertension, race, smoking status, and so on. In many applications, we wish to assess the extent to which a set of candidate variables are related to a particular dependent variable and investigate their relative importance.

In multiple regression analysis, we consider applications involving a single continuous dependent variable, Y, and multiple independent variables, denoted X_1, X_2, and so on. The form of the multiple linear regression equation is

$$Y = \beta_0 + \beta_1 X_1 + \beta_2 X_2 + \cdots + \beta_p X_p + \varepsilon \qquad (10.8)$$

where Y is the dependent variable

X_1 to X_p are the independent variables

β_0 is the intercept (i.e., the value of Y when $X_1 = X_2 = \cdots = X_p = 0$)

β_i $(i = 1, \ldots, p)$ are the slope coefficients, also called the regression parameters (i.e., the expected change in Y relative to a 1-unit change in X_i)

ε is the random error

NOTE: The dependent variable, Y, is a continuous variable. The independent variables, X_i, can be continuous variables or dichotomous (sometimes called *indicator*) variables. In the following example we consider both continuous independent variables (e.g., age) and indicator variables (e.g., smoking status, where 1 = smoker, 0 = nonsmoker).

The formulas used to estimate the intercept and slope coefficients are computationally complex. We therefore restrict our attention to interpreting a multiple regression analysis performed in SAS. Interested readers can refer to *Applied Regression Analysis and Other Multivariable Methods*, 2nd ed. by Kleinbaum, D. G., Kupper, L. L., and Muller, K. E. (1988), PWS-Kent Publishing Company, Boston, MA, for a more complete discussion of multiple regression analysis. Here we present only a single example as a means of illustrating the conceptual framework of the application in a basic sense. Consider the following example.

SAS EXAMPLE 10.3 **Multiple Linear Regression Analysis for Systolic Blood Pressure**

We used SAS to analyze a large data set ($n = 5078$). The dependent variable is systolic blood pressure (SBP) and we consider three independent variables: AGE (a continuous variable, measured in years), MALE (an indicator variable, coded 1 for males and 0 for females), and SMOKER (an indicator variable, coded 1 for smokers and 0 for nonsmokers). In the following we estimated a multiple regression equation using SAS. A brief interpretation appears after the output.

SAS Output for Example 10.3

The REG Procedure
Model: MODEL1
Dependent Variable: SBP

Analysis of Variance

Source	DF	Sum of Squares	Mean Square	F Value	Pr > F
Model	3	446821	148940	493.03	<.0001
Error	5074	1532804	302.08991		
Corrected Total	5077	1979625			

Root MSE	17.38073	R-Square	0.2257
Dependent Mean	129.60339	Adj R-Sq	0.2253
Coeff Var	13.41071		

Parameter Estimates

Variable	DF	Parameter Estimate	Standard Error	t Value	DF	Pr > |t|
Intercept	1	90.57147	1.12386	80.59	1	<.0001
age	1	0.77398	0.02094	36.96	1	<.0001
male	1	4.39800	0.49022	8.97	1	<.0001
smoker	1	-1.84484	0.50366	-3.66	1	0.0003

Interpretation of SAS Output for Example 10.3

The SAS Reg procedure generates an ANOVA table used to test whether the regression is significant or not and then provides estimates of the regression parameters (e.g., estimates of the intercept and regression slopes). The ANOVA table is set up exactly like the ANOVA tables we used in analysis of variance applications to test the equality of k treatment means. In multiple regression analysis, the total sums of squares represents the variation in the dependent variable Y. The total variation is partitioned into two components, labeled Model and Error. The Model sums of squares, also referred to as the regression sums of squares, reflects the variation in Y accounted for by the regression equation. In multiple regression analysis, the ANOVA table is used to perform a global test—in particular, to test if the collection of variables is significant. The p value (<0.0001) is used to test whether the set of independent variables considered is significant—here, whether AGE, MALE, and SMOKER, considered simultaneously, are significant in explaining variation in SBP.

The next part of the regression output includes estimates of the regression parameters. The estimate of the intercept is 90.57 and is the expected systolic blood pressure if all of the independent variables are zero, that is, if AGE = 0 (which is unreasonable), MALE = 0 (which is the code for female), and SMOKER = 0 (which is the code for a nonsmoker). The estimate of the regression parameter associated with AGE is 0.77. A 1-year increase in AGE is associated with a 0.77-unit increase in SBP, holding the other variables in the equation constant. The estimate of the regression parameter associated with MALE is 4.40. Because MALE is an indicator variable, the effect is interpreted as follows. On average, males (MALE = 1) have SBPs 4.40 units higher than females (MALE = 0), holding the other variables constant. Smoking status is interpreted in a similar fashion. The estimate of the regression parameter associated with SMOKER is -1.84. On average, smokers (SMOKER = 1) have SBPs 1.84 units lower than nonsmokers (SMOKER = 0), holding the other variables constant. We should be cautious interpreting this effect of smoking, as smoking status may be related to other behaviors and smoking, per se, may not be associated with lower systolic blood pressure. Each of these parameter estimates is adjusted for the other independent variables in the model. They reflect the impact of each independent variable on SBP after considering the other variables.

SAS produces two-sided p values to test if the intercept and regression coefficients are significantly different from zero. Again, it is usually not of interest to test if the intercept is significantly different from zero, but it is of interest to test if the other coefficients are different from zero. Here, $p < 0.001$ for each independent variable, indicating that each of the variables is highly significant. In this example, the sample size is very large, which accounts, in part, for the highly significant results.

It is often of interest to determine the relative importance of variables in a multiple regression analysis. This is determined by the magnitude of the t statistics (or associated p values). One cannot determine relative importance based on the magnitude of the parameter estimates, as the estimates are affected by the scales on which variables are measured. In this example, age is the most important (most significant) independent variable, followed by gender and then smoking status. These three variables account for, or explain, 22.6% of the variation in the dependent variable SBP. ▪

10.4 Logistic Regression Analysis

In logistic regression analysis, we consider applications involving a single dependent variable, Y, which is dichotomous (i.e., Success versus Failure). The technique is discussed in detail in Chapter 11; here we present a brief overview for comparison to linear regression analysis. Suppose in Example 10.3 the dependent variable was not systolic blood pressure (a continuous variable), but instead diagnosis of hypertension (hypertensive or not, a dichotomous variable). Logistic regression applications can involve one or several independent variables, denoted X_1, X_2, and so on. The form of the logistic regression equation is

$$\ln\left\{\frac{p}{(1-p)}\right\} = \beta_0 + \beta_1 X_1 + \beta_2 X_2 + \cdots + \beta_p X_p + \varepsilon \qquad (10.9)$$

where Y is the dichotomous dependent variable (success or failure)
p is the proportion of successes
X_1 to X_p are the independent variables
β_0 is the intercept
β_i $(i = 1, \ldots, p)$ are the slope coefficients, also called the regression parameters
ε is the random error

NOTES: The left-hand side of the equation displays the dependent or outcome variable in a specific form. The quantity $p/(1-p)$ is the "odds" of possessing the event. The expression $\ln\{p/(1-p)\}$ is called the "log odds" or the "logit" of Y. The slope coefficients, β_i $(i = 1, \ldots, p)$, reflect the change in the logit or log odds of Y relative to a 1 unit change in X_i.

The dependent variable, Y, is a dichotomous variable. The independent variables X_i, can be continuous variables or dichotomous (sometimes called *indicator*) variables. In Example 10.4 we consider both continuous independent variables (e.g., age) and indicator variables (e.g., smoking status, where 1 = smoker, 0 = nonsmoker).

The formulas to estimate the intercept and slope coefficients are computationally complex. We again restrict our attention to interpreting a logistic regression analysis performed in SAS. Consider the following example.

SAS EXAMPLE 10.4 Multiple Logistic Regression Analysis for Hypertension

We used SAS to analyze a large data set ($n = 5078$). The dependent variable is a dichotomous variable (HTN, coded 1 for patients classified as hypertensive and 0 otherwise) and we consider three independent variables: AGE (a continuous variable, measured in years), MALE (an indicator variable, coded 1 for males and 0 for females), and SMOKER (an indicator variable, coded for smokers and 0 for nonsmokers). In the following we estimated a logistic regression equation using SAS. A brief interpretation appears after the output.

SAS Output for Example 10.4

The LOGISTIC Procedure
Response Profile

Ordered Value	HTN	Total Frequency
1	1	349
2	0	4729

```
                Probability modeled is HTN=1.
                   Model Convergence Status
           Convergence criterion (GCONV=1E-8) satisfied.
                    Model Fit Statistics
                        Intercept      Intercept and
           Criterion      Only           Covariates
           AIC          2544.410          2246.882
           SC           2550.943          2273.013
           -2 Log L     2542.410          2238.882

        Testing Global Null Hypothesis: BETA=0
        Test                Chi-Square    DF    Pr > ChiSq
        Likelihood Ratio     303.5282     3      <.0001
        Score                291.3059     3      <.0001
        Wald                 259.4685     3      <.0001
                    The LOGISTIC Procedure
```

```
        Analysis of Maximum Likelihood Estimates
                            Standard        Wald
Parameter   DF    Estimate    Error     Chi-Square    Pr > ChiSq
Intercept    1     -7.1813    0.3371     453.9220       <.0001
age          1      0.0654    0.00534    149.6551       <.0001
male         1      1.2628    0.1254     101.4887       <.0001
smoker       1      0.9520    0.1187      64.3556       <.0001
```

```
                Odds Ratio Estimates
                    Point        95% Wald
            Effect  Estimate   Confidence Limits
            age      1.068      1.056     1.079
            male     3.535      2.765     4.520
            smoker   2.591      2.053     3.269
```

```
Association of Predicted Probabilities and Observed Responses
        Percent Concordant      77.0      Somers' D    0.550
        Percent Discordant      22.1      Gamma        0.555
        Percent Tied             0.9      Tau-a        0.070
        Pairs                1650421      c            0.775
```

Interpretation of SAS Output for Example 10.4

The SAS Logistic procedure first displays the numbers of subjects classified in each of the two response categories. In this example, 349 subjects are hypertensive and 4729 are not. SAS then indicates that the model is set up to predict the probability that a person is hypertensive (HTN = 1). The next sections of the output are entitled "Model Fit Statistics" and "Testing Global Null Hypothesis: BETA = 0." The statistics are used for testing whether the collection of variables considered are significant and for comparing models. In this application, we considered three independent variables. The statistic labeled "−2 log L" for model containing intercept only (2542.410) represents a measure of the overall variation in the dependent variable. This quantity is similar to the total sum of squares in a multiple regression analysis. The Chi-Square for Covariates (303.528) is computed by taking the difference between −2 log L for model containing intercept only and −2 log L for model with intercept and covariates. This statistic is used to perform a global test of significance of the set of independent variables considered. In Example 10.4, $p < 0.0001$, so AGE, MALE, and SMOKER considered simultaneously, are significant in explaining variation in hypertensive status.

The next part of the regression output includes estimates of the regression parameters. The estimate of the intercept is −7.1813. The estimate of the regression parameter associated with AGE is 0.0654. A 1-year increase in AGE is associated with a 0.0654-unit increase in the logit or log odds of Y. SAS also produces odds ratios for each independent variable (computed by $\exp(\beta_i)$) The odds ratio for AGE is estimated as 1.068. The odds of having hypertension are 1.068 times higher with every additional year of age, holding the other variables constant. The regression parameter associated with MALE is 1.2628. Because MALE is an indicator variable, the effect is interpreted as follows. On average, the logit or log odds of Y is 1.2628 times higher for males (MALE = 1) as compared to females (MALE = 0). Smoking status is interpreted in a similar fashion. The estimate of the regression parameter associated with SMOKER is 0.9520. On average, smokers (SMOKER = 1) are more likely to be hypertensive than nonsmokers. The odds ratio for MALE is 3.535, so males are 3.535 times more likely to have hypertension than females (odds of being hypertensive are 3.535 times higher for males as compared to females), holding the other variables constant. The odds ratio for SMOKER is 2.591, so smokers are more likely to have hypertension than nonsmokers (odds of being hypertensive are 2.591 times higher for smokers as compared to nonsmokers), holding the other variables constant. Each of these parameter estimates and estimates of odds ratios is adjusted for the other independent variables in the model. They reflect the impact of each independent variable on hypertensive status after considering the other variables in the model.

SAS produces two-sided p values to test if the intercept and regression coefficients are significantly different from zero. Again, it is usually not of interest to test if the intercept is significantly different from zero, but it is of interest to test if the other coefficients are different from zero. Here, $p < 0.0001$ for each independent variable, indicating that each of the variables is highly significant. In this example, the sample size is very large, which accounts, in part, for the highly significant results.

It is often of interest to determine the relative importance of variables in a multiple logistic regression analysis. This is determined by the magnitude of the Wald chi-square statistics (or associated p values). One cannot determine relative importance based on the magnitude of the parameter estimates, as the estimates are affected by the scales on which variables are measured. In this example, age is the most important (most significant) independent variable, followed by gender and then smoking status. It is not possible to compute R^2 (10.7) for a logistic regression to describe how much variation in the dependent variable is explained by the independent variables. In logistic regression, we use the c statistic for a similar purpose. The c statistic in Example 10.4 is 0.775 and represents the extent to which the actual values of the dependent variable and the predicted values (generated by the estimated model) agree. Values exceeding 0.7 are generally considered adequate.

A more detailed discussion of logistic regression analysis is contained in Chapter 11. ■

10.5 Key Formulas

Application	Notation/Formula	Description
Estimate sample correlation coefficient	$r = \dfrac{\mathrm{Cov}(X, Y)}{\sqrt{\mathrm{Var}(X)\mathrm{Var}(Y)}}$	quantifies the nature and extent of linear association between X and Y
Test H_0: $\rho = 0$	$t = r\sqrt{\dfrac{n-2}{1-r^2}}, \quad \mathrm{df} = n-2$	test for significant correlation between X and Y
Simple linear regression equation	$Y = \beta_0 + \beta_1 X + \varepsilon$	see (10.5) for least squares estimates of regression parameters
Estimate R^2	$R^2 = \dfrac{SS_{\text{model}}}{SS_{\text{total}}} = \dfrac{SS_{\text{regression}}}{SS_{\text{total}}}$	proportion of variation in dependent variable explained by independent variable(s)
Multiple linear regression equation	$Y = \beta_0 + \beta_1 X_1 + \beta_2 X_2 + \cdots + \beta_p X_p + \varepsilon$	continuous dependent variable Y, continuous or dichotomous independent variables X_i
Multiple logistic regression equation	$\ln\left\{\dfrac{p}{(1-p)}\right\}$ $= \beta_0 + \beta_1 X_1 + \beta_2 X_2 + \cdots + \beta_p X_p + \varepsilon$	dichotomous dependent variable Y, p is the proportion of successes, continuous or dichotomous independent variables X_i (see Chapter 11)

10.6 Statistical Computing

Following are the SAS programs used to generate a scatter diagram and to estimate correlations between variables, a simple linear regression equation, a multiple regression equation, and a logistic regression equation. The SAS procedures and brief descriptions of their use are noted in the header to each example. Notes are provided to the right of the SAS programs (in blue) for orientation purposes and are not part of the programs. In addition, the blank lines in the programs are solely to accommodate the notes. Blank lines and spaces can be used throughout SAS programs to enhance readability. A summary of the SAS procedures used in the examples is provided at the end of this section.

SAS EXAMPLE 10.1 **Scatter Diagram, Correlation, and Simple Linear Regression Analysis**
Assess the Relationship Between Body Mass Index and Systolic Blood Pressure (Example 10.1)

Suppose we are interested in the relationship between body mass index (computed as the ratio of weight in kilograms to height in meters squared) and systolic blood pressure in males 50 years of age. A random sample of 10 males 50 years of age is selected and their weights, heights, and systolic blood pressures are measured. Their weights and heights are transformed into body mass index scores and are given in the following table. In this analysis, the independent (or predictor) variable is body mass index, and the dependent (or outcome) variable is systolic blood pressure. Generate a scatter diagram to assess the relationship between body mass index and systolic blood pressure using SAS. In addition, estimate the correlation between body mass index and systolic blood pressure and the regression equation relating body mass index to systolic blood pressure using SAS.

X = Body Mass Index	Y = Systolic Blood Pressure
18.4	120
20.1	110
22.4	120
25.9	135
26.5	140
28.9	115
30.1	150
32.9	165
33.0	160
34.7	180

Program Code

`options ps=62 ls=80;`	Formats the output page to 62 lines in length and 80 columns in width
`data in;`	Beginning of Data Step
`  input bmi sbp;`	Inputs two variables **bmi** and **sbp** (both continuous variables).
`cards;`	Beginning of Raw Data section.
`18.4 120`	actual observations (value of **bmi** and
`20.1 110`	**sbp** on each line)
`22.4 120`	
`25.9 135`	
`26.5 140`	
`28.9 115`	
`30.1 150`	
`32.9 165`	
`33.0 160`	
`34.7 180`	
`run;`	
`proc plot;`	Procedure call. Proc Plot generates a scatter diagram for two continuous variables.
`  plot sbp*bmi;`	Specification of analytic variables. First variable specified is plotted on the vertical axis (*y*).
`run;`	End of procedure section.
`proc corr cov;`	Procedure call. Proc Corr estimates correlation coefficients and tests their significance. The Cov option produces a covariance matrix.
`  var bmi sbp;`	Specification of analytic variables.
`run;`	End of procedure section.
`proc reg;`	Procedure call. Proc Reg estimates regression parameters and tests significance.
`  model sbp=bmi;`	Specification of regression model. The format is dependent (**sbp**) = independent variable(s) (**bmi**).
`run;`	End of procedure section. ■

SAS EXAMPLE 10.2 Correlation and Simple Linear Regression Analysis

Assess the Relationship Between Number of Hours of Exercise per Week and Systolic Blood Pressure (Example 10.2)

Consider the application described in Example 10.1. Suppose for the same sample, we also recorded the number of hours of vigorous exercise in a typical week. We wish to investigate the relationship between the number of hours of exercise per week and systolic blood pressure in males 50 years of age. In this analysis, the independent (or predictor) variable is number of hours of exercise per week and the dependent (or response) variable is systolic blood pressure. Estimate the correlation between the number of hours of exercise and systolic blood pressure and the regression equation relating the number of hours of exercise to systolic blood pressure using SAS.

X = Number of Hours of Exercise per Week	Y = Systolic Blood Pressure
4	120
10	110
2	120
3	135
3	140
5	115
1	150
2	165
2	160
0	180

Program Code

```options ps=62 ls=80;```	Formats the output page to 62 lines in length and 80 columns in width
```data in;```	Beginning of Data Step
``` input exercise sbp;```	Inputs two variables *exercise* and *sbp* (both continuous variables).
```cards;```	Beginning of Raw Data section.
```4 120```	actual observations (value of *exercise*
```10 110```	and *sbp* on each line)
```2 120```	
```3 135```	
```3 140```	
```5 115```	
```1 150```	
```2 165```	
```2 160```	
```0 180```	
```run;```	

```
proc corr;
```
Procedure call. Proc Corr estimates correlation coefficients and tests their significance.

```
 var exercise sbp;
```
Specification of analytic variables.

```
run;
```
End of procedure section.

```
proc reg;
```
Procedure call. Proc Reg estimates regression parameters and tests their significance.

```
 model sbp=exercise;
```
Specification of regression model. The format is dependent variable (*sbp*) = independent variable(s) (*exercise*).

```
run;
```
End of procedure section. ▪

SAS EXAMPLE 10.3 Multiple Regression Analysis

Assess the Effects of Age, Gender, and Smoking Status, Considered Simultaneously, on Systolic Blood Pressure (Example 10.3)

In the following we use SAS to analyze a large data set ($n = 5078$). The dependent variable is systolic blood pressure (SBP) and we consider three independent variables: AGE (a continuous variable, measured in years), MALE (an indicator variable, coded 1 for males and 0 for females), and SMOKER (an indicator variable, coded 1 for smokers and 0 for nonsmokers). We estimated a multiple regression equation using SAS—the data are abbreviated.

Program Code

```
options ps=62 ls=80;
```
Formats the output page to 62 lines in length and 80 columns in width

```
data in;
  input sbp age male smoker;
```
Beginning of Data Step
Inputs four variables *sbp, age, male,* and *smoker.*

```
cards;
120 55 1 0
110 40 0 0
 .
 .
 .
140 35 1 1
run;
```
Beginning of Raw Data section.
actual observations (value of *sbp, age, male,* and *smoker* on each line)

```
proc reg;
```
Procedure call. Proc Reg estimates regression parameters and tests their significance.

```
 model sbp=age male smoker;
```
Specification of regression model. The format is dependent variable (*sbp*) = independent variable(s) (*age, male,* and *smoker*).

```
run;
```
End of procedure section. ▪

SAS EXAMPLE 10.4 Logistic Regression Analysis

Assess the Effects of Age, Gender, and Smoking Status, Considered Simultaneously, on Hypertensive Status (Example 10.4)

In the following we use SAS to analyze a large data set ($n = 5078$). The dependent variable is a dichotomous variable (HTN, coded 1 for patients classified as hypertensive and 0 otherwise) and we consider three independent variables: AGE (a continuous variable, measured in years), MALE (an indicator variable, coded 1 for males and 0 for females), and SMOKER (an indicator variable, coded 1 for smokers and 0 for nonsmokers). We estimated a logistic regression equation using SAS—the data are abbreviated.

Program Code

```
options ps=62 ls=80;
```
Formats the output page to 62 lines in length and 80 columns in width

```
data in;
  input htn age male smoker;
```
Beginning of Data Step
Inputs four variables *htn*, *age*, *male*, and *smoker*.

```
cards;
0 55 1 0
0 40 0 0
.
.
.
1 35 1 1
run;
proc logistic descending;
```
Beginning of Raw Data section.
actual observations (value of *htn*, *age*, *male*, and *smoker* on each line)

Procedure call. Proc Logistic estimates logistic regression parameters and tests their significance. The descending option indicates that the value 1 is the outcome of interest (the value 0 is the comparison).

```
  model htn=age male smoker;
```
Specification of regression model. The format is dependent variable (*htn*) = independent variable(s) (*age*, *male*, and *smoker*).

```
run;
```
End of procedure section.

10.6.1 Summary of SAS Procedures

The SAS procedures for correlation and regression analysis are summarized in the following table. Specific options can be requested in these procedures to produce specific results. The options are shown in italics. Users should refer to the examples in this section for complete descriptions of the procedures and specific options.

Procedure	Sample Procedure Call	Description
proc plot	proc plot; plot y*x;	Generates a scatter diagram for two continuous variables with Y on the vertical axis and X on the horizontal axis.
proc corr	proc corr *cov*; var y x1 x2 x3 x4;	Produces a correlation matrix for specified variables. Matrix includes estimates of correlations between variables and associated significance tests. Cov option generates a covariance matrix.
proc reg	proc reg; model y = x1 x2 x3 x4;	Estimates a linear regression model relating dependent variable Y to independent variables X_1, X_2, X_3, X_4.
proc logistic	proc logistic *descending*; model y = x1 x2 x3 x4;	Estimates a logistic regression model relating dichotomous dependent variable Y to independent variables X_1, X_2, X_3, X_4. The descending option considers the response with the higher numerical code the outcome of interest (e.g., 1 = outcome of interest, 0 = comparison).

10.7 Analysis of Framingham Heart Study Data

The Framingham data set includes data collected from the original cohort. Participants contributed up to three examination cycles of data. Here we analyze data collected in the first examination cycle (called the period = 1 examination) and use SAS Proc Corr to investigate correlations between body mass index (BMI), number of cigarettes smoked per day, and systolic blood pressure. We then develop a simple linear regression model relating systolic blood pressure to BMI and a multiple linear regression model relating systolic blood pressure to BMI, age, gender, number of cigarettes smoked per day, and whether participants are on antihypertensive medications or not. For this analysis we exclude persons who are underweight (BMI < 18.5) because analysis has shown that there may be a different relationship between very low BMI and other risk factors. We also create an indicator variable for male gender. The SAS code to create the analytic data set along with the procedure calls is shown next.

Framingham Data Analysis—SAS Code

```
data fhs;
 set in.frmgham;
 if period=1;

if bmi<18.5 then delete;

if sex=1 then male=1;
else if sex=2 then male=0;
run;
```

```
proc corr data=fhs;
 var sysbp bmi cigpday;
run;

proc reg data=fhs;
 model sysbp=bmi;
run;

proc reg data=fhs;
 model sysbp=bmi age male bpmeds cigpday;
run;
```

Framingham Data Analysis—SAS Output

The CORR Procedure

3 Variables: SYSBP BMI CIGPDAY

Simple Statistics

Variable	N	Mean	Std Dev	Sum	Minimum	Maximum
SYSBP	4358	133.06436	22.36517	579895	83.50000	295.00000
BMI	4358	25.95387	4.01749	113107	18.52000	56.80000
CIGPDAY	4326	8.96163	11.95879	38768	0	70.00000

Simple Statistics

Variable	Label
SYSBP	Systolic BP mmHg
BMI	Body Mass Index (kr/(M*M)
CIGPDAY	Cigarettes per day

Pearson Correlation Coefficients
Prob > |r| under H0: Rho=0
Number of Observations

	SYSBP	BMI	CIGPDAY
SYSBP Systolic BP mmHg	1.00000 4358	0.32353 <.0001 4358	-0.09910 <.0001 4326
BMI Body Mass Index (kr/(M*M)	0.32353 <.0001 4358	1.00000 4358	-0.09824 <.0001 4326
CIGPDAY Cigarettes per day	-0.09910 <.0001 4326	-0.09824 <.0001 4326	1.00000 4326

The first part of the correlation output contains summary statistics on the three variables. SAS then produces the correlations between pairs of variables. For each pair, SAS produces the correlation, a *p* value to test if the correlation is significantly different from zero, and then the number of subjects available (i.e., the number of subjects who have complete data on both variables). What is the nature of the correlation between BMI and systolic blood pressure? Is it in the expected direction? Is it statistically significant? What is the nature of the correlation between the number of cigarettes smoked per day and systolic blood pressure? Is it in the expected direction? Is it statistically significant?

The following is a simple linear regression analysis relating BMI to systolic blood pressure. What is the estimate of the slope? How is the slope interpreted? What is the expected systolic blood pressure for a person with BMI = 25?

```
                    The REG Procedure
                     Model: MODEL1
        Dependent Variable: SYSBP Systolic BP mmHg

                  Analysis of Variance
```

		Sum of	Mean		
Source	DF	Squares	Square	F Value	Pr > F
Model	1	228114	228114	509.24	<.0001
Error	4356	1951261	447.94797		
Corrected Total	4357	2179375			

Root MSE	21.16478	R-Square	0.1047
Dependent Mean	133.06436	Adj R-Sq	0.1045
Coeff Var	15.90567		

```
                  Parameter Estimates
```

			Parameter	Standard	
Variable	Label	DF	Estimate	Error	t Value
Intercept	Intercept	1	86.32004	2.09608	41.18
BMI	Body Mass Index (kr/(M*M)	1	1.80105	0.07981	22.57

```
                  Parameter Estimates
```

Variable	Label	DF	Pr >	t	
Intercept	Intercept	1	<.0001
BMI	Body Mass Index (kr/(M*M)	1	<.0001

The following is a multiple linear regression analysis relating age, gender, BMI, antihypertensive treatment, and the number of cigarettes smoked per day to systolic blood pressure. Is the set of predictors statistically significant? How much variation in systolic blood pressure is explained by this set of predictors? Assess the slope coefficients—are they all in the expected direction? What is the relative importance of the risk factors? Do men or women have higher systolic blood pressures, adjusting for age, BMI, number of cigarettes smoked, and antihypertensive medication?

```
                    The REG Procedure
                     Model: MODEL1
           Dependent Variable: SYSBP Systolic BP mmHg
```

Analysis of Variance

Source	DF	Sum of Squares	Mean Square	F Value	Pr > F
Model	5	573039	114608	316.14	<.0001
Error	4260	1544325	362.51768		
Corrected Total	4265	2117364			

Root MSE	19.03990	R-Square	0.2706
Dependent Mean	132.99672	Adj R-Sq	0.2698
Coeff Var	14.31607		

Parameter Estimates

Variable	Label	DF	Parameter Estimate	Standard Error	t Value
Intercept	Intercept	1	51.24242	2.50258	20.48
AGE	Age (years) at examination	1	0.87136	0.03481	25.03
MALE		1	-2.38027	0.62292	-3.82
BMI	Body Mass Index (kr/(M*M)	1	1.47203	0.07407	19.87
BPMEDS	Anti-hypertensive meds Y/N	1	23.80633	1.65356	14.40
CIGPDAY	Cigarettes per day	1	0.03689	0.02633	1.40

Parameter Estimates

Variable	Label	DF	Pr > |t|
Intercept	Intercept	1	<.0001
AGE	Age (years) at examination	1	<.0001
MALE		1	0.0001
BMI	Body Mass Index (kr/(M*M)	1	<.0001
BPMEDS	Anti-hypertensive meds Y/N	1	<.0001
CIGPDAY	Cigarettes per day	1	0.1613

10.8 Problems

1. Data were collected from a random sample of eight patients currently undergoing treatment for hypertension. Each subject reported the average number of cigarettes smoked per day and each was assigned a numerical value reflecting their risk of cardiovascular disease (CVD). The risk assessments were computed by physicians and based on blood pressure, cholesterol level, and exercise status. The risk assessments ranged from 0 to 100, with higher values indicating increased risk.

Number of Cigarettes:	0	2	6	8	12	0	2	20
Risk of CVD:	12	20	50	68	75	8	10	80

   a. Compute the correlation between number of cigarettes and risk of CVD.

   b. Based on this sample, is there evidence of a significant correlation between number of cigarettes and risk of CVD?

   c. Compute the equation of the line that best fits the data to predict risk of CVD from the number of cigarettes (i.e., risk of CVD = dependent variable).

2. Consider the following data reflecting lengths of stay in the hospital (recorded in days) and the total charge (in $000s) for six patients undergoing a minor surgical procedure:

Length of Stay:	5	7	9	10	12	15
Total Charge:	6	5	7.2	8	9.4	7.9

   Consider length of stay as the independent and total charge as the dependent variable.

   a. Describe the relationship between length of stay and total charge using a scatter diagram.

   b. Compute the sample correlation coefficient.

   c. Compute the regression equation.

   d. Estimate the total charge for an individual who stays 11 days in the hospital.

   e. Suppose we compare two patients and one stays 3 days longer in the hospital than the other. What is the expected difference in total charges between these patients?

3. Consider a study assessing the quality of life (QOL) of patients with arthritis. The following figure describes the relationship between QOL and the duration of arthritis, measured in years.

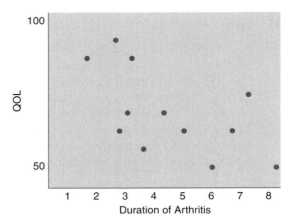

The mean QOL score is 75.8, with a standard deviation of 6.3. The mean duration of arthritis is 4 years, with a standard deviation of 0.7 years. The covariance between QOL and duration is -2.9.

a. What is the nature of the relationship between duration of arthritis and QOL based on the figure? Describe briefly.

b. Estimate the sample correlation coefficient.

c. Compute the equation of the line that best describes the relationship between duration of arthritis and QOL.

d. Interpret the estimated slope.

4. Consider the study described in Problem 3. Suppose that we investigate the relationship between age and the severity of arthritis (measured on a scale from 0 to 100, with higher scores indicative of more severe disease). The following summary statistics are available on the total sample ($n = 175$):

Characteristic	Mean	SD
Age	57.7	3.8
Severity score	59.8	19.5

a. The point estimate for the correlation between age and severity score is 0.36 ($p = 0.0001$). Is there evidence of a significant correlation between age and severity score among all patients?

b. Estimate the equation of the line that best describes the relationship between age and severity score (consider severity score as the dependent variable).

c. What is the expected severity score for an individual 60 years of age?

5. An analysis is performed to investigate the relationship between cardiovascular exercise and percent body fat. A sample of 50 subjects is

involved, and the number of hours of cardiovascular exercise over the previous week and percent body fat are measured on each subject. Summary statistics are shown here:

Variable	n	Mean	SD
# Hours of cardiovascular exercise	50	3.7	1.9
Percent body fat	50	28.5	5.8

a. Suppose the sample correlation coefficient is $r = -0.48$. Is there evidence of a significant correlation? Run the appropriate test at $\alpha = 0.05$.

b. Suppose that the investigation involved 20 men and 30 women and separate correlation analyses were performed that produced the following results: $r_{men} = -0.17$ ($p = 0.4748$), $r_{women} = -0.59$ ($p = 0.0006$). Describe the relationships between exercise and percent body fat in men and women.

c. Summary statistics for the 20 men and 30 women are

Variable	Men Mean (SD)	Women Mean (SD)
# Hours of cardiovascular exercise	4.7 (2.2)	2.5 (1.4)
Percent body fat	20.1 (3.1)	31.6 (8.1)

Estimate the regression equations relating the number of hours of exercise to percent body fat for men and women (separately). (Let Y = percent body fat.)

d. What is the expected percent body fat for a male who exercises 2 hours per week?

e. What is the expected percent body fat for a female who exercises 2 hours per week?

6. An investigation is performed to understand the relationship between age and satisfaction with medical care. Each individual in the investigation is asked to rate satisfaction with medical care on a scale of 0 to 100, with 100 denoting complete satisfaction. Other data, including sociodemographic characteristics (age, gender, race) are also recorded on each individual. A total of 200 individuals are involved in the investigation, and the following results were obtained: $r = 0.43$ ($p = 0.0001$), satisfaction $= 45.2 + 0.9$ age.

a. Based on the correlation, are older or younger individuals more likely to be more satisfied with medical care? (Be brief.)

b. Is the correlation between age and satisfaction significant? Justify.

c. Estimate the satisfaction rating of a 50-year-old individual.

7. Anecdotal evidence suggests that there is an inverse relationship between alcohol consumption and medication adherence (measured as percent of prescribed doses taken). A study is run involving $n = 50$ subjects, and data are measured on each subject reflecting the number of alcoholic drinks consumed in the week prior to study enrollment. The sample correlation coefficient between the number of alcoholic drinks consumed and medication adherence is -0.47.

a. Is there evidence of a significant correlation between the number of alcoholic drinks consumed and medication adherence? Run the appropriate test at $\alpha = 0.05$.

b. Using the following information, estimate the equation of the line that best describes the relationship between the number of alcoholic drinks consumed and medication adherence. The mean number of alcoholic drinks consumed (per week) is 14, with a standard deviation of 4.5. The mean medication adherence is 78.5, with a standard deviation of 13.5. Consider medication adherence as the dependent variable.

c. What is the expected medication adherence for a person who does not drink alchohol?

8. A study was conducted on a random sample of 15 undergraduates to assess whether there is a relationship between stress and GPA. Stress was measured on a scale of 0 to 100, with higher scores indicative of more stress. Descriptive statistics were generated in SAS and are given here.

Correlation Analysis
2 'VAR' Variables: STRESS GPA
Covariance Matrix DF = 14

	STRESS	GPA
STRESS	1075.666667	-11.328571
GPA	-11.328571	0.226857

Simple Statistics

Variable	N	Mean	Std Dev	Sum	Minimum	Maximum
STRESS	15	54.66667	32.79736	820.00000	5.00000	100.00000
GPA	15	2.76000	0.47630	41.40000	2.00000	3.90000

a. Compute the sample correlation coefficient.

b. Is there evidence of a significant correlation between stress and GPA? Run the appropriate test at $\alpha = 0.05$.

c. Compute the equation of the line that best describes the relationship between stress and GPA. Assume that GPA is the dependent variable.

d. What is the expected GPA for a person with a stress score of 80?

SAS Problems

Use SAS to solve the following problems.

1. Data were collected from a random sample of eight patients currently undergoing treatment for hypertension. Each subject reported the average number of cigarettes smoked per day and each was assigned a numerical value reflecting risk of cardiovascular disease (CVD). The risk assessments were computed by physicians and based on blood pressure, cholesterol level, and exercise status. The risk assessments ranged from 0 to 100, with higher values indicating increased risk.

Number of Cigarettes:	0	2	6	8	12	0	2	20
Risk of CVD:	12	20	50	68	75	8	10	80

Use SAS to generate a scatter diagram, to estimate the correlation between variables, and to test if the correlation is significant. In addition, estimate a simple linear regression equation and compute R^2.

2. Consider the following data reflecting lengths of stay in the hospital (recorded in days) and the total charge (in \$000s) for six patients undergoing a minor surgical procedure:

Length of Stay:	5	7	9	10	12	15
Total Charge:	6	5	7.2	8	9.4	7.9

Consider length of stay as the independent and total charge as the dependent variable and use SAS to generate a scatter diagram, to estimate the correlation between variables, and to test if the correlation is significant. In addition, estimate a simple linear regression equation and compute R^2.

Descriptive Statistics
(Ch. 2)

Probability
(Ch. 3)

Sampling Distributions
(Ch. 4)

Statistical Inference
(Chapters 5–13)

OUTCOME VARIABLE	GROUPING VARIABLE(S)/ PREDICTOR(S)	ANALYSIS	CHAPTER(S)
Continuous	—	Estimate μ; Compare μ to Known, Historical Value	5/12
Continuous	Dichotomous (2 groups)	Compare Independent Means (Estimate/Test $(\mu_1 - \mu_2)$) or the Mean Difference(μ_d)	6/12
Continuous	Discrete (> 2 groups)	Test the Equality of k Means using Analysis of Variance ($\mu_1 = \mu_2 = \cdots = \mu_k$)	9/12
Continuous	Continuous	Estimate Correlation or Determine Regression Equation	10/12
Continuous	Several Continuous or Dichotomous	Multiple Linear Regression Analysis	10
Dichotomous	—	Estimate p; Compare p to Known, Historical Value	7
Dichotomous	Dichotomous (2 groups)	Compare Independent Proportions (Estimate/Test $(p_1 - p_2)$)	7/8
Dichotomous	Discrete (>2 groups)	Test the Equality of k Proportions (Chi-Square Test)	7
Dichotomous	Several Continuous or Dichotomous	Multiple Logistic Regression Analysis	11
Discrete	Discrete	Compare Distributions Among k Populations (Chi-Square Test)	7
Time to Event	Several Continuous or Dichotomous	Survival Analysis	13

Logistic Regression Analysis

In Chapter 8 we introduced several effect measures used to compare risks in two populations. We presented estimation and statistical inference procedures for crude comparisons and a technique for estimation and statistical inference adjusting for one categorical confounder variable. In Chapter 10 we presented simple linear regression techniques used to estimate the linear equation describing the relationship between two continuous variables. We also introduced multiple linear regression techniques, which are used when the continuous outcome variable is linearly related to a set of independent variables.

In this chapter we describe logistic regression analysis, which can be used to model the effect of one or several independent variables on the risk of a dichotomous outcome. In Section 11.1 we introduce the logistic model, and in Section 11.2 we focus on statistical inference for situations with a single independent variable. In Section 11.3 we extend our discussion to the multiple logistic model, in which a single dichotomous outcome variable is modeled as a function of a set of independent variables. We briefly describe the use of the receiver operating characteristic (ROC) curve as a measure of the goodness-of-fit of logistic regression models in Section 11.4, and we summarize key formulas and present statistical computing applications in Sections 11.5 and 11.6, respectively. In Section 11.7 we use data from the Framingham Heart Study to illustrate the applications presented here.

As in linear regression, our goal is to estimate the regression coefficients in a model, given a sample of (X, Y) pairs. In the case of logistic regression, the Xs can be continuous or dichotomous, but the Ys are generally coded as 0 (for those who do not have the event) or 1 (for those who do have the event).

11.1 The Logistic Model

The simple logistic model is based on a linear relationship between the natural logarithm (ln) of the odds of an event and a continuous independent variable. The form of this relationship is as follows:

$$L = \ln(o) = \ln\left(\frac{p}{1-p}\right) = \beta_0 + \beta_1 X + \varepsilon \tag{11.1}$$

where Y is the dichotomous event of interest, coded 0/1 for failure/success
p is the proportion of successes
o is the odds of the event
L is the ln(odds of event)
X is the independent variable
β_0 is the intercept
β_1 is the regression coefficient
ε is the random error

The relationship between X and L is linear:

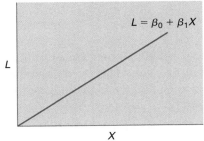

$$L = \beta_0 + \beta_1 X$$

Recall from Chapter 8 that if p is the probability of the event, then the odds of the event are

$$\text{Odds} = o = \frac{p}{(1 - p)}$$

We defined $L = \ln(\text{odds of event } Y)$, sometimes called the "log odds" or "logit" of Y. We can write L in terms of p, Probability$(Y = 1)$, as follows:

$$L = \ln(o) = \ln\left(\frac{p}{(1 - p)}\right)$$

We can then use the laws of exponents and logs and some algebra to express p (the proportion of successes or risk of the event) in terms of L:

$$e^L = o$$

$$e^L = \frac{p}{(1 - p)}$$

$$p = e^L(1 - p)$$

$$p = e^L - pe^L$$

$$p + pe^L = e^L$$

$$p(1 + e^L) = e^L$$

$$p = \frac{e^L}{(1 + e^L)}$$

This is called the logistic function and its graph is as follows. Notice that p, the probability of the event, increases from 0 to 1.

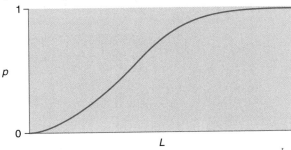

Logistic function: $p = \dfrac{e^L}{(1 + e^L)}$ \hfill (11.2)

11.2 Statistical Inference for Simple Logistic Regression

The logistic regression model (11.1) may be written in terms of p, the risk of event Y, using equations (11.1) and (11.2). We assume that L is a linear function of X, and we substitute (11.1) into the logistic function (11.2).

$$p = \frac{e^{\beta_0 + \beta_1 X + \varepsilon}}{(1 + e^{\beta_0 + \beta_1 X + \varepsilon})} \tag{11.3}$$

As in linear regression, our goal is to estimate the regression coefficients β and β_1, given a sample of (X, Y) pairs. Here, as in the linear regression framework, X can be continuous or dichotomous. However, the Y is not continuous as in linear regression; rather, it is coded 0 (for those who do not have the event) or 1 (for those who do have the event). Unfortunately, the technique used in linear regression to estimate the regression coefficients cannot be applied to the logistic regression case. The iterative maximum likelihood estimation process used to estimate coefficients is computationally complex and is beyond the scope of this book. Here we restrict our attention to interpretation of the logistic model estimated by SAS.

SAS Example 11.1 Logistic Regression Relating White Blood Count to Coronary Abnormalities

Recall the clinical trial described in Example 8.1 in which patients with Kawasaki syndrome were treated with gamma globulin (GG = 1) or with the standard treatment (GG = 0) and the primary outcome was the development of coronary abnormalities (CA). A possible explanation for the effect of treatment with gamma globulin on the development of CA is that it reduces the elevated white blood count (WBC) early in the course of the disease and that WBC is related to CA. This example addresses the relationship between WBC and CA. The data set contains a total of $n = 168$ observations; each participant has a continuous value for WBC and a dichotomous value (0 or 1) for the outcome, CA. The following is a subset of the output generated by SAS Proc Logistic. A brief interpretation follows the output.

SAS Output for Example 11.1

```
               The LOGISTIC Procedure
                  Model Information
        Data Set                      WORK.ONE
        Response Variable             CA
        Number of Response Levels     2
        Number of Observations        156
        Model                         binary logit
        Optimization Technique        Fisher's scoring
```

Response Profile

Ordered Value	CA	Total Frequency
1	1	25
2	0	131

Probability modeled is CA=1.

NOTE: 12 observations were deleted due to missing values for the response or explanatory variables.

The LOGISTIC Procedure

Analysis of Maximum Likelihood Estimates

Parameter	DF	Estimate	Standard Error	Wald Chi-Square	Pr > ChiSq
Intercept	1	-3.3848	0.5838	33.6120	<.0001
WBC	1	0.1253	0.0362	11.9835	0.0005

Interpretation of SAS Output for Example 11.1

We coded the variable, CA, to represent the development of CA and specified that the event of interest is CA $= 1$. SAS reports this under "Probability modeled is CA $= 1$." Among the 168 patients, 12 were missing the WBC measure and SAS notes that 12 observations were deleted due to missing values. Thus the analysis is based on $n = 156$. The results of the logistic regression estimation procedure are given under "Analysis of Maximum Likelihood Estimates." The estimated coefficients are in the column labeled "Estimate" and are $\hat{\beta}_0 = -3.385$ and $\hat{\beta}_1 = 0.125$.

SAS also provides the p value associated with the test $H_0: \beta_1 = 0$ in the column labeled "Pr > ChiSq." In this case, $p < 0.0005$, so we reject H_0 and conclude that there is significant evidence that WBC is linearly related to the log odds of CA. ▪

Now that the coefficients have been estimated, we can estimate the risk, $\hat{p}$, of the event Y, given a specific value of X, by substituting estimates of β_0 and β_1 into equation (11.3) as follows:

$$\hat{p} = \frac{e^{\hat{\beta}_0 + \hat{\beta}_1 X}}{(1 + e^{\hat{\beta}_0 + \hat{\beta}_1 X})} \tag{11.4}$$

Consider a person with $X = x_a$. We estimate the risk of Y given $X = x_a$ as

$$\hat{p}_a = \frac{e^{\hat{\beta}_0 + \hat{\beta}_1 x_a}}{1 + e^{\hat{\beta}_0 + \hat{\beta}_1 x_a}}$$

For example, in SAS Example 11.1,

$$\hat{p} = \frac{e^{-3.385 + 0.125(\text{WBC})}}{(1 + e^{-3.385 + 0.125(\text{WBC})})}$$

The risk of CA for a patient with WBC = 10 is

$$\hat{p} = \frac{e^{-3.385 + 0.125(10)}}{(1 + e^{-3.385 + 0.125(10)})}$$

$$= \frac{e^{-2.135}}{(1 + e^{-2.135})}$$

$$= 0.106$$

We can also use the estimate of β_1 to estimate the odds of the event for specified values of X and the odds ratio comparing the odds of the event for people with different values of X. Recall that the logistic model is based on the linear relationship between X and the log odds: $\ln(o) = L = \beta_0 + \beta_1 X$. Thus, the estimated odds are

$$\hat{o} = e^{\hat{L}} = e^{\hat{\beta}_0 + \hat{\beta}_1 X} \tag{11.5}$$

Consider two people with different values of X, one with $X = x_a$ and one with $X = x_b$. The odds of the event given $X = x_a$ are $\hat{o}_a = e^{\hat{\beta}_0 + \hat{\beta}_1 X_a}$ and, similarly, for $X = x_b$, the odds are $\hat{o}_b = e^{\hat{\beta}_0 + \hat{\beta}_1 X_b}$. For example, the odds of CA given WBC are

$$\hat{o} = e^{\hat{L}} = e^{\hat{\beta}_0 + \hat{\beta}_1 X} = e^{-3.385 + 0.125(\text{WBC})}$$

For a patient with WBC = 10, the odds of CA are

$$\hat{o} = e^{-3.385 + 0.125(10)} = e^{-2.135} = 0.118$$

The odds ratio comparing the odds of an event for two people, one with $X = x_a$ and one with $X = x_b$, is

$$\hat{\text{OR}} = \frac{e^{\hat{\beta}_0 + \hat{\beta}_1 x_a}}{e^{\hat{\beta}_0 + \hat{\beta}_1 x_b}}$$

Recall some of the properties of exponents:

$$e^{A+B} = e^A e^B$$
$$e^{A-B} = e^A / e^B$$
$$e^{AB} = (e^A)^B \tag{11.6}$$

The estimate of the odds ratio,

$$\hat{OR} = \frac{e^{\hat{\beta}_0 + \hat{\beta}_1 x_a}}{e^{\hat{\beta}_0 + \hat{\beta}_1 x_b}}$$

can be written as

$$\hat{OR} = e^{(\hat{\beta}_0 + \hat{\beta}_1 x_a) - (\hat{\beta}_0 + \hat{\beta}_1 x_b)}$$

which is equivalent to

$$\hat{OR} = e^{\hat{\beta}_1 (x_a - x_b)}$$

The odds ratio comparing the odds of the event for a person $X = x_a$ compared to one with $X = x_b$ is

$$\hat{OR} = e^{\hat{\beta}_1 (x_a - x_b)} \tag{11.7}$$

In SAS Example 11.1, the estimate of the odds ratio comparing a person with WBC = 15 to a person with WBC = 10 is

$$\hat{OR} = e^{\hat{\beta}_1 (x_a - x_b)} = e^{0.1253(15-10)} = e^{0.1253(5)} = e^{0.6265} = 1.87$$

Thus the odds of CA is 1.87 times higher for every 5-unit increase in WBC. Notice that this depends only on the difference in the X values $(x_a - x_b)$, not on their actual values. Thus the estimated odds ratio comparing one person with WBC = 10 to another person with WBC = 5 is also equal to 1.87, as is the odds ratio comparing any two people whose WBC values are 5 units apart.

The formula for a 95% confidence interval around the odds ratio is

$$\left(e^{(\hat{\beta}_1 - 1.96 s.e.(\hat{\beta}_1))(x_a - x_b)}, \ e^{(\hat{\beta}_1 + 1.96 s.e.(\hat{\beta}_1))(x_a - x_b)} \right) \tag{11.8}$$

where $s.e.(\hat{\beta}_1)$ is the standard error of $(\hat{\beta}_1)$. The calculation of $s.e.(\hat{\beta}_1)$ is beyond the scope of this book, but it is produced by SAS in the following sections. In SAS Example 11.1, the standard error of $\hat{\beta}_1$, $s.e.(\hat{\beta}_1) = 0.0362$. Thus, using (11.8), the 95% confidence interval for the odds ratio comparing the odds of CA in children with Kawasaki syndrome whose WBC are 5 units apart is as follows:

$$\left(e^{(\hat{\beta}_1 - 1.96 s.e.(\hat{\beta}_1))(x_a - x_b)}, \ e^{(\hat{\beta}_1 + 1.96 s.e.(\hat{\beta}_1))(x_a - x_b)} \right)$$
$$= \left(e^{(0.1253 - 1.96(0.0362))(5)}, \ e^{(0.1253 + 1.96(0.0362))(5)} \right)$$
$$= \left(e^{(0.2717)}, \ e^{(0.9813)} \right)$$
$$= (1.31, 2.67)$$

Thus, we conclude that the odds ratio comparing the odds of CA in one child with Kawasaki syndrome whose WBC is 5 units higher than another child is 1.87 and that the 95% confidence interval for the odds ratio is (1.31, 2.67).

In SAS Example 11.1, the odds ratio comparing two people with WBC values 1 unit apart is $\hat{OR} = e^{\hat{\beta}_1} = e^{0.125} = 1.13$. The 95% confidence interval i

$$\left(e^{(\hat{\beta}_1 - 1.96s.e.(\hat{\beta}_1))(x_a - x_b)}, e^{(\hat{\beta}_1 + 1.96s.e.(\hat{\beta}_1))(x_a - x_b)}\right)$$

$$= \left(e^{(0.1253 - 1.96(0.0362))(1)}, e^{(0.1253 + 1.96(0.0362))(1)}\right)$$

$$= \left(e^{(0.0543)}, e^{(0.1963)}\right)$$

$$= (1.056, 1.217)$$

SAS automatically provides the odds ratio (and the associated 95% confidence interval) comparing the odds of the event for two people with X value 1 unit apart $(x_a - x_b = 1)$. This is $\hat{OR} = e^{\hat{\beta}_1(x_a - x_b)} = e^{\hat{\beta}_1(1)} = e^{\hat{\beta}_1}$. The label i simply "Odds Ratio Estimates," but it is important to remember that this i the estimate of the odds ratio comparing people exactly 1 unit apart.

SAS Output for Example 11.1 (Continued)

The LOGISTIC Procedure

Analysis of Maximum Likelihood Estimates

Parameter	DF	Estimate	Standard Error	Wald Chi-Square	Pr > ChiSq
Intercept	1	-3.3848	0.5838	33.6120	<.0001
WBC	1	0.1253	0.0362	11.9835	0.0005

Odds Ratio Estimates

Effect	Point Estimate	95% Wald Confidence Limits	
WBC	1.133	1.056	1.217

In clinical trials, X is usually a dichotomous variable representing mem bership in one treatment group or another. For example, $X = 1$ could denote the treatment group, and $X = 0$ could denote the control group. Suppose tha X is dichotomous (0 or 1) and we use (11.7) to estimate the odds ratio. The estimate of the odds ratio comparing those with $X = 1$ to those with $X = ($ reduces to

$$\hat{OR} = e^{\hat{\beta}_1(1-0)} = e^{\hat{\beta}_1(1)} = e^{\hat{\beta}_1}$$

In this situation, where X is dichotomous, the null hypothesis, $H_0: \beta_1 = 0$, car be phrased, equivalently, as $H_0: e^{\beta} = 1$, or $H_0: OR = 1$.

SAS EXAMPLE 11.2 **Logistic Regression Relating Treatment to Coronary Abnormalities**

We now use SAS Proc Logistic to estimate the probabilities and odds of the development of coronary abnormalities (CA) in children with Kawasaki syndrome treated with gamma globulin (GG = 1) as compared to the standard treatment (GG = 0).

SAS Output for Example 11.2

Model Information

Data Set	WORK.ONE
Response Variable	CA
Number of Response Levels	2
Number of Observations	167
Model	binary logit
Optimization Technique	Fisher's scoring

Response Profile

Ordered Value	CA	Total Frequency
1	1	26
2	0	141

Probability modeled is CA=1.

NOTE: 1 observation was deleted due to missing values for the response or explanatory variables.

The LOGISTIC Procedure

Analysis of Maximum Likelihood Estimates

Parameter	DF	Estimate	Standard Error	Wald Chi-Square	Pr > ChiSq
Intercept	1	-1.0986	0.2520	19.0094	<.0001
gg	1	-1.6487	0.5257	9.8370	0.0017

Odds Ratio Estimates

Effect	Point Estimate	95% Wald Confidence Limits	
gg	0.192	0.069	0.539

Interpretation of SAS Output for Example 11.2

The estimated coefficients are in the column labeled "Estimate" and are $\hat{\beta}_0 = -1.099$ and $\hat{\beta}_1 = -1.649$. The p value associated with the test $H_0: \beta_1 = 0$ is $p = 0.0017$, so we reject H_0 and conclude that there is significant evidence that treatment (gamma globulin versus standard care) is associated with the development of CA.

The odds ratio comparing children with Kawasaki syndrome treated with gamma globulin (GG $= 1$) to those treated with the standard treatment (GG $= 0$) with respect to the development of coronary abnormalities (CA) is given here as 0.19, with 95% confidence interval (0.069, 0.539). Note that the p value associated with the test $H_0: \beta_1 = 0$ is also the p value associated with the test $H_0: OR = 1$. Here, this p value is $p = 0.0017$, so we reject H_0 and conclude that there is significant evidence that the odds ratio is not equal to 1. ■

Recall that we used these data in Example 8.1 and estimated the odds ratio using equation (8.6). This estimate will be identical to that obtained using equation (11.8). In fact, we obtained the same result as we do here: $\hat{OR} = 0.19$. In Chapter 8, we used the formula given in Table 8.2 to estimate the 95% confidence interval for the odds ratio; in this chapter we provide an estimate of the confidence interval that assumes the logistic model. The difference in estimated confidence intervals will be very slight. Using Table 8.2, we estimated the 95% confidence interval as (0.069, 0.539), which, in this case, is identical to the estimate provided by SAS.

SAS does not automatically provide an estimate of the relative risk as it does the odds ratio. To estimate the relative risk, RR, comparing a patient with $X = x_a$ to one with $X = x_b$, we must first estimate the individual probabilities using (11.4).

$$\hat{RR} = \hat{p}_a / \hat{p}_b = \frac{\left(\dfrac{e^{\hat{\beta}_0 + \hat{\beta}_1 x_a}}{1 + e^{\hat{\beta}_0 + \hat{\beta}_1 x_a}} \right)}{\left(\dfrac{e^{\hat{\beta}_0 + \hat{\beta}_1 x_b}}{1 + e^{\hat{\beta}_0 + \hat{\beta}_1 x_b}} \right)} \tag{11.9}$$

In SAS Example 11.1, the estimated regression coefficients were $\hat{\beta}_0 = -3.385$ and $\hat{\beta}_1 = 0.125$, and the estimated risk of CA given WBC was $\hat{p} = \dfrac{e^{-3.385+0.125(\text{WBC})}}{(1 + e^{-3.385+0.125(\text{WBC})})}$. We estimated the risk of CA for a patient with WBC $= 10$ to be $\hat{p}_{10} = 0.106$. Similarly, the estimate of the risk of CA for a patient with WBC $= 5$ was $\hat{p}_5 = 0.060$. Thus, the estimated relative risk of CA for a patient with WBC $= 10$ as compared to a patient with WBC $= 5$ is $\hat{RR} = (\hat{p}_{10} / \hat{p}_5) = (0.106/0.060) = 1.77$.

Remember that the odds ratio comparing a patient with $X = x_a$ to one with $X = x_b$ depends only on the difference $(x_a - x_b)$, not on the actual values

x_a and x_b. The relative risk comparing those with $X = x_a$ to those with $X = x_b$, however, does depend on the actual values x_a and x_b.

In SAS Example 11.1, the estimated risk of CA for a patient with WBC = 15 is $\hat{p}_{15} = 0.181$. Therefore, the relative risk of CA comparing patients with WBC = 15 to those with WBC = 10 is $\hat{RR} = (\hat{p}_{15}/\hat{p}_{10}) = (0.181/0.106) = 1.71$. An increase of 5 units in WBC is associated with a relative risk $\hat{RR} = 1.77$ if the WBC values are 5 and 10, but is associated with a relative risk $\hat{RR} = 1.71$ if the WBC values are 10 and 15.

Now consider the situation in SAS Example 11.2 in which the comparison is of patients in two treatment groups, of those with $X = 1$ to those with $X = 0$. We can modify (11.9) slightly to estimate the relative risk of the event in patients with $X = 1$ as compared to those with $X = 0$.

$$\hat{RR} = \hat{p}_1/\hat{p}_0 = \frac{\left(\dfrac{e^{\hat{\beta}_0 + \hat{\beta}_1}}{1 + e^{\hat{\beta}_0 + \hat{\beta}_1}} \right)}{\left(\dfrac{e^{\hat{\beta}_0}}{1 + e^{\hat{\beta}_0}} \right)} \qquad (11.10)$$

In SAS Example 11.2, the relative risk of CA for patients treated with gamma globulin as compared to those on the standard treatment is estimated as follows from the SAS output.

$$\hat{RR} = \hat{p}_1/\hat{p}_0 = \frac{\left(\dfrac{e^{\hat{\beta}_0 + \hat{\beta}_1}}{1 + e^{\hat{\beta}_0 + \hat{\beta}_1}} \right)}{\left(\dfrac{e^{\hat{\beta}_0}}{1 + e^{\hat{\beta}_0}} \right)} = \frac{\left(\dfrac{e^{-1.099 - 1.649}}{1 + e^{-1.099 - 1.649}} \right)}{\left(\dfrac{e^{-1.099}}{1 + e^{-1.099}} \right)}$$

$$= (0.060/0.250) = 0.24$$

The estimated relative risk of CA for patients treated with gamma globulin as compared to those on the standard treatment is $\hat{RR} = 0.24$. This may be interpreted as the risk of CA among patients treated with gamma globulin is less than a quarter the risk for those on the standard treatment. Recall that this is the estimate we obtained in Chapter 8 using (8.5).

As discussed in Chapter 8, the odds ratio may be used to estimate the relative risk if the prevalence of the disease is low (the overall risk is small). Here we see that it is much easier to obtain the estimate of the odds ratio from the results of a logistic regression than it is to obtain an estimate of the relative risk.

II.3 Multiple Logistic Regression

As in the case of linear regression, logistic regression techniques may be generalized to models with more than one independent variable. The methods used to estimate coefficients, standard errors, and p values are beyond the scope of this book, but we present some examples of multiple logistic regression in this section using SAS. The general multiple logistic regression model is

$$p = \frac{e^{\beta_0 + \beta_1 X_1 + \beta_2 X_2 + \cdots + \beta_k X_k + \varepsilon}}{(1 + e^{\beta_0 + \beta_1 X_1 + \beta_2 X_2 + \cdots + \beta_k X_k + \varepsilon})} \tag{11.11}$$

where p is the probability of the event and $X_1, X_2, \ldots, X_k$ are independent variables. The independent variables may be dichotomous or continuous.

SAS EXAMPLE 11.3 **Multiple Logistic Regression Relating White Blood Count and Treatment to Coronary Abnormalities**

Suppose we want to use the sample described in SAS Example 11.2 to assess the effect of treatment with gamma globulin on CA but we are concerned that white blood count is a potential confounder. Although patients were randomized to one of the two treatment groups, it turns out that the mean WBC in patients treated with gamma globulin was significantly lower than the mean WBC in patients on the standard treatment. Thus, the investigators were concerned that the patients treated with gamma globulin were less sick than those on the standard treatment and that the observed impact of the gamma globulin treatment might not be real. The following output is a multiple logistic regression in which the outcome is the dichotomous variable CA and the two independent variables are the dichotomous treatment variable, GG, and the continuous variable, WBC.

SAS Output for Example 11.3

The LOGISTIC Procedure

Analysis of Maximum Likelihood Estimates

Parameter	DF	Estimate	Standard Error	Wald Chi-Square	Pr > ChiSq
Intercept	1	-2.6352	0.6562	16.1283	<.0001
gg	1	-1.3152	0.5496	5.7272	0.0167
WBC	1	0.1048	0.0383	7.4781	0.0062

Odds Ratio Estimates

Effect	Point Estimate	95% Wald Confidence Limits	
gg	0.268	0.091	0.788
WBC	1.111	1.030	1.197

Interpretation of SAS Output for Example 11.3

In SAS Example 11.2, we estimated the *crude* odds ratio comparing patients treated with gamma globulin to patients on standard treatment. The estimated OR is $\hat{OR} = 0.19$ with $p = 0.0017$. The odds ratio estimated here is the odds ratio comparing patients treated with gamma globulin to patients on standard treatment, *adjusted* for white blood count. The estimated OR is $\hat{OR} = 0.27$ with $p = 0.0167$. As suspected, part of the observed effect of gamma globulin may have been due to the lower initial WBC in patients treated with gamma globulin. Thus, we see the estimated OR is closer to 1 after adjustment for WBC. The crude estimate indicates that gamma globulin reduces the odds by just over 80% (the crude $\hat{OR} = 0.19$), while the adjusted $\hat{OR}$ of 0.27 indicates that gamma globulin reduces the odds by 73%. Although the adjustment appears to reduce the impact of gamma globulin, the effect is still quite important and the hypothesis of no effect is rejected with $p = 0.0167$. ■

Another application of multiple logistic regression is in model prediction. The multiple logistic regression model can be used to predict probabilities of an event for subjects with specific characteristics (i.e., values of the independent variables included in the model).

SAS EXAMPLE 11.4 Multiple Logistic Regression Relating White Blood Count and Hemoglobin to Coronary Abnormalities

Suppose we want to use the sample described in SAS Example 11.1 to predict the probability of developing CA as a function of both white blood count and hemoglobin. The following output is based on a multiple logistic regression in which the outcome is the dichotomous variable, CA, and the two independent variables are the continuous variables, WBC and HEM.

SAS Output for Example 11.4

```
                  The LOGISTIC Procedure


                     Model Information


        Data Set                      WORK.ONE
        Response Variable             CA
        Number of Response Levels     2
        Number of Observations        151
        Model                         binary logit
        Optimization Technique        Fisher's scoring
```

Response Profile

Ordered Value	CA	Total Frequency
1	1	25
2	0	126

Probability modeled is CA=1.

NOTE: 17 observations were deleted due to missing values for the response or explanatory variables.

Model Convergence Status

Convergence criterion (GCONV=1E-8) satisfied.

Model Fit Statistics

Criterion	Intercept Only	Intercept and Covariates
AIC	137.532	124.420
SC	140.549	133.472
-2 Log L	135.532	118.420

Testing Global Null Hypothesis: BETA=0

Test	Chi-Square	DF	Pr > ChiSq
Likelihood Ratio	17.1120	2	0.0002
Score	19.1517	2	<.0001
Wald	14.1978	2	0.0008

The LOGISTIC Procedure

Analysis of Maximum Likelihood Estimates

Parameter	DF	Estimate	Standard Error	Wald Chi-Square	Pr > ChiSq
Intercept	1	1.2859	2.2545	0.3253	0.5684
HEM	1	-0.4272	0.2078	4.2294	0.0397
WBC	1	0.1135	0.0376	9.0948	0.0026

```
                        Odds Ratio Estimates

                      Point              95% Wald
        Effect       Estimate        Confidence Limits

        HEM           0.652          0.434          0.980
        WBC           1.120          1.041          1.206
```

```
Association of Predicted Probabilities and Observed Responses

    Percent Concordant       75.0    Somers' D      0.504
    Percent Discordant       24.6    Gamma          0.506
    Percent Tied              0.5    Tau-a          0.140
    Pairs                    3150    c              0.752
```

Interpretation of SAS Output for Example 11.4

We first consider the overall null hypothesis that all the β coefficients in (11.11) are zero. SAS provides three tests of this hypothesis; we recommend the *likelihood ratio test*. In this example, the likelihood ratio test statistic $\chi^2 = 17.11$, with 2 df and the associated $p < 0.0002$. Therefore, we reject H_0 and conclude that at least one of the regression coefficients is not equal to zero. We then look at the individual tests $H_0: \beta_1 = 0$ and $H_0: \beta_2 = 0$, where β_1 and β_2 are the coefficients associated with HEM and WBC, respectively. We reject $H_0: \beta_1 = 0$, with $p = 0.0397$, and conclude that hemoglobin is significantly associated with the development of CA, even after adjusting for white blood count. We also reject $H_0: \beta_2 = 0$, with $p = 0.0026$, and conclude that white blood count is significantly associated with the development of CA, even after adjusting for hemoglobin. In fact, we conclude that hemoglobin and white blood count each make an independent contribution to the risk of CA. ■

We now turn to the prediction of the risk of CA given hemoglobin and white blood count. In SAS Example 11.1, we used logistic regression to estimate the probability of CA given WBC. The estimated probability was

$$\hat{p} = \frac{e^{-3.385+0.125(\text{WBC})}}{(1 + e^{-3.385+0.125(\text{WBC})})}$$

We used this to estimate the risk of CA for a patient with WBC = 10 and obtained the estimate $\hat{p} = 0.106$.

The output for SAS Example 11.4 allows us to estimate the probability of CA given both white blood count and hemoglobin.

$$\hat{p} = \frac{e^{1.286-0.427(\text{HEM})+0.114(\text{WBC})}}{(1 + e^{1.286-0.427(\text{HEM})+0.114(\text{WBC})})}$$

Now, suppose WBC $= 10$ and HEM $= 10$. We estimate the risk of CA by substituting these values for WBC and HEM into the equation.

$$\hat{p} = \frac{e^{1.286-0.427(10)+0.114(10)}}{(1 + e^{1.286-0.427(10)+0.114(10)})}$$

$$= \frac{e^{-1.844}}{(1 + e^{-1.844})}$$

$$= 0.137$$

Similarly, we can estimate the risk of CA given WBC $= 10$ and HEM $= 12$, and obtain the estimated risk $\hat{p} = 0.063$. Notice that as HEM increases, the risk of CA decreases. This can be seen from the negative sign of the coefficient, β_1, associated with HEM. In contrast, β_2 is positive, indicating that the risk of CA increases as WBC increases.

The odds ratio describing the impact of a 1-unit increase in the independent variable on the risk of the event, adjusting for the other independent variables, is automatically displayed. In this example, an increase of 1 unit in HEM is associated with a 35% decrease in the odds of CA ($\hat{OR} = 0.65$). An increase of 1 unit in WBC is associated with a 12% increase in the odds of CA ($\hat{OR} = 1.12$).

11.4 Area under the ROC Curve

We use maximum likelihood estimation to estimate the coefficients in logistic regression models as opposed to the least squares estimation used in linear regression models. One application of logistic regression analysis is the comparison of risks between groups. We use the estimated coefficients to estimate odds ratios and relative risks. Another application of logistic regression is in prediction. The estimated coefficients may be used to estimate or predict probabilities of the event for subjects with specified characteristics (i.e., values on the independent variables included in the model). In this application, we may also want to assess the extent to which the set of independent variables is associated with the event.

It is relatively easy to compare pairs of observed and predicted values in the linear regression framework, as they are both measured on the same scale. For example, pairs $(Y, \hat{Y})$ can be compared by simple subtraction, $(Y - \hat{Y})$ or by squaring the difference, $(Y - \hat{Y})^2$. A summary over the Y values in the sample can be made by summing the squares of the differences (called the error sums of squares, denoted SSE) or by calculating $R^2 = \sum(\hat{Y} - \bar{Y})^2 / \sum(Y - \bar{Y})^2$. In linear regression modeling, R^2 may be interpreted as the percent of variability in Y that can be explained by the set of independent variables. This gives an idea of how well the selected model fits or how close the predicted values ($\hat{Y}$) are to the observed values, Y.

Unfortunately, this statistic has no obvious interpretation in the logistic regression setting and depends on the overall event prevalence. Consider pairs of observed and predicted values, $(Y, \hat{p})$. The Y values are all equal to either 0 or 1 and the $\hat{p}$ values are all between 0 and 1. Clearly, if $\hat{p}$ is equal to or close to 1 for an individual who had the event ($Y = 1$), we would say that the model was successful in predicting that individual's risk. However, what if $\hat{p} = 0.8$ or 0.25? Suppose that the model only yields the following predicted probabilities: 0, 0.06, 0.25, and 1.00. Suppose also that all the individuals who had the event had $\hat{p} = 0.25$ and those who did not have the event had $\hat{p} = 0.06$. The model seems to distinguish those who did and did not have the event even though the individual $\hat{p}$ values are not particularly close to the observed Y values. We would like a summary measure of the goodness-of-fit that takes into account whether the model distinguishes those who do and do not have the outcome.

Recall in SAS Example 11.2 that the risk of CA in patients treated with gamma globulin was estimated using logistic regression to be $\hat{p} = 0.25$ and the estimated risk of CA in patients on the standard treatment was $\hat{p} = 0.06$. Suppose we decide to classify individuals in terms of predicting event status by using a cutoff in predicted probability. We predict that individuals with $\hat{p} > 0.06$ will have the event and assign them the predicted value $\hat{Y} = 1$. We predict that individuals with $\hat{p} \leq 0.06$ will not have the event and assign them the predicted value $\hat{Y} = 0$.

Five of the 26 patients who did develop CA ($Y = 1$) had been treated with gamma globulin and have $\hat{p} = 0.06$; the other 21 were on standard treatment and have $\hat{p} = 0.25$. Thus, if we apply a cutoff of 0.06 and decide that patients with $\hat{p} > 0.06$ are predicted to have CA, then we have correctly predicted event status in 21 of the 26 patients who actually did have the event. This is called the *true positive rate*, or *sensitivity*. In this example, the sensitivity is $21/26 = 0.808$.

Conversely, 78 of the 141 patients who did not develop CA ($Y = 0$) had been on standard treatment and have $\hat{p} = 0.25$. If we again apply a cutoff of 0.06 (assigning patients with $\hat{p} > 0.06$ to have $\hat{Y} = 1$, and those with $\hat{p} \leq 0.06$ to have $\hat{Y} = 0$), then we have correctly predicted event status in 78 of the 141 patients who actually did not have the event. This is called the *true negative rate*, or *specificity*. In this example, the specificity is $78/141 = 0.553$.

Now consider the cutoff of 0 (individuals with $\hat{p} > 0$ will be assigned $\hat{Y} = 1$). Since all the $\hat{p}$ values are either $= 0.06$ or 0.25, all the patients have $\hat{p} > 0$ and thus all the patients will be assigned $\hat{Y} = 1$. The sensitivity $= 26/26 = 1$, and specificity $= 0/141 = 0$. The other extreme is the situation in which the cutoff is 1, all the patients are assigned $\hat{Y} = 0$, the sensitivity is 0, and the specificity is 1. Any other cutoffs will produce the same sensitivity-specificity combination as one of these three cutoffs. For example, any cutoff between 0 and 0.06 will have sensitivity and specificity 1 and 0, respectively. Cutoffs between 0.06 and 0.25 will have sensitivity and specificity 0.808 and 0.553, respectively, and cutoffs between 0.25 and 1 will have sensitivity and specificity 0 and 1, respectively.

Models with only one dichotomous independent variable produce only two possible predicted probabilities: individuals with $X = 0$ have predicted probability $\hat{p}_0$, and those with $X = 1$ have predicted probability $\hat{p}_1$. For example, the only possible predicted values in the example were $\hat{p}_0 = 0.25$ and $\hat{p}_1 = 0.06$. As a result, there is only one cutoff (in addition to cutoffs of 0 and 1) that produces distinct values of sensitivity and specificity. Models with one continuous independent variable or more than one independent variable all have more possible values for $\hat{p}$, and there may be many cutoffs that produce distinct values of sensitivity and specificity.

A measure of goodness-of-fit often used to evaluate the fit of a logistic regression model is based on the simultaneous measure of sensitivity and specificity for all possible cutoff points. First, we calculate sensitivity and specificity pairs for each possible cutoff point and plot sensitivity on the y axis by (1 − specificity) on the x axis. This curve is called the *receiver operating characteristic* (ROC) curve, and the area under the curve, the "*area under the ROC curve*," is a summary of the sensitivities and specificities over all possible cutoff points. It ranges from 0.5 to 1.0, with larger values indicative of better fit. The following figure shows an application in which the area under the ROC curve (the area to the right under the curve) is equal to 0.68.

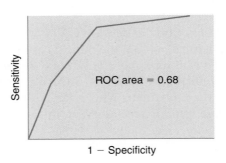

The following figure shows an application in which the area under the ROC curve is 0.5. When the area under the ROC curve is 0.5, the logistic model is said to classify events and nonevents simply by chance or at random.

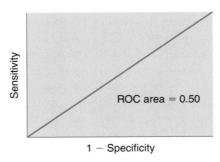

SAS EXAMPLE 11.5 Area Under the ROC Curve

Proc Logistic produces the "c" statistic automatically in the output of a logistic regression analysis; this is equal to the area under the ROC curve. We can compare the models used in SAS Examples 11.2, 11.3, and 11.4, each of which was used to predict the development of CA. Recall that the independent variables in SAS Examples 11.2, 11.3, and 11.4 were {gamma globulin alone}, {gamma globulin plus white blood count}, and {white blood count plus hemoglobin}, respectively.

SAS Output for Example 11.2 (Continued)

The LOGISTIC Procedure

Analysis of Maximum Likelihood Estimates

Parameter	DF	Estimate	Standard Error	Wald Chi-Square	Pr > ChiSq
Intercept	1	-1.0986	0.2520	19.0094	<.0001
gg	1	-1.6487	0.5257	9.8370	0.0017

Association of Predicted Probabilities and Observed Responses

Percent Concordant	44.7	Somers' D	0.361
Percent Discordant	8.6	Gamma	0.677
Percent Tied	46.7	Tau-a	0.095
Pairs	3666	c	0.680

SAS Output for Example 11.3 (Continued)

The LOGISTIC Procedure

Analysis of Maximum Likelihood Estimates

Parameter	DF	Estimate	Standard Error	Wald Chi-Square	Pr > ChiSq
Intercept	1	-2.6352	0.6562	16.1283	<.0001
gg	1	-1.3152	0.5496	5.7272	0.0167
WBC	1	0.1048	0.0383	7.4781	0.0062

```
                      Odds Ratio Estimates

                     Point              95% Wald
         Effect    Estimate        Confidence Limits

         gg          0.268        0.091          0.788
         WBC         1.111        1.030          1.197
```

Association of Predicted Probabilities and Observed Responses

```
         Percent Concordant      75.5     Somers' D     0.518
         Percent Discordant      23.8     Gamma         0.521
         Percent Tied             0.7     Tau-a         0.140
         Pairs                   3275     c             0.759
```

SAS Output for Example 11.4 (Continued)

The LOGISTIC Procedure

Analysis of Maximum Likelihood Estimates

Parameter	DF	Estimate	Standard Error	Wald Chi-Square	Pr > ChiSq
Intercept	1	1.2859	2.2545	0.3253	0.5684
HEM	1	-0.4272	0.2078	4.2294	0.0397
WBC	1	0.1135	0.0376	9.0948	0.0026

Association of Predicted Probabilities and Observed Responses

```
         Percent Concordant      75.0     Somers' D     0.504
         Percent Discordant      24.6     Gamma         0.506
         Percent Tied             0.5     Tau-a         0.140
         Pairs                   3150     c             0.752
```

Interpretation of SAS Output for Example 11.4 (Continued)

The logistic regression model used to predict the development of CA based on treatment with gamma globulin alone (SAS Example 11.2) has $c = 0.680$. The addition of white blood count to the model increases c to 0.759 (SAS Example 11.3). Thus the model that includes white blood count fits better, as measured by c, the area under the ROC curve.

This model in SAS Example 11.4, which predicts the development of CA based on the combination of white blood count and hemoglobin, has $c = 0.752$.

11.5 Key Formulas

Application	Notation/Formula	Description
Logistic function	$L = \beta_0 + \beta_1 X + \varepsilon$ $p = \dfrac{e^L}{(1 + e^L)}$	$L = \ln(\text{odds of event } Y)$ Y is the dichotomous event of interest X is the independent variable β_0 is the intercept β_1 is the coefficient ε is the random error
Logistic regression model	$p = \dfrac{e^{\beta_0 + \beta_1 X + \varepsilon}}{(1 + e^{\beta_0 + \beta_1 X + \varepsilon})}$	
Estimated logistic regression equation	$\hat{p} = \dfrac{e^{\hat{\beta}_0 + \hat{\beta}_1 X}}{(1 + e^{\hat{\beta}_0 + \hat{\beta}_1 X})}$	
Estimate of the odds given X	$\hat{o} = e^{\hat{\beta}_0 + \hat{\beta}_1 X}$	
Estimate of the odds ratio	$\hat{OR} = e^{\hat{\beta}_1(x_a - x_b)}$	compares odds of the event for those with $X = x_a$ to those with $X = x_b$
95% confidence interval for OR	$\left(e^{(\hat{\beta}_1 - 1.96s.e.(\hat{\beta}_1))(x_a - x_b)}, \right.$ $\left. e^{(\hat{\beta}_1 + 1.96s.e.(\hat{\beta}_1))(x_a - x_b)} \right)$	
Estimate of the OR in the special case where $x_a = 1$ and $x_b = 0$	$\hat{OR} = e^{\hat{\beta}_1(1-0)} = e^{\hat{\beta}_1(1)} = e^{\hat{\beta}_1}$	
Estimate of the relative risk	$\hat{RR} = \hat{p}_a / \hat{p}_b = \dfrac{\left(\dfrac{e^{\hat{\beta}_0 + \hat{\beta}_1 x_a}}{1 + e^{\hat{\beta}_0 + \hat{\beta}_1 x_a}} \right)}{\left(\dfrac{e^{\hat{\beta}_0 + \hat{\beta}_1 x_b}}{1 + e^{\hat{\beta}_0 + \hat{\beta}_1 x_b}} \right)}$	compares the risks of the event for those with $X = x_a$ to those with $X = x_b$
Estimate of the RR in the special case where $x_a = 1$ and $x_b = 0$	$\hat{RR} = \hat{p}_1 / \hat{p}_0 = \dfrac{\left(\dfrac{e^{\hat{\beta}_0 + \hat{\beta}_1}}{1 + e^{\hat{\beta}_0 + \hat{\beta}_1}} \right)}{\left(\dfrac{e^{\hat{\beta}_0}}{1 + e^{\hat{\beta}_0}} \right)}$	

11.6 Statistical Computing

Following are the SAS programs used to perform logistic regression analysis. The SAS procedures and brief descriptions are noted in the header to each example. Notes are provided to the right of the SAS programs (in blue) for orientation purposes and are not part of the programs. In addition, the blank lines in the programs are solely to accommodate the notes. Blank lines and

spaces can be used throughout SAS programs to enhance readability. A sum
mary of the SAS procedures used in the examples is provided at the end of thi
section.

SAS EXAMPLE 11.1 **Estimate Relative Risk and Odds Ratios in Logistic Regression Model**
Estimate Relative Risk and Odds Ratio of CA Comparing Patients with
Kawasaki Syndrome Who Have Different White Blood Counts
(Example 11.1)

A trial of gamma globulin in the treatment of children with Kawasaki syn
drome randomized approximately half of the patients to receive gamma glob
ulin plus aspirin; the other half received the standard treatment of aspirin
The outcome of interest was the development of coronary abnormalities (CA
within 7 weeks of treatment. A possible explanation for the effect of treat
ment with gamma globulin on CA is that it reduces the elevated white bloo
count (WBC) early in the course of the disease and that WBC is related to CA
Use SAS to estimate a simple logistic regression model relating WBC to th
development of CA.

Program Code

`options ps=62 ls=80;`	Formats the output page to 62 lines in length and 80 columns in width
`data in;`	Beginning of Data Step
`   input gg wbc ca;`	Inputs three variables, **gg** (noGG or GG), **wbc** (white blood count), and **ca** (CA or noCA)
`cards;`	Beginning of Raw Data section.
`0 9.4 0`	actual observations (value of **group**, **wbc**, and **event** on each line)
`0 20.4 1`	
`0 8.7 0`	
`.`	
`1 5.7 0`	
`run;`	
`proc logistic descending;`	Procedure call. Proc logistic provides estimates of
`  model ca=wbc;`	the coefficients in a logistic regression model. The procedure is set up for outcomes with value of 1 or 2 instead of 0 and 1. The option "descending" ensures that outcomes of 1 are counted as events and outcomes of 0 are counte as nonevents. Proc logistic also provides estimates of the odds ratio and 95% confidence limits comparing the odds of the event (ca) for two people with a difference of 1 unit (in wbc).
`run;`	End of procedure section

SAS EXAMPLE 11.2 **Estimate Relative Risk and Odds Ratios in Logistic Regression Model**
Estimate Relative Risk and Odds Ratio of CA Comparing GG to no GG (Example 11.2)

A trial of gamma globulin in the treatment of children with Kawasaki syndrome randomized approximately half of the patients to receive gamma globulin plus aspirin; the other half received the standard treatment of aspirin. The outcome of interest was the development of coronary abnormalities (CA) within 7 weeks of treatment. Use SAS to estimate the effect of treatment on development of CA.

Program Code

`options ps=62 ls=80;`	Formats the output page to 62 lines in length and 80 columns in width
`data in;`	Beginning of Data Step
`  input gg wbc ca;`	Inputs three variables, **gg** (noGG or GG), **wbc** (white blood count), and **ca** (CA or noCA)
`cards;`	Beginning of Raw Data section.
`0 9.4 0`	actual observations (value of **group**, **wbc**, and **event** on each
`0 20.4 1`	line)
`0 8.7 0`	
`.`	
`.`	
`.`	
`1 5.7 0`	
`run;`	
`proc logistic descending;`	Procedure call. Proc logistic provides estimates of the
`  model ca=gg;`	coefficients in a logistic regression model. The procedure is set up for outcomes with values of 1 or 2 instead of 0 and 1. The option "descending" ensures that outcomes of 1 are counted as events and outcomes of 0 are counted as nonevents. Proc logistic also provides estimates of the odds ratio and 95% confidence limits comparing the odds of the event (ca) in those with gg=1 as compared to those with gg=0
`run;`	End of procedure section ■

SAS EXAMPLE 11.3 **Estimate Adjusted Relative Risk and Odds Ratios in Logistic Regression Model**
Estimate the Odds Ratio Comparing Patients on Gamma Globulin to Those on Standard Treatment with Respect to CA, Adjusted for WBC (Example 11.3)

Suppose we want to use the sample described in SAS Example 11.2 to assess the effect of treatment with gamma globulin on CA but we are concerned that white blood count is a potential confounder. Use SAS to estimate a multiple logistic regression model where the outcome is the dichotomous variable, CA, and the two independent variables are the dichotomous grouping variable, GG, and the continuous variable, WBC.

Program Code

`options ps=62 ls=80;`	Formats the output page to 62 lines in length and 80 columns in width
`data in;`	Beginning of Data Step
`  input gg wbc ca;`	Inputs three variables, **gg** (noGG or GG), **wbc** (white blood count), and **ca** (CA or noCA)
`cards;`	Beginning of Raw Data section.
`0 9.4 0`	actual observations (value of **group**, **wbc**, and
`0 20.4 1`	**event** on each line)
`0 8.7 0`	
`.`	
`.`	
`.`	
`1 5.7 0`	
`run;`	
`proc logistic descending;`	Procedure call. Proc logistic provides estimates of
`  model ca=gg wbc;`	the coefficients in a logistic regression model. Proc Logistic also provides estimates of the odds ratio and 95% confidence limits comparing the odds of the event (ca) in those with gg=1 as compared to those with gg=0, adjusted for wbc.
`run;`	End of procedure section

SAS EXAMPLE 11.4 **Estimate a Multiple Logistic Regression Model**

Perform a Multiple Logistic Regression, Predicting the Risk of Developing CA Given Both Hemoglobin and White Blood Count (Example 11.4)

Suppose we want to use the sample described in SAS Example 11.2 to predict the probability of developing CA as a function of both white blood count and hemoglobin. Use SAS to estimate a multiple logistic regression model where the outcome is the dichotomous variable, CA, and the two independent variables are the continuous variables WBC and HEM.

Program Code

```
options ps=62 ls=80;
```
Formats the output page to 62 lines in length and 80 columns in width

```
data in;
   input ca wbc hem;
```
Beginning of Data Step

Inputs three variables, **ca** (CA or noCA) **wbc** (white blood count), and **hem** (hemoglobin).

```
cards;
0 9.4 11.0
1 20.4 10.1
0 8.7 10.0
.

.
0 5.7 10.2
run;
proc logistic descending;
  model ca=wbc hem;

run;
```

Beginning of Raw Data section.

actual observations (value of **group**, **wbc**, and **event** on each line)

Procedure call. Proc logistic provides estimates of the coefficients in a multiple logistic regression model.

End of procedure section. ▪

11.6.1 Summary of SAS Procedures

The SAS procedure for logistic regression analysis is summarized in the following table. Specific options can be requested in this procedure to produce specific results. These options are shown in italics. Users should refer to the examples in this section for complete descriptions of the procedure and specific options.

Procedure	Sample Procedure Call	Description

proc logistic	proc logistic *descending*;
	    model y = x1 x2 x3 x4/rl;
	    units x1 = d;
		Estimates a logistic regression model relating dichotomous dependent variable Y to independent variables X_1, X_2, X_3, X_4. The descending option considers the response with the higher numerical code the outcome of interest (e.g., 1 = outcome of interest, 0 = comparison). The units option produces CI for the odds ratios relative to a difference of d units (e.g., $d = 5$).

11.7 Analysis of Framingham Heart Study Data

The Framingham data set includes data collected from the original cohort. Participants contributed up to three examination cycles of data. Here we analyze data collected in the first examination cycle (called the period = 1

examination) and use SAS Proc Logistic to investigate predictors of inci
dent hypertension. The candidate predictor variables are age, gender, and
body mass index. For this analysis, we exclude persons who are underweight
(BMI < 18.5) because analysis has shown that there may be a different
relationship between very low BMI and other risk factors. We also create an
indicator variable for male gender and two variables to represent BMI cate
gories. The two BMI variables represent overweight and obese classifications.
When they are included in the model together, we can estimate the effect of
each of these BMI categories compared to normal-weight persons (called the
referent group) on incident hypertension. The SAS code to create the analytic
data set along with the procedure calls is shown next.

Framingham Data Analysis—SAS Code

```
data fhs;
 set in.frmgham;
 if period=1;

if bmi<18.5 then delete;

if sex=1 then male=1;
else if sex=2 then male=0;

if 25.0 le bmi lt 30.0 then overwt=1; else overwt=0;
if bmi ge 30.0 then obese=1; else obese=0;
run;


proc logistic descending data=fhs;
 model hyperten=age male bmi;
run;


proc logistic descending data=fhs;
 model hyperten=age male bmi;
 units age=10 bmi=5;
run;


proc logistic descending data=fhs;
 model hyperten=age male overwt obese;
 units age=10;
run;
```

Framingham Data Analysis—SAS Output

The LOGISTIC Procedure
Model Information

Data Set	WORK.FHS
Response Variable	HYPERTEN Incident Hypertension
Number of Response Levels	2
Number of Observations	4358
Model	binary logit
Optimization Technique	Fisher's scoring

Response Profile

Ordered Value	HYPERTEN	Total Frequency
1	1	3210
2	0	1148

Probability modeled is HYPERTEN=1.

Model Convergence Status
Convergence criterion (GCONV=1E-8) satisfied.

Model Fit Statistics

Criterion	Intercept Only	Intercept and Covariates
AIC	5027.711	4606.015
SC	5034.091	4631.534
-2 Log L	5025.711	4598.015

Testing Global Null Hypothesis: BETA=0

Test	Chi-Square	DF	Pr > ChiSq
Likelihood Ratio	427.6957	3	<.0001
Score	378.3059	3	<.0001
Wald	350.6524	3	<.0001

The LOGISTIC Procedure

Analysis of Maximum Likelihood Estimates

Parameter	DF	Estimate	Standard Error	Wald Chi-Square	Pr > ChiSq
Intercept	1	-5.4069	0.3419	250.0608	<.0001
AGE	1	0.0519	0.00440	138.6171	<.0001
MALE	1	-0.2496	0.0738	11.4306	0.0007
BMI	1	0.1582	0.0113	196.4913	<.0001

```
              Odds Ratio Estimates
                 Point              95% Wald
    Effect      Estimate        Confidence Limits
     AGE          1.053         1.044       1.062
     MALE         0.779         0.674       0.900
     BMI          1.171         1.146       1.198
```

Association of Predicted Probabilities and Observed Responses

```
    Percent Concordant      69.7    Somers' D    0.397
    Percent Discordant      29.9    Gamma        0.399
    Percent Tied             0.4    Tau-a        0.154
    Pairs                3685080    c            0.699
```

Wald Confidence Interval for Adjusted Odds Ratios

```
Effect         Unit     Estimate    95% Confidence Limits
AGE          1.0000      1.053       1.044       1.062
MALE         1.0000      0.779       0.674       0.900
BMI          1.0000      1.171       1.146       1.198
```

Is the model significant? How significant is each predictor? Is the effect of each predictor in the expected direction? The odds ratios are often reporte as the measures of effect. SAS produces odds ratios relative to a 1-un increase in each predictor. For example, each additional year of age associated with a 5% increase in risk of hypertension (estimate $OR = 1.053$). Each additional increase of 1 unit of BMI is associated with 17% increase in risk of hypertension. In the following logistic regressio model, SAS produces the estimates of the OR and associated 95% conf dence intervals relative to a 10-year increase in age and a 5-unit increase i BMI. These unit increases are specified by the user (see the preceding SA program).

```
                  The LOGISTIC Procedure
                     Model Information
Data Set                      WORK.FHS
Response Variable             HYPERTEN         Incident Hypertension
Number of Response Levels     2
Number of Observations        4358
Model                         binary logit
Optimization Technique        Fisher's scoring
```

```
                   Response Profile
          Ordered                     Total
          Value      HYPERTEN      Frequency
             1           1            3210
             2           0            1148
```

Probability modeled is HYPERTEN=1.

```
            Model Convergence Status
   Convergence criterion (GCONV=1E-8) satisfied.
```

```
              Model Fit Statistics
                                    Intercept
                         Intercept      and
          Criterion        Only      Covariates
          AIC            5027.711     4606.015
          SC             5034.091     4631.534
          -2 Log L       5025.711     4598.015
```

```
     Testing Global Null Hypothesis: BETA=
   Test                Chi-Square    DF    Pr > ChiSq
   Likelihood Ratio     427.6957      3      <.0001
   Score                378.3059      3      <.0001
   Wald                 350.6524      3      <.0001
```

The LOGISTIC Procedure

Analysis of Maximum Likelihood Estimates

Parameter	DF	Estimate	Standard Error	Wald Chi-Square	Pr > ChiSq
Intercept	1	-5.4069	0.3419	250.0608	<.0001
AGE	1	0.0519	0.00440	138.6171	<.0001
MALE	1	-0.2496	0.0738	11.4306	0.0007
BMI	1	0.1582	0.0113	196.4913	<.0001

Odds Ratio Estimates

Effect	Point Estimate	95% Wald Confidence Limits	
AGE	1.053	1.044	1.062
MALE	0.779	0.674	0.900
BMI	1.171	1.146	1.198

```
Association of Predicted Probabilities and Observed Responses
      Percent Concordant        69.7      Somers' D   0.397
      Percent Discordant        29.9      Gamma       0.399
      Percent Tied               0.4      Tau-a       0.154
      Pairs                  3685080      c           0.699


      Wald Confidence Interval for Adjusted Odds Ratios

   Effect      Unit    Estimate    95% Confidence Limits
   AGE      10.0000       1.680        1.541        1.831
   BMI       5.0000       2.206        1.975        2.464
```

The odds ratios above can be interpreted as follows. Ten years of aging is
associated with an increase in risk of hypertension of 68%. An increase of 5
units of BMI is associated with more than a twofold increase in risk of hypertension. In the next model, we consider BMI categories; the two indicator
variables reflect overweight and obese categories, and the referent category is
normal weight. An interpretation of the effect of BMI is given after the
output.

```
                    The LOGISTIC Procedure
                      Model Information
Data Set                        WORK.FHS
Response Variable               HYPERTEN         Incident Hypertension
Number of Response Levels       2
Number of Observations          4358
Model                           binary logit
Optimization Technique          Fisher's scoring


                      Response Profile
              Ordered                    Total
              Value    HYPERTEN       Frequency
                  1           1            3210
                  2           0            1148


         Probability modeled is HYPERTEN=1.


              Model Convergence Status
    Convergence criterion (GCONV=1E-8) satisfied.
```

Model Fit Statistics

Criterion	Intercept Only	Intercept and Covariates
AIC	5027.711	4634.628
SC	5034.091	4666.527
-2 Log L	5025.711	4624.628

Testing Global Null Hypothesis: BETA=0

Test	Chi-Square	DF	Pr > ChiSq
Likelihood Ratio	401.0833	4	<.0001
Score	367.6993	4	<.0001
Wald	330.8209	4	<.0001

The LOGISTIC Procedure
Analysis of Maximum Likelihood Estimates

Parameter	DF	Estimate	Standard Error	Wald Chi-Square	Pr > ChiSq
Intercept	1	-1.9005	0.2163	77.1786	<.0001
AGE	1	0.0528	0.00440	143.6058	<.0001
MALE	1	-0.2189	0.0738	8.7967	0.0030
OVERWT	1	0.7001	0.0770	82.5950	<.0001
OBESE	1	1.7752	0.1599	123.2305	<.0001

Odds Ratio Estimates

Effect	Point Estimate	95% Wald Confidence Limits	
AGE	1.054	1.045	1.063
MALE	0.803	0.695	0.928
OVERWT	2.014	1.732	2.342
OBESE	5.901	4.313	8.073

Association of Predicted Probabilities and Observed Responses

Percent Concordant	68.8	Somers' D	0.385
Percent Discordant	30.3	Gamma	0.388
Percent Tied	0.9	Tau-a	0.149
Pairs	3685080	c	0.692

```
        Wald Confidence Interval for Adjusted Odds Ratios
    Effect           Unit      Estimate      95% Confidence Limits
    AGE            10.0000       1.695         1.555        1.847
```

Persons who are overweight are 2.014 times more likely to develop hypertension as compared to persons of normal weight; persons who are obese are 5.901 times more likely to develop hypertension as compared to normal-weight persons, adjusting for age and gender.

It is sometimes of interest to compare different models in terms of their fit, and SAS produces a number of statistics for this purpose. One such statistic is the AIC statistic, a smaller value of which indicates better fit. Which model is better, the one with continuous BMI or the one with BMI categories?

11.8 Problems

1. A placebo-controlled clinical trial of a new treatment for chronic pain was performed on 200 patients in a pain clinic: 100 patients were given the new treatment and 100 were given a placebo. A pain questionnaire was administered to all 200 patients 1 week later. Based on the questionnaire, patients were classified as having moderate to severe pain (pain = 1) or mild or no pain (pain = 0).

   a. Use the following output from a logistic regression to estimate the probability of pain in patients on placebo (newtreat = 0).
   b. Use the following output from a logistic regression to estimate the probability of pain in patients on the new treatment (newtreat = 1).
   c. Estimate the relative risk of pain comparing those on the new treatment to those on placebo.
   d. Compare this to the estimated odds ratio provided in the output.
   e. Does the odds ratio provide a reasonable estimate of the relative risk?

The LOGISTIC Procedure

Analysis of Maximum Likelihood Estimates

Parameter	DF	Estimate	Standard Error	Wald Chi-Square	Pr > ChiSq
Intercept	1	-1.2657	0.2414	27.4888	<.0001
newtreat	1	-0.8251	0.4005	4.2435	0.0394

Odds Ratio Estimates

Effect	Point Estimate	95% Wald Confidence Limits	
newtreat	0.438	0.200	0.961

In Problems 2–4, suppose we have 30-day follow-up data on 350 ischemic stroke patients and want to investigate whether the risk of recurrent stroke and/or death (RD) depends on the type of stroke. You classify patients according to initial stroke type—having a cerebral embolism (CE = 1) or not (CE = 0)—and perform a series of logistic regression analyses.

2. First, consider the crude relationship between CE and RD. The following output is produced by SAS.

The LOGISTIC Procedure

Analysis of Maximum Likelihood Estimates

Parameter	DF	Estimate	Standard Error	Wald Chi-Square	Pr > ChiSq
Intercept	1	-2.8034	0.5149	29.6390	<.0001
ce	1	1.8651	0.6479	8.2874	0.0040

Odds Ratio Estimates

Effect	Point Estimate	95% Wald Confidence Limits	
ce	6.457	1.814	22.986

a. Use the output to estimate the odds ratio, provide a 95% confidence interval, and test $H_0: OR = 1$.

b. What is the risk of RD for CE patients?

c. What is the risk of RD for non-CE patients?

d. Is the risk of RD the same for CE and non-CE patients? Estimate the relative risk of RD.

3. Next, consider the relationship between age and RD. The following output is produced by SAS.

The LOGISTIC Procedure

Analysis of Maximum Likelihood Estimates

Parameter	DF	Estimate	Standard Error	Wald Chi-Square	Pr > ChiSq
Intercept	1	-8.0798	8.1749	0.9769	0.3230
age	1	0.0869	0.1149	0.5714	0.4497

Odds Ratio Estimates

Effect	Point Estimate	95% Wald Confidence Limits	
age	1.091	0.871	1.366

a. What is the odds ratio comparing the odds of RD in patients whose ages are 1 year apart? Provide a 95% confidence interval and test H_0: $OR = 1$.

b. What is the risk of RD for a patient aged 65?

c. What is the risk of RD for a patient aged 66?

d. Estimate the relative risk of RD comparing patients who are 65 and 66.

e. How does this compare with the odds ratio given in the output?

f. What is the risk of RD for a patient aged 75?

g. Estimate the relative risk of RD comparing patients who are 75 to those who are 65.

4. Finally, consider the relationship between CE and RD, adjusted for age.

The LOGISTIC Procedure

Analysis of Maximum Likelihood Estimates

Parameter	DF	Estimate	Standard Error	Wald Chi-Square	Pr > ChiSq
Intercept	1	-15.3151	9.4983	2.5999	0.1069
ce	1	2.0684	0.6822	9.1919	0.0024
age	1	0.1751	0.1318	1.7654	0.1840

Odds Ratio Estimates

Effect	Point Estimate	95% Wald Confidence Limits	
ce	7.912	2.078	30.129
age	1.191	0.920	1.542

a. Use the output to estimate the odds ratio comparing the odds of RD in patients with CE to those without CE, adjusted for age. Provide a 95% confidence interval and test $H_0: OR = 1$.

b. How do these adjusted results differ from the crude results in Problem 2a?

5. A clinical trial was designed to investigate the effect of a new treatment on the course of disease among pediatric patients with a particular infectious disease. Fifty boys and fifty girls were randomized to receive the new treatment (newtreat = 1) or the standard treatment (newtreat = 0), and the outcome was hospitalization (hospital = 1 or 0).

a. What is the odds ratio comparing patients treated with the new treatment to patients receiving standard treatment with respect to the odds of hospitalization? Test $H_0: OR = 1$.

The LOGISTIC Procedure

Analysis of Maximum Likelihood Estimates

Parameter	DF	Estimate	Standard Error	Wald Chi-Square	Pr > ChiSq
Intercept	1	-0.5754	0.2083	7.6273	0.0057
newtreat	1	-0.9410	0.3334	7.9660	0.0048

Odds Ratio Estimates

Effect	Point Estimate	95% Wald Confidence Limits	
newtreat	0.390	0.203	0.750

b. What is the odds ratio comparing boys treated with the new treatment to boys receiving standard treatment with respect to the odds of hospitalization? Test $H_0: OR = 1$.

```
-------------------- gender=boy --------------------
```

Analysis of Maximum Likelihood Estimates

Parameter	DF	Estimate	Standard Error	Wald Chi-Square	Pr > ChiSq
Intercept	1	-0.0800	0.2831	0.0800	0.7774
newtreat	1	-1.0726	0.4356	6.0626	0.0138

Odds Ratio Estimates

Effect	Point Estimate	95% Wald Confidence Limits	
newtreat	0.342	0.146	0.803

c. What is the odds ratio comparing girls treated with the new treatment to girls receiving standard treatment with respect to the odds of hospitalization? Test $H_0: OR = 1$.

```
-------------------- gender=girl --------------------
```

Analysis of Maximum Likelihood Estimates

Parameter	DF	Estimate	Standard Error	Wald Chi-Square	Pr > ChiSq
Intercept	1	-1.1527	0.3311	12.1175	0.0005
newtreat	1	-0.8397	0.5468	2.3581	0.1246

Odds Ratio Estimates

Effect	Point Estimate	95% Wald Confidence Limits	
newtreat	0.432	0.148	1.261

d. Does the new treatment have the same effect on girls and boys?

SAS Problems

Use SAS to solve the following problems.

1. A clinical trial was conducted to compare a new therapy for HIV to a standard therapy with respect to CD4 cell counts and incident opportunistic infections. A total of 30 subjects with diagnosed HIV were enrolled in the trial, randomized to receive standard or new therapy, and studied for 3 months. The following are data on age and OI (presence of opportunistic infection during the study period), coded 0 or 1 for absent or present, respectively.

Standard Therapy Group

Age	23	34	25	29	33	35	31	26	29	20	31	37	28	45	49
OI	0	1	0	0	0	1	1	1	1	1	1	1	0	1	1

New Therapy Group

Age	30	32	40	37	38	28	47	49	50	43	41	38	37	36	34
OI	0	0	0	0	0	0	0	1	1	0	1	1	0	0	0

a. Use logistic regression to estimate the odds ratio comparing the therapies with respect to risk of opportunistic infection.

b. Provide a 95% confidence interval for the odds ratio.

c. Test the appropriate hypothesis.

d. Use your output to provide estimates of the risk of opportunistic infection in each of the therapy groups.

e. Estimate the relative risk of opportunistic infection comparing the new therapy to the standard therapy.

f. Perform a separate logistic regression to estimate the odds ratio comparing the effect of therapy on the risk of opportunistic infection, adjusted for age. Test the appropriate hypothesis.

Descriptive Statistics
(Ch. 2)

Probability
(Ch. 3)

Sampling Distributions
(Ch. 4)

Statistical Inference
(Chapters 5–13)

OUTCOME VARIABLE	GROUPING VARIABLE(S)/ PREDICTOR(S)	ANALYSIS	CHAPTER(S)
Continuous	—	Estimate μ, Compare μ to Known, Historical Value	5/12
Continuous	Dichotomous (2 groups)	Compare Independent Means (Estimate/Test $(\mu_1 - \mu_2)$) or the Mean Difference (μ_d)	6/12
Continuous	Discrete (>2 groups)	Test the Equality of k Means Using Analysis of Variance $(\mu_1 = \mu_2 = \cdots = \mu_k)$	9/12
Continuous	Continuous	Estimate Correlation or Determine Regression Equation	10/12
Continuous	Several Continuous or Dichotomous	Multiple Linear Regression Analysis	10
Dichotomous	—	Estimate p; Compare p to Known, Historical Value	7
Dichotomous	Dichotomous (2 groups)	Compare Independent Proportions (Estimate/Test $(p_1 - p_2)$)	7/8
Dichotomous	Discrete (>2 groups)	Test the Equality of k Proportions (Chi-Square Test)	7
Dichotomous	Several Continuous or Dichotomous	Multiple Logistic Regression Analysis	11
Discrete	Discrete	Compare Distributions Among k Populations (Chi-Square Test)	7
Time to Event	Several Continuous or Dichotomous	Survival Analysis	13

Nonparametric Tests

12

In Chapters 5, 6, and 9 we presented techniques for tests of hypothesis concerning one, two (independent and dependent, matched or paired), and more than two population means. Valid application of these tests and procedures requires specific assumptions. These tests assume that the characteristic under investigation is approximately normally distributed or rely on large samples for the application of the Central Limit Theorem. If the samples are small and the analytic variable is clearly not normally distributed, we violate the assumptions for valid application of the procedures. In such cases, alternative methods are required. The techniques we presented in Chapters 5, 6, and 9 are called *parametric* procedures, as they are based on assumptions regarding the distributional form of the analytic variable (e.g., that the analytic variable follows a normal distribution). Methods that do not require such assumptions are called *nonparametric* procedures. Here we present four nonparametric procedures analogous to the two dependent samples test, the two independent samples test, the $k > 2$ independent samples test, and correlation analysis. The hypotheses tested with nonparametric procedures are more general than hypotheses we tested with parametric procedures. For example, the parametric test for two independent means is of the form H_0: $\mu_1 = \mu_2$. The nonparametric analog tests for equality of medians in the two distributions.

In Sections 12.1 and 12.2 we present nonparametric tests for two dependent samples. In Section 12.3 we present a technique for the two independent samples test. In Section 12.4 we present a technique for the $k > 2$ independent samples test, and in Section 12.5 we present a nonparametric approach to correlation analysis. We summarize key formulas in Section 12.6, and in Section 12.7 we display the statistical computing programs used to generate the nonparametric analyses presented in this chapter. In Section 12.8 we use data from the Framingham Heart Study to illustrate the applications presented here.

12.1 The Sign Test (Two Dependent Samples Test)

Recall the two dependent (also called matched or paired) samples procedure we presented in Chapter 6. In the examples we discussed, a single random sample of subjects was selected from the population of interest, and two measurements were taken on each subject. Because the measurements were dependent, we calculated differences between measurements and performed a test on the mean difference (e.g., H_0: $\mu_d = 0$). When the sample is small and/or if the differences are not normally distributed, we consider a nonparametric test. One popular nonparametric test for two dependent samples is the Sign test. The null hypothesis in the Sign test is that the median difference is zero. We illustrate the test using an example.

EXAMPLE 12.1

Test for Mean Difference in Systolic Blood Pressures Using Sign Test

Suppose we are investigating a new drug hypothesized to lower systolic blood pressure. We select a random sample of subjects and record their resting systolic blood pressure at baseline (i.e., prior to the investigation). Each subject is then given the new drug, and resting systolic blood pressure is measured again after 4 weeks of drug treatment. The data are shown in the following table. Based on the data, does it appear that the new drug lowers systolic blood pressure?

Subject Identification Number	Baseline Systolic Blood Pressure	Post-Treatment Systolic Blood Pressure
1	166	138
2	135	120
3	189	176
4	180	180
5	156	160
6	142	150
7	176	152
8	156	140
9	164	160
10	142	130

In the Sign test, as we did with the parametric test in Chapter 6, we focus on differences between measurements. In this application, we are investigating whether there is a significant reduction in systolic blood pressure following drug treatment. In the following table we display the differences between systolic blood pressures (baseline–post-treatment blood pressures). In the rightmost column of the table, we record the sign of the difference (+ or −, or 0 if there is no difference).

Subject Identification Number	Baseline Systolic Blood Pressure	Post-Treatment Systolic Blood Pressure	Difference (Baseline–Post-Treatment)	Sign of Difference
1	166	138	28	+
2	135	120	15	+
3	189	176	13	+
4	180	180	0	0
5	156	160	−4	−
6	142	150	−8	−
7	176	152	24	+
8	156	140	16	+
9	164	160	4	+
10	142	130	12	+

The Sign test is based on the binomial distribution. There are a total of 10 difference scores (one for each subject in the sample). If the drug has no effect on systolic blood pressure, we expect the post-treatment systolic blood pressures to be the same as the baseline pressures. Because there are many factors that affect blood pressure, expecting identical results is unrealistic. If the drug has no effect, we expect some subjects' post-treatment systolic blood pressures to be higher than their baseline pressures (negative differences) and some subjects' post-treatment systolic blood pressures to be lower than their baseline pressures (positive differences). If the drug has no effect, we expect these differences to be small, and with respect to the signs of the differences, we expect to see about five + and five − signs (or 50% in each direction).

In Example 12.1 we observed seven (out of ten) + signs. Is a total of seven + signs indicative of a drug effect (here a + sign indicates a difference in the hypothesized direction, i.e., a lowering of systolic blood pressure)? The exact significance of the test is determined from the binomial distribution (discussed in Chapter 3). The null hypothesis is that, for each person, the probability of a + sign is 0.5. We therefore consider a binomial distribution with $n = 10$ (because there are 10 subjects, or trials) and $p = 0.5$. The following values are found in Table B.1 in the Appendix.

Number of Successes, x	$P(X = x \mid n = 10, p = 0.5)$
0	0.0010
1	0.0098
2	0.0439
3	0.1172
4	0.2051
5	0.2461
6	0.2051
7	0.1172
8	0.0439
9	0.0098
10	0.0010

The question of interest is, *How likely is it to observe as many as seven or more successes out of ten when the probability of success is 0.5?* The *p* value for the test statistic (seven successes or seven + signs out of ten) is the probability of observing seven or more successes. (Recall the *p* value is defined as the probability of observing a test statistic as more extreme. In Example 12.1, the *p* value is $P(X \geq 7) = P(X = 7) + P(X = 8) + P(X = 9) + P(X = 10) = 0.1172 + 0.0439 + 0.0098 + 0.0010 = 0.1719$. We reject H_0 if the p value is small (i.e., 0.05 or less). In Example 12.1, we do not reject H_0. We do not have significant evidence, $p = 0.1719$, to show that the drug lowers systolic blood pressure. ■

There are several options for handling observations in which the difference is zero. We can ignore the zero (i.e., not assign a sign). Another alternative is to count a zero difference as $0.5+$ and $0.5-$. Had we used this strategy, we would have counted $7.5 +$ signs in Example 12.1. The p value for the test would then have been $P(X \geq 7.5) = P(X = 8) + P(X = 9) + P(X = 10) = 0.0439 + 0.0098 + 0.0010 = 0.0547$, which is marginally significant.

Note that we performed a one-sided test with the alternative hypothesis that the drug lowers systolic blood pressure. The p value corresponding to a two-sided test with the alternative hypothesis that the drug either raises or lowers systolic blood pressure is simply twice the one-sided p value. In our example, the two-sided p value is $P(X \geq 7 \text{ or } X \leq 3) = 2P(X \geq 7) = 2(0.1719) = 0.3438$.

The analysis of the data presented in Example 12.1 was based solely on the signs ($+$ or $-$) of the differences in blood pressures from baseline to post-treatment. In the parametric test, we also computed differences but focused on the magnitude of those differences. Recall, our test statistic was based on $\overline{X}_d$, the mean of the difference scores. In the Sign test we do not capture the magnitude of the differences, only the direction. For example, if a particular patient has a baseline systolic blood pressure of 150 and a post-treatment blood pressure of 149, we count that observation as evidence in favor of the alternative hypothesis (lowering of blood pressure) because the difference is positive ($+$). Suppose a second patient has a baseline systolic blood pressure of 150 and a post-treatment blood pressure of 129, we again count this observation as evidence in favor of the alternative hypothesis. In the Sign test, there is no distinction between these subjects, when in fact the second has a much more substantial reduction in blood pressure. Because we are basing the Sign test on limited information (only the sign of the difference in measurements), this nonparametric test often has lower power than competing procedures. A second nonparametric procedure for two dependent samples is described in the next section. This procedure incorporates the magnitude of the differences in measurements.

12.2 The Wilcoxon Signed-Rank Test (Two Dependent Samples Test)

The Wilcoxon Signed-Rank test is a second nonparametric alternative for two dependent matched or paired samples. To perform the Wilcoxon Signed-Rank test we compute differences in measurements as we did to perform the Sign test. However, here we also take into account the relative magnitude of these differences. The null hypothesis is that the median difference is zero. We illustrate the test using the data we presented in Example 12.1.

EXAMPLE 12.2

Test for Mean Difference in Systolic Blood Pressures Using Signed-Rank Test

Consider the data presented in Example 12.1. Again, the question of interest is whether there is significant evidence that the new drug lowers systolic blood pressure. The data are shown here along with the difference scores computed by subtracting the post-treatment systolic blood pressures from the baseline pressures.

Subject Identification Number	Baseline Systolic Blood Pressure	Post-Treatment Systolic Blood Pressure	Difference (Baseline–Post-Treatment)
1	166	138	28
2	135	120	15
3	189	176	13
4	180	180	0
5	156	160	−4
6	142	150	−8
7	176	152	24
8	156	140	16
9	164	160	4
10	142	130	12

In the Wilcoxon Signed-Rank test we assign ranks to the *absolute values* of the difference scores (see the third column of the following table). We assign a 1 to the smallest absolute difference, 2 to the next smallest, and so on, up to n. For now, we will ignore the case with no difference, although there are alternative methods for handling these cases. If there are ties in the absolute values of the differences, then the mean rank is assigned to both. For example, subjects 5 and 9 had absolute differences of 4 units. These are the first and second smallest differences, so we assign a rank of 1.5 to each. The next (third) smallest absolute difference is measured in subject 6, who is assigned a rank of 3. The ranking continues until all nonzero differences are ranked. Once the ranks are assigned to the absolute differences, we then reattach the signs of the differences (+ or −) to the ranks (see the right-most column of the table).

Subject Identification Number	Difference (Baseline– Post-Treatment)	Ranks of Absolute Values of Differences	Signed Ranks
1	28	9	+9
2	15	6	+6
3	13	5	+5
4	0	—	—
5	−4	1.5	−1.5
6	−8	3	−3
7	24	8	+8
8	16	7	+7
9	4	1.5	+1.5
10	12	4	+4

If the drug has no effect on systolic blood pressures, we expect about half of the post-treatment systolic blood pressures to be higher than the baseline pressures and half of the post-treatment pressures to be lower than the baseline pressures. In addition, we expect the magnitudes of the increases to be about the same as the magnitudes of the decreases. In terms of the signed ranks, if the drug has no effect, we expect the sum of the positive ranks to be approximately equal to the sum of the negative ranks.

The test statistic in the Wilcoxon Signed-Rank test is the sum of the positive ranks, called T. If all the differences are negative, then all the signs will be negative, so all the signed ranks will be negative and T will equal 0. The other extreme is all positive differences, which will yield all positive signed ranks and T will therefore be the sum $1 + 2 + 3 + 4 + \cdots + n = n(n + 1)/2$ (where n represents the number of ranked observations, i.e., the number of observations with nonzero differences). Thus, the sum of positive ranks, T, ranges from 0 to $n(n + 1)/2$. The median value is $n(n + 1)/4$. In Example 12.2, the observed sum of the positive ranks is $T = 40.5$. The maximum possible value of the sum of positive ranks is $9(9 + 1)/2 = 45$, and the median is $9(9 + 1)/4 = 22.5$. The observed test statistic, $T = 40.5$, is very close to the theoretical maximum (i.e., it falls in the tail of the distribution). To draw a conclusion in the test, we compare the observed test statistic to an appropriate critical value. Because the observed test statistic is large, we would expect a very small p value and therefore would likely reject H_0. There are tables of critical values for this test, but one can use the normal approximation to the distribution instead, which is what we illustrate here. SAS runs the Wilcoxon Signed-Rank test and produces a p value based on a normal approximation to the distribution of T. Specifically, SAS converts the sum of positive ranks, T, to a Z score, and then produces a p value from the standard normal distribution. The Z score (12.1) is computed by subtracting the median, $n(n+1)/4$, and dividing by the standard error, which is $\sqrt{\dfrac{n(n+1)(2n+1)}{24}}$

$$Z = \frac{T - \dfrac{n(n+1)}{4}}{\sqrt{\dfrac{n(n+1)(2n+1)}{24}}} \qquad (12.1$$

In Example 12.2,

$$Z = \frac{40.5 - \dfrac{9(9+1)}{4}}{\sqrt{\dfrac{9(9+1)(2(9)+1)}{24}}} = \frac{18}{8.44} = 2.13$$

The one sided p value is $P(Z \geq 2.13) = 1 - 0.9834 = 0.0166$. Based on the Wilcoxon Signed-Rank test, $p = 0.0166 < 0.05$; we therefore reject H_0: The medians are equal in favor of the alternative, H_1: The median systolic blood pressure is lower post-treatment as compared to baseline.

SAS EXAMPLE 12.2 Test for Mean Difference in Systolic Blood Pressures Using Signed-Rank Test in SAS

SAS performs the Wilcoxon Signed-Rank test in its Proc Univariate. We use Proc Univariate in Chapter 2 to generate summary statistics for continuous variables. The following output was generated by SAS on the difference variable (i.e., differences between baseline and post-treatment systolic blood pressures). A brief interpretation appears after the output.

SAS Output for Example 12.2

```
              The UNIVARIATE Procedure
                 Variable:   diff
                    Moments
N                        10    Sum Weights              10
Mean                     10    Sum Observations        100
Std Deviation     11.785113    Variance          138.888889
Skewness         -0.0712764    Kurtosis          -0.9438912
Uncorrected SS         2250    Corrected SS           1250
Coeff Variation   117.85113    Std Error Mean    3.72677996

              Basic Statistical Measures
        Location                    Variability
   Mean      10.00000    Std Deviation        11.78511
   Median    12.50000    Variance            138.88889
   Mode        .         Range                36.00000
                         Interquartile Range  16.00000
```

```
                  Tests for Location: Mu0=0
        Test              -Statistic-       -----p Value------
        Student's t     t  2.683282       Pr > |t|     0.0251
        Sign            M       2.5       Pr >= |M|    0.1797
        Signed Rank     S        18       Pr >= |S|    0.0313

                     Tests for Normality
Test                      --Statistic---      -----p Value------
Shapiro-Wilk              W    0.962454       Pr < W        0.8135
Kolmogorov-Smirnov       D    0.167379       Pr > D       >0.1500
Cramer-von Mises         W-Sq  0.035094       Pr > W-Sq    >0.2500
Anderson-Darling         A-Sq  0.209068       Pr > A-Sq    >0.2500

                  Quantiles (Definition 5)
                     Quantile        Estimate
                     100% Max           28.0
                     99%                28.0
                     95%                28.0
                     90%                26.0
                     75% Q3             16.0
                     50% Median         12.5
                     25% Q1              0.0

                  The UNIVARIATE Procedure
                      Variable:  diff
                  Quantiles (Definition 5)
                     Quantile       Estimate
                     10%               -6.0
                     5%                -8.0
                     1%                -8.0
                     0% Min            -8.0

                  Extreme Observations
          ----Lowest----         ----Highest---
          Value      Obs         Value       Obs
            -8        6            13          3
            -4        5            15          2
             0        4            16          8
             4        9            24          7
            12       10            28          1
```

Interpretation of SAS Output for Example 12.2

The output for the Wilcoxon Signed-Rank test is in the third section of the output. SAS produces the numerator of the test statistic in (12.1) and gives

"Signed Rank S = 18," which is computed by subtracting the median = 22.5 from $T = 40.5$ ($S = 40.5 - 22.5 = 18$). SAS then gives a two-sided p value "Pr >= $|S| = 0.0313$," which is based on the normal approximation. (SAS applies a correction factor to formula (12.1)—see also SAS Example 12.3.) If a one-sided test is desired (as is the case in Example 12.2), we divide $p = 0.0313/2 = 0.016$. Based on the observed p value, $p = 0.016$ (<0.05), we reject H_0: The medians are equal in favor of the alternative, H_1: The median systolic blood pressure is lower post-treatment as compared to baseline.

The Signed-Rank test uses more information in the data than the Sign test in that it incorporates the *relative* magnitude of the values through ranks. Note that the Signed-Rank test rejected the two-sided null hypothesis, with $p = 0.0313$, whereas the Sign test did not reject the same null hypothesis, with $p = 0.3438$. Ranks are particularly useful in the presence of outliers. However, tests based on ranks do not capture the *absolute* magnitude of the differences (in the two dependent samples case) as compared to parametric tests such as the two dependent samples *t* test.

In the next section of the output (just below the results of the Signed-Rank test), SAS produces several tests for normality. The null hypothesis is H_0: Differences follow a normal distribution. We use the Shapiro–Wilk test, with test statistic $W = 0.962454$ and p value $= 0.8135$. We would not reject H_0 based on the observed p value; therefore, we do not have significant evidence to show that the data do not follow a normal distribution. This test can be useful in assessing whether a parametric test (which assumes that the analytic variable follows a normal distribution) or a nonparametric test should be applied. In this example, we could use the parametric test, as there is no evidence that the differences are not normally distributed. ■

12.3 The Wilcoxon Rank Sum Test (Two Independent Samples Test)

We now present a nonparametric test for two independent samples. In these applications, we have two independent populations defined based on a specific attribute of the subjects under study (e.g., gender) or based on the study design (e.g., some patients are assigned to receive Drug A while others receive Drug B). The parametric procedure tests the equality of population means and assumes large samples ($n_i > 30$, $i = 1, 2$) or, if the sample sizes are small, that the analytic variable under investigation is approximately normally distributed. If these assumptions are not met, a nonparametric test might be appropriate. A popular nonparametric test comparing two independent samples is the Wilcoxon Rank Sum test, in which the null hypothesis is the equality of medians. This test is equivalent to the nonparametric Mann–Whitney U test. We illustrate the test using an example.

EXAMPLE 12.3

Test for Difference in Mean Health Status Between Treatments Using Wilcoxon Rank Sum Test

Suppose we wish to compare two competing treatments for the management of adult-onset diabetes. A total of eight subjects agree to participate in the investigation and are randomly assigned to one of the competing treatments. After following the prescribed treatment regimen for 6 weeks, we assess the patients' self-reported health status. Patients are asked to rate their current health on an ordinal scale from 0 to 20, with higher scores reflecting better health. To anchor the scale, the following instruction is provided: Subjects who feel that their health is poor should report a score of 0, and subjects who feel that their health is excellent should report a score of 20. The test of interest is a two-sided test (i.e., Are self-reported health status scores different between treatment groups?). The data are

Self-Reported Health Status	
Treatment 1	Treatment 2
0	8
7	10
11	12
16	15

In this application we have small samples and the analytic variable is ordinal. Therefore, we consider a nonparametric test. To perform the Wilcoxon Rank Sum test, we pool the data from the two groups and order the values from lowest to highest (i.e., from lowest self-reported health status to highest). We then assign ranks to the values in increasing order. We assign a 1 to the lowest value, 2 to the next lowest, and so on, up to $N = n_1 + n_2$. When there are ties, the mean ranks are assigned (similar to the procedure we followed with the Signed-Rank test). The following table contains the ranks of the values:

Ranks	
Treatment 1	Treatment 2
1	3
2	4
5	6
8	7

If there is no difference between treatments, we expect to see some low ranks and some high ranks in each group. If there is a difference between treatments, we expect to see clustering of lower ranks in one group and higher ranks in the other.

The Wilcoxon Rank Sum test statistic is S, the smaller of the sums of the ranks in the groups. The sum of all ranks is $N(N+1)/2$. For Example 12.3 the sum of all ranks is $8(8+1)/2 = 36$. If there is no difference between treatments, we expect the sums of the ranks to be about 18 in each group In the most extreme situation (for $N = 8$), the four smallest values would fall in one group, producing ranks in that group of 1, 2, 3, and 4, and the smaller sum of ranks would be equal to $S = 10$ ($S = 1 + 2 + 3 + 4$). In Example 12.3, the sum of ranks in Treatment 1 is 16 and the sum of ranks in Treatment 2 is 20. The smaller sum is $S = 16$. Is that significantly different from the expected sum (if there were no difference between treatments of 18?

To draw a conclusion in the test, we compare the observed sum to an appropriate critical value. Again, we will use SAS to run the test. SAS runs the Wilcoxon Rank Sum test and produces a p value based on a normal approximation. Specifically, SAS converts the smaller sum of ranks, S, to a Z score and then produces a p value from the standard normal distribution. The Z score (12.2) is computed by subtracting the mean, $n_1(n_1 + n_2 + 1)/2$, and dividing by the standard error, which is $\sqrt{\dfrac{n_1 n_2 (n_1 + n_2 + 1)}{12}}$.

$$Z = \frac{S - \dfrac{n_1(n_1 + n_2 + 1)}{2}}{\sqrt{\dfrac{n_1 n_2 (n_1 + n_2 + 1)}{12}}} \qquad (12.2)$$

In Example 12.3,

$$Z = \frac{16 - \dfrac{4(4 + 4 + 1)}{2}}{\sqrt{\dfrac{(4)4(4 + 4 + 1)}{12}}} = \frac{-2}{3.46} = -0.58$$

The one-sided p value is $P(Z \le -0.58) = 0.2810$. The two-sided p value = $2(0.2810) = 0.5620$. Based on the Wilcoxon Rank Sum test, we would not reject H_0. We do not have significant evidence to show a difference between treatment with respect to self-reported health status because $p = 0.5620 > 0.05$.

SAS EXAMPLE 12.3 **Test for Difference in Mean Health Status Between Treatments Using Wilcoxon Rank Sum Test in SAS**

SAS performs the Wilcoxon Rank Sum test in its Proc Npar1way. The following output was generated by SAS. A brief interpretation appears after the output.

SAS Output for Example 12.3

```
                 The NPAR1WAY Procedure
        Wilcoxon Scores (Rank Sums) for Variable hlthstat
                   Classified by Variable trt


               Sum of      Expected      Std Dev       Mean
   trt    N    Scores      Under H0      Under H0      Score
   ----------------------------------------------------------
   1      4    16.0          18.0       3.464102        4.0
   2      4    20.0          18.0       3.464102        5.0


                  Wilcoxon Two-Sample Test
               Statistic               16.0000
               Normal Approximation
               Z                       -0.4330
               One-Sided Pr < Z         0.3325
               Two-Sided Pr > |Z|       0.6650


               t Approximation
               One-Sided Pr < Z         0.3390
               Two-Sided Pr > |Z|       0.6780

        Z includes a continuity correction of 0.5.


                     Kruskal-Wallis Test
               Chi-Square               0.3333
               DF                            1
               Pr > Chi-Square          0.5637
```

Interpretation of SAS Output for Example 12.3

For the Wilcoxon Rank Sum test, SAS produces the sum of the ranks (labeled "Sum of Scores") in each treatment group. SAS then gives the expected sums and the standard deviation (assuming no difference between treatments) and then the mean rank in each group. SAS then shows the sum of the smaller ranks ($S = 16$) and the corresponding Z score. It applies a correction of ½ to formula (12.2) in the standardization as follows:

$$Z = \frac{S - \dfrac{n_1(n_1 + n_2 + 1)}{2} + \dfrac{1}{2}}{\sqrt{\dfrac{n_1 n_2(n_1 + n_2 + 1)}{12}}}$$

For Example 12.3, SAS computes $Z = -0.4330$ (with the correction) and gives a two-sided p value of 0.6650. Based on the Wilcoxon Rank Sum test, we would not reject H_0 because $p = 0.6650 > 0.05$. We do not have significant evidence to show a difference between treatments with respect to self-reported health status.

The Rank Sum test provides a comparison of the relative magnitude of values in the two groups but does not use the actual observed values—as does the two independent samples (t or Z) test. Just below the results of the Rank Sum test, SAS provides an approximate p value for the two independent samples t test for means (Proc Ttest in SAS). For Example 12.3, SAS gives "t Approximation Pr > $|Z| = 0.6780$." Had we run a two independent samples test for equality of means we would not have rejected $H_0: \mu_1 = \mu_2$ because $p = 0.6780 > 0.05$. Note that this is an approximation to the t test.

12.4 The Kruskal–Wallis Test (k Independent Samples Test)

We now present a nonparametric procedure for the k independent samples test. This procedure is the nonparametric analog to analysis of variance (ANOVA), discussed in Chapter 9. A popular nonparametric test for the k independent samples test is the Kruskal–Wallis test. Like the Wilcoxon Signed Rank and Rank Sum tests, the Kruskal–Wallis test is based on assigning ranks to the observed values and then comparing the observed sums of ranks to what would be expected if there were no difference among groups. The computations involved in the Kruskal–Wallis test are similar to those in the Wilcoxon Rank Sum test but are complicated by the fact that there are more groups involved. We illustrate the application of the Kruskal–Wallis test using SAS for the sample data in the next example.

EXAMPLE 12.4

Test for Difference in Mean Symptom Scores Between Treatments Using Kruskal–Wallis Test

Suppose we wish to compare four treatments for seasonal allergies. A total of 20 subjects agree to participate in the investigation and are randomly assigned to one of the four competing treatments. After following the prescribed treatment regimen for 2 weeks, we assess the subjects' status. The outcome variable in this application is an index score based on three distinct symptoms. At the end of treatment, subjects are asked if they are currently experiencing any (or all) of the following symptoms: scratchy throat, itchy eyes, runny nose. Each subject responds "yes" or "no" to each of the three symptoms. The index score is the sum of affirmative responses. The range of scores is 0 (no symptoms) to (all three symptoms). The data are shown in the following table:

Treatment 1	Treatment 2	Treatment 3	Treatment 4
0	2	0	2
0	2	0	3
1	3	1	2
2	3	1	3
3	2	1	3

Is there is a significant difference among the treatments with respect to symptom scores? Here again, we have small samples and an analytic variable with limited response options. Therefore, we consider a nonparametric test. ■

SAS EXAMPLE 12.4 Test for Difference in Mean Symptom Scores Between Treatments Using Kruskal–Wallis Test in SAS

SAS performs the Kruskal–Wallis test in its Proc Npar1way. The following output was generated by SAS. A brief interpretation appears after the output.

SAS Output for Example 12.4

```
                    The NPAR1WAY Procedure
          Wilcoxon Scores (Rank Sums) for Variable symptoms
                     Classified by Variable trt
                 Sum of      Expected      Std Dev        Mean
 trt    N       Scores      Under H0      Under H0       Score
 --------------------------------------------------------------
  1     5        40.50        52.50      11.062026        8.10
  2     5        69.50        52.50      11.062026       13.90
  3     5        24.50        52.50      11.062026        4.90
  4     5        75.50        52.50      11.062026       15.10

          Average scores were used for ties.
                  Kruskal-Wallis Test
             Chi-Square           10.7013
             DF                         3
             Pr > Chi-Square       0.0135
```

Interpretation of SAS Output for Example 12.4

For the Kruskal–Wallis test, SAS produces the sum of the ranks (labeled "Sum of Scores") in each treatment group. SAS then gives the expected sums and the standard deviation (assuming no difference among treatments) and then the mean rank in each group. It then gives a test statistic—in this case, a chi-square statistic—and a corresponding p value. For Example 12.4, SAS computes $\chi^2 = 10.7013$, which has 3 degrees of freedom (number of groups − 1), and a *p* value = 0.0135. Based on the Kruskal–Wallis test, we reject H_0 because $p = 0.0135 < 0.05$. We have significant evidence of a difference among the treatments with respect to median symptom scores. ▪

12.5 Spearman Correlation (Correlation Between Variables)

In Chapter 10 we presented a formula for the sample correlation coefficient, $r (r = \text{Cov}(X, Y)/\sqrt{\text{Var}(X)\text{Var}(Y)})$. The correlation coefficient quantifies the nature and strength of the linear association between X and Y. Extreme values can have a substantial impact on the value of the sample correlation coefficient. When data are subject to extremes, an alternative measure of correlation between variables is based on ranks. The correlation based on ranks is called the Spearman correlation. We illustrate the computation of the Spearman correlation using an example.

EXAMPLE 12.5

Spearman Correlation Between Number of Cigarettes Smoked and Aerobic Exercise

Suppose we wish to assess the relationship between the number of cigarettes smoked per day and the number of hours of aerobic exercise per week. A total of 12 subjects agree to participate in the investigation, and we measure the typical number of cigarettes smoked per day and the number of hours of exercise in a typical week on each subject. The data are shown next.

Raw Scores	
X = Number of Cigarettes per Day	Y = Number of Hours of Exercise per Week
20	0
0	0
20	1
10	2
5	3
4	5
3	5
5	6
0	3
0	4
0	7
0	8

The first step in the analysis is to replace the raw *X* and *Y* scores with ranks. The ranks are assigned for each variable, considered separately, as shown in the following table. In this example, there are several instances of ties in raw scores. When scores are tied, the mean rank is applied to each of the tied values.

	Ranks
Rx = Rank of Number of Cigarettes per Day	*Ry = Rank of Number of Hours of Exercise per Week*
11.5	1.5
3	1.5
11.5	3
10	4
8.5	5.5
7	8.5
6	8.5
8.5	10
3	5.5
3	7
3	11
3	12

The Spearman correlation is computed using the same formula we used in Chapter 10, based on the ranks. In the formula *Rx* and *Ry* are the ranks of *X* and *Y*, respectively:

$$r_s = \frac{\text{Cov}(Rx, Ry)}{\sqrt{\text{Var}(Rx)\text{Var}(Ry)}} \tag{12.3}$$

We now calculate the components for r_s.

We first compute the variance of *Rx*: $\text{Var}(Rx) = \sum(Rx - \overline{Rx})^2/(n - 1)$. The following table summarizes the computations:

Rx = Rank of Number of Cigarettes per Day	(Rx − R̄x)	(Rx − R̄x)²
11.5	5.0	25.00
3	−3.5	12.25
11.5	5.0	25.00
10	3.5	12.25
8.5	2.0	4.00
7	0.5	0.25
6	−0.5	0.25
8.5	2.0	4.00
3	−3.5	12.25
3	−3.5	12.25
3	−3.5	12.25
3	−3.5	12.25
R̄x = 6.5	0	132.0

So, $\text{Var}(Rx) = \sum (Rx - \overline{Rx})^2/(n-1) = 132.0/11 = 12.0$.

We now compute the variance of Ry: $\text{Var}(Ry) = \sum (Ry - \overline{Ry})^2/(n-1)$. The following table summarizes the computations:

Ry = Rank of Number of Hours of Exercise per Week	(Ry − R̄y)	(Ry − R̄y)²
1.5	−5.0	25.00
1.5	−5.0	25.00
3	−3.5	12.25
4	−2.5	6.25
5.5	−1.0	1.00
8.5	2.0	4.00
8.5	2.0	4.00
10	3.5	12.25
5.5	−1.0	1.00
7	0.5	0.25
11	4.5	20.25
12	5.5	30.25
R̄y = 6.5	0	141.50

So, $\text{Var}(Ry) = \sum(Ry - \overline{Ry})^2/(n-1) = 141.50/11 = 12.86$.

Finally, we compute the covariance of Rx and Ry: $\text{Cov}(Rx, Ry) = \sum(Rx - \overline{Rx})(Ry - \overline{Ry})/(n-1)$. The following table summarizes the computations:

$(Rx - \overline{Rx})$	$(Ry - \overline{Ry})$	$(Rx - \overline{Rx})(Ry - \overline{Ry})$
5.0	−5.0	−25.00
−3.5	−5.0	17.50
5.0	−3.5	−17.50
3.5	−2.5	−8.75
2.0	−1.0	−2.00
0.5	2.0	1.00
−0.5	2.0	−1.00
2.0	3.5	7.00
−3.5	−1.0	3.50
−3.5	0.5	−1.75
−3.5	4.5	−15.75
−3.5	5.5	−19.25
		−62.0

So, $\text{Cov}(Rx, Ry) = \sum(Rx - \overline{Rx})(Ry - \overline{Ry})/(n-1) = -62.0/11 = -5.64$.

Substituting into (12.3):

$$r_s = \frac{\text{Cov}(Rx, Ry)}{\sqrt{\text{Var}(Rx)\text{Var}(Ry)}} = \frac{-5.64}{\sqrt{(12.05)(12.86)}} = -0.453$$

Based on the sign and the magnitude of r_s, there is a moderately strong, inverse association between the number of cigarettes smoked per day and the number of hours of aerobic exercise per week. ■

SAS EXAMPLE 12.5 Spearman Correlation Between Number of Cigarettes Smoked and Aerobic Exercise Using SAS

Users can request that SAS compute a correlation based on ranks by specifying the Spearman option in Proc Corr. Before computing the rank correlation, we generated a scatter diagram using Proc Plot. The following output was generated by SAS. A brief interpretation appears after the output.

SAS Output for Example 12.5

```
              Plot of exercise*cigarett.  Legend: A = 1 obs, B = 2 obs, etc.
exercise |
         |
      8  +   A
         |
         |
         |
         |
      7  +   A
         |
         |
         |
         |
      6  +                       A
         |
         |
         |
         |
      5  +                 A
         |
         |
         |
         |
      4  +   A             A
         |
         |
         |
         |
      3  +   A             A
         |
         |
         |
         |
      2  +                               A
         |
         |
         |
         |
      1  +                                                             A
         |
         |
         |
         |
      0  +   A                                                         A
         |
         ---+------------+------------+------------+------------+--
            0            5           10           15           20
                                 cigarett
```

```
                      The CORR Procedure
                2 Variables:     cigarett exercise
                       Simple Statistics
Variable     N      Mean    Std Dev    Median    Minimum    Maximum
cigarett    12   5.58333   7.39113    3.50000          0   20.00000
exercise    12   3.66667   2.64002    3.50000          0    8.00000

            Spearman Correlation Coefficients, N = 12
                 Prob > |r| under H0: Rho=0
                              cigarett        exercise
               cigarett        1.00000        -0.45366
                                                0.1385
               exercise       -0.45366         1.00000
                                0.1385
```

Interpretation of SAS Output for Example 12.5

The scatterplot shows the inverse relationship between the number of hours of exercise per week and the number of cigarettes smoked per day. The Corr Procedure first generates summary statistics on the raw scores of the variables specified. For example, the mean number of hours of exercise per week in the sample is 3.67 and the mean number of cigarettes smoked per day is 5.58. Because we requested a correlation based on ranks (Spearman correlation), SAS makes this note in the header to the correlation matrix. The Spearman correlation is estimated at -0.45 and the two-sided p value $= 0.1385$. The correlation is not significantly different from zero, $p = 0.1385 > 0.05$. ▪

12.6 Key Formulas

Application	Notation/Formula	Description
Two dependent samples test	$Z = \dfrac{T - \dfrac{n(n+1)}{4}}{\sqrt{\dfrac{n(n+1)(2n+1)}{24}}},$ where $T = $ sum of positive ranks	normal approximation for Signed-Rank test
Two independent samples test	$Z = \dfrac{S - \dfrac{n_1(n_1 + n_2 + 1)}{2}}{\sqrt{\dfrac{n_1 n_2(n_1 + n_2 + 1)}{12}}},$ where $S = $ smaller sum of ranks	normal approximation for Rank Sum test
Rank correlation	$r_s = \dfrac{\text{Cov}(Rx, Ry)}{\sqrt{\text{Var}(Rx)\text{Var}(Ry)}}$	Spearman correlation based on ranks

12.6.1 Guidelines for Determining When to Use a Nonparametric Procedure

There are no "rules" for determining when it is appropriate to use a nonpara
metric procedure instead of a parametric one. Substantial work has been done t
show the robustness of many parametric procedures in the presence of violation
of the normality assumption. The following are guidelines that may be useful i
determining when it might be appropriate to employ a nonparameteric test:

■ When substantive knowledge of the analytic variable suggests
nonnormality. Some variables clearly do not follow a normal distribution
(e.g., ordinal variables with few response options); analyses focused on
these variables are candidates for nonparametric procedures.

■ Observed nonnormality in the sample data. Visual inspection of the
distribution of a variable might suggest that the variable is highly
skewed. Comparison of measures of central tendency, such as the mean
and median, which are equal in symmetric distributions, can help
determine the extent of skewness. Situations in which the standard
deviation is much larger than the mean also suggest nonnormality. A
formal test for normality (such as one of the tests available in Proc
Univariate) might indicate that a variable does not follow a normal
distribution. (These tests have been shown to be very sensitive and migh
suggest nonnormality when in fact the data are not substantially differer
from normal, so they should be interpreted with caution.) In all of these
cases, nonparametric procedures might be appropriate.

12.7 Statistical Computing

Following are the SAS programs used to conduct the nonparametric tests fc
two dependent samples, two independent samples, and k independent sample
Also included is the SAS program used to estimate a correlation based on rank
The SAS procedures and brief descriptions of their use are noted in the header t
each example. Notes are provided to the right of the SAS programs (in blue) fc
orientation purposes and are not part of the programs. In addition, blank line
in the programs are solely to accommodate the notes. Blank lines and spaces ca
be used throughout SAS programs to enhance readability. A summary of th
SAS procedures used in the examples is provided at the end of this section.

SAS EXAMPLE 12.2 Wilcoxon Signed-Rank Test: Two Dependent Samples

*Test to Determine If New Drug Lowers Systolic Blood Pressure
(Example 12.2)*

Suppose we are investigating a new drug hypothesized to lower systolic bloo
pressure. We select a random sample of subjects and record their resting sys
tolic blood pressure at baseline (i.e., prior to the investigation). Each subjec
is then given the new drug, and resting systolic blood pressure is agai

measured after 4 weeks of drug treatment. The data are shown in the following table. Based on the data, does it appear that the new drug lowers systolic
blood pressure? Run a Wilcoxon Signed-Rank test using SAS.

Subject Identification Number	Baseline Systolic Blood Pressure	Post-Treatment Systolic Blood Pressure
1	166	138
2	135	120
3	189	176
4	180	180
5	156	160
6	142	150
7	176	152
8	156	140
9	164	160
10	142	130

Program Code

`options ps=62 ls=80;`	Formats the output page to 62 lines in length and 80 columns in width
`data in;`	Beginning of Data Step
`  input baseline post_trt;`	Inputs two variables, **baseline** and **post_trt**, for each subject.
`diff=baseline-post_trt;`	Compute the difference between blood pressures (**diff**).
`cards;`	Beginning of Raw Data section.
`166 138`	actual observations
`135 120`	
`189 176`	
`180 180`	
`156 160`	
`142 150`	
`176 152`	
`156 140`	
`164 160`	
`142 130`	
`run;`	
`proc univariate normal;`	Procedure call. Proc Univariate generates summary statistics and the Wilcoxon Signed-Rank test. The normal option requests a test for normality.
`  var diff;`	Specification of analytic variable (**diff**).
`run;`	End of procedure section.

▪

SAS EXAMPLE 12.3 Wilcoxon Rank Sum Test: Two Independent Samples

Test for Difference in Treatments with Respect to Health Status (Example 12.3)

We wish to compare two competing treatments for the management of adult-onset diabetes. A total of eight subjects agree to participate in the investigation and are randomly assigned to one of the competing treatments. After subjects follow the prescribed treatment regimen for 6 weeks, we assess their self-reported health status. Subjects are asked to rate their current health using an ordinal scale with the following response options: Excellent, Very Good, Good, Fair, or Poor. Investigators often assign numerical values to ordinal responses and analyze these values as if they were continuous. The assignment of numerical values can be made in a variety of ways. Suppose we assign increasing numerical values to the response options as follows Poor = 0, Fair = 5, Good = 10, Very Good = 15, and Excellent = 20. Here higher values indicate better self-reported health status. Are self-reported health status scores different between treatment groups? Run a Wilcoxon Signed-Rank test using SAS.

Self-Reported Health Status	
Treatment 1	Treatment 2
0	8
7	10
11	12
16	15

Program Code

`options ps=62 ls=80;`	Formats the output page to 62 lines in length and 80 columns in width
`data in;`	Beginning of Data Step
`  input trt hlthstat;`	Inputs two variables, **trt** and **hlthstat**, for each subject.
`cards;`	Beginning of Raw Data section.
`1 0`	actual observations
`1 7`	
`1 11`	
`1 16`	
`2 8`	
`2 10`	
`2 12`	
`2 15`	
`run;`	

```
proc npar1way wilcoxon;
```
Procedure call. Proc Npar1way runs nonparametric tests. We request a Wilcoxon Rank Sum test by specifying the wilcoxon option.

```
    class trt;
```
Specification of grouping variable (**trt**).

```
    var hlthstat;
```
Specification of analytic variable (**hlthstat**).

```
run;
```
End of procedure section. ▪

SAS EXAMPLE 12.4 Kruskal–Wallis Test: *k* Independent Samples

Test for Difference Among Treatments with Respect to Symptom Scores (Example 12.4)

Suppose we wish to compare four treatments for seasonal allergies. A total of 20 subjects agree to participate in the investigation and are randomly assigned to one of the four competing treatments. After subjects follow the prescribed treatment regimen for 2 weeks, we assess their status. The outcome variable in this application is an index score based on three distinct symptoms. At the end of treatment, subjects are asked if they are currently experiencing any (or all) of the following symptoms: scratchy throat, itchy eyes, runny nose. Each subject responds "yes" or "no" to each of the three symptoms. This index score is the sum of affirmative responses. The range of scores is 0 (no symptoms) to 3 (all three symptoms). Is there a significant difference among the treatments with respect to symptom scores? Run a Kruskal–Wallis test using SAS.

Treatment 1	*Treatment 2*	*Treatment 3*	*Treatment 4*
0	2	0	2
0	2	0	3
1	3	1	2
2	3	1	3
3	2	1	3

Program Code

```
options ps=62 ls=80;
```
Formats the output page to 62 lines in length and 80 columns in width

```
data in;
```
Beginning of Data Step

```
  input trt symptoms;
```
Inputs two variables, **trt** and **symptoms**, for each subject.

```
cards;
1 0
1 0
1 1
1 2
1 3
2 2
2 2
2 3
2 3
2 2
3 0
3 0
3 1
3 1
3 1
4 2
4 3
4 2
4 3
4 3
run;

proc npar1way wilcoxon;


  class trt;
  var symptoms;

run;
```

Beginning of Raw Data section.
actual observations

Procedure call. Proc Npar1way runs nonparametric tests. When there are more than two comparison groups, the Kruskal–Wallis test is run.
Specification of grouping variable (**trt**).
Specification of analytic variable (**symptoms**).
End of procedure section. ■

SAS Example 12.5 Spearman (Rank) Correlation

Assess Relationship Between Number of Cigarettes Smoked per Day and Number of Hours of Exercise per Week (Example 12.5)

Suppose we wish to assess the relationship between the number of cigarettes smoked per day and the number of hours of aerobic exercise per week. A total of 12 subjects agree to participate in the investigation, and we measure the average number of cigarettes smoked per day and the number of hours of exercise in a typical week on each subject. Estimate the Spearman correlation using SAS.

Raw Scores

X = Number of Cigarettes per Day	Y = Number of Hours of Exercise per Week
20	0
0	0
20	1
10	2
5	3
4	5
3	5
5	6
0	3
0	4
0	7
0	8

Program Code

`options ps=62 ls=80;`	Formats the output page to 62 lines in length and 80 columns in width
`data in;`	Beginning of Data Step
`  input cigarett exercise;`	Inputs two variables, **cigarett** and **exercise**, for each subject.
`cards;`	Beginning of Raw Data section.
`20 0`	actual observations

```
0 0
20 1
10 2
5 3
4 5
3 5
5 6
0 3
0 4
0 7
0 8
run;
```

`proc plot;`	Procedure call. Proc Plot generates a scatter diagram.
`  plot exercise*cigarett;`	Specification of analytic variables; **exercise** is plotted on the vertical axis and **cigarett** on the horizontal.
`run;`	End of procedure section.
`proc corr spearman;`	Procedure call. Proc Corr runs a correlation analysis. The Spearman option requests that the correlation be based on ranks.
`  var exercise cigarett;`	Specification of analytic variables.
`run;`	End of procedure section.

12.7.1 Summary of SAS Procedures

The SAS procedures for nonparametric analysis are outlined in the following table. Specific options can be requested in these procedures to generate specific tests or analyses. The options are shown in italics. Users should refer to the examples in this section for complete descriptions of the procedure and specific options.

Procedure	Sample Procedure Call	Description
proc univariate	proc univariate *normal;* var diff;	Runs a Wilcoxon Signed-Rank test. The normal option produces a test for normality. The analytic variable is the difference between measures in dependent samples.
proc npar1way	proc npar1way *wilcoxon;* class group; var x;	Runs nonparametric tests for equality of medians among independent groups. The wilcoxon option requests the Wilcoxon (ranks-based) test. When the group variable is dichotomous, a Wilcoxon Rank Sum test is run; when the group variable has $k > 2$ levels a Kruskal–Wallis test is run.
proc corr	proc corr *spearman;* var x y;	Runs a correlation analysis. The Spearman option requests that the correlation be based on ranks.

12.8 Analysis of Framingham Heart Study Data

The Framingham data set includes data collected from the original cohort. Participants contributed up to three examination cycles of data. First we analyze data collected in the first examination cycle (called the period = 1 examination) and use SAS Proc Npar1way to test for differences in medians between two and more than two independent groups. We then construct a data set that contains risk factors measured at period 1 and then again at period 2 (approximately 6 years later) and evaluate changes in risk factors over time using the nonparametric procedures for two dependent samples implemented through Proc Univariate.

Framingham Data Analysis—SAS Code

```
data fhs;
   set in.frmgham;
   if period=1;
run;


proc sort data=fhs;
   by sex;
run;


proc univariate normal data=fhs;
   var glucose;
   by sex;
   where diabetes=1;
run;


proc npar2way wilcoxon data=fhs;
   class sex;
   var glucose;
   where diabetes=1;
run;


proc ttest data=fhs;
   class sex;
   var glucose;
   where diabetes=1;
run;
```

Framingham Data Analysis—SAS Output

------------------------------- SEX=M -------------------------------

The UNIVARIATE Procedure
Variable: GLUCOSE (Casual Glucose mg/dL)

Moments

N	57	Sum Weights	57
Mean	168.824561	Sum Observations	9623
Std Deviation	78.748724	Variance	6201.36153
Skewness	0.98724434	Kurtosis	0.50420161
Uncorrected SS	1971875	Corrected SS	347276.246
Coeff Variation	46.6453005	Std Error Mean	10.4305233

Basic Statistical Measures

Location		Variability	
Mean	168.8246	Std Deviation	78.74872
Median	150.0000	Variance	6201
Mode	120.0000	Range	321.00000
		Interquartile Range	99.00000

Tests for Location: Mu0=0

Test	-Statistic-	-----p Value------	
Student's t	t 16.18563	Pr > |t|	<.0001
Sign	M 28.5	Pr >= |M|	<.0001
Signed Rank	S 826.5	Pr >= |S|	<.0001

Tests for Normality

Test	--Statistic---	-----p Value------	
Shapiro-Wilk	W 0.91455	Pr < W	0.0007
Kolmogorov-Smirnov	D 0.123195	Pr > D	0.0301
Cramer-von Mises	W-Sq 0.196426	Pr > W-Sq	0.0056
Anderson-Darling	A-Sq 1.325553	Pr > A-Sq	<0.0050

Quantiles (Definition 5)

Quantile	Estimate
100% Max	394
99%	394
95%	332
90%	292
75% Q3	207

```
--------------------------- SEX=M ------------------------------
```

The UNIVARIATE Procedure
Variable: GLUCOSE (Casual Glucose mg/dL)

Quantiles (Definition 5)

Quantile	Estimate
50% Median	150
25% Q1	108
10%	80
5%	75
1%	73
0% Min	73

Extreme Observations

----Lowest----		----Highest---	
Value	Obs	Value	Obs
73	46	297	23
73	3	325	17
75	28	332	51
78	15	370	54
80	58	394	39

Missing Values

Missing Value	Count	All Obs	----Percent Of----- Missing Obs
.	2	3.39	100.00

```
------------------------------ SEX=F ------------------------------
```

The UNIVARIATE Procedure
Variable: GLUCOSE (Casual Glucose mg/dL)

Moments

N	59	Sum Weights	59
Mean	169.915254	Sum Observations	10025
Std Deviation	91.0915205	Variance	8297.66511
Skewness	0.92774764	Kurtosis	0.00307055
Uncorrected SS	2184665	Corrected SS	481264.576
Coeff Variation	53.6099722	Std Error Mean	11.8591059

                    Basic Statistical Measures
        Location   Variability
    Mean   169.9153   Std Deviation   91.09152
    Median   137.0000   Variance   8298
    Mode   107.0000   Range   347.00000
                               Interquartile Range   128.00000

NOTE: The mode displayed is the smallest of 3 modes with a count of 2

                    Tests for Location: Mu0=0
        Test   -Statistic-   -----p Value------
        Student's t   t   14.32783   Pr > |t| <.0001
        Sign   M   29.5   Pr >= |M| <.0001
        Signed Rank   S   885   Pr >= |S| <.0001

                    Tests for Normality
    Test   --Statistic---   -----p Value------
    Shapiro-Wilk   W   0.905032   Pr < W   0.0002
    Kolmogorov-Smirnov   D   0.171072   Pr > D   <0.0100
    Cramer-von Mises   W-Sq 0.333946   Pr > W-Sq   <0.0050
    Anderson-Darling   A-Sq 1.910492   Pr > A-Sq   <0.0050

                    Quantiles (Definition 5)
                    Quantile   Estimate
                    100% Max   394
                    99%   394
                    95%   368

------------------------------ SEX=F ------------------------------

                The UNIVARIATE Procedure
        Variable: GLUCOSE   (Casual Glucose mg/dL)

                    Quantiles (Definition 5)
                    Quantile   Estimate
                    90%   320
                    75% Q3   235
                    50% Median   137
                    25% Q1   107
                    10%   78
                    5%   57
                    1%   47
                    0% Min   47

Extreme Observations

----Lowest----		----Highest---	
Value	Obs	Value	Obs
47	27	348	55
55	2	366	19
57	43	368	54
63	18	386	30
66	21	394	38

Missing Values

		----Percent Of-----	
Missing Value	Count	All Obs	Missing Obs
.	3	4.84	100.00

The NPAR1WAY Procedure

Wilcoxon Scores (Rank Sums) for Variable GLUCOSE
Classified by Variable SEX

SEX	N	Sum of Scores	Expected Under H0	Std Dev Under H0	Mean Score
M	57	3388.50	3334.50	181.070365	59.447368
F	59	3397.50	3451.50	181.070365	57.584746

Average scores were used for ties.

Wilcoxon Two-Sample Test

Statistic	3388.5000

Normal Approximation
Z	0.2955
One-Sided Pr > Z	0.3838
Two-Sided Pr > |Z|	0.7676

t Approximation
One-Sided Pr > Z	0.3841
Two-Sided Pr > |Z|	0.7682

Z includes a continuity correction of 0.5.

Kruskal-Wallis Test

Chi-Square	0.0889
DF	1
Pr > Chi-Square	0.7655

The TTEST Procedure

Statistics

Variable	SEX	N	Lower CL Mean	Mean	Upper CL Mean	Lower CL Std Dev	Std Dev
GLUCOSE	M	57	147.93	168.82	189.72	66.484	78.749
GLUCOSE	F	59	146.18	169.92	193.65	77.112	91.092
GLUCOSE	Diff (1-2)		-32.46	-1.091	30.275	75.477	85.252

Statistics

Variable	SEX	Upper CL Std Dev	Std Err	Minimum	Maximum
GLUCOSE	M	96.605	10.431	73	394
GLUCOSE	F	111.31	11.859	47	394
GLUCOSE	Diff (1-2)	97.959	15.833		

T-Tests

Variable	Method	Variances	DF	t Value	Pr > |t|
GLUCOSE	Pooled	Equal	114	-0.07	0.9452
GLUCOSE	Satterthwaite	Unequal	113	-0.07	0.9451

Equality of Variances

Variable	Method	Num DF	Den DF	F Value	Pr > F
GLUCOSE	Folded F	58	56	1.34	0.2758

We used SAS to first generate descriptive statistics on GLUCOSE levels in male and female participants with diabetes. Is the distribution of glucose levels approximately normal for men and women? We then ran a Wilcoxon Rank Sum test to compare median glucose levels for male and female diabetics. Are the medians similar or different? For comparison purposes, we also ran a *t* test comparing mean glucose levels. How do the nonparametric and parametric tests compare? Which test is appropriate here?

Framingham Data Analysis—SAS Code

```
data fhs1;
   set in.frmgham;
   if period=1;

glucose1=glucose;
keep randid sex glucose1 diabetes;
run;

data fhs2;
   set in.frmgham;
   if period=2;

glucose2=glucose;
keep randid glucose2;
run;

proc sort data=fhs1; by randid; run;
proc sort data=fhs2; by randid; run;

data fhs12;
   merge fhs1(in=a)  fhs2(in=b);
   by randid;
   if a and b;

diffglucose=glucose2-glucose1;
run;

proc univariate normal data=fhs12;
   var diffglucose;
run;
```

We created two data sets, called fhs1 and fhs2, which contain the glucose data measured at periods 1 and 2, respectively. We then merged them into a single data set so that the period 1 and period 2 values are together (one SAS record per participant). In the merged data set, we created a difference score by subtracting the glucose measured at period 1 from the glucose measured at period 2. The difference reflects how much the glucose level changed over time (specifically, how it increased from period 1 to period 2). In the following, we used SAS Proc Univariate to test for differences in glucose levels over time among participants with diabetes. Here we perform a nonparametric test.

Framingham Data Analysis—SAS Output

The UNIVARIATE Procedure
Variable: diffglucose

Moments

N	71	Sum Weights	71
Mean	-11.492958	Sum Observations	-816
Std Deviation	64.8745764	Variance	4208.71066
Skewness	-0.7233025	Kurtosis	0.68490171
Uncorrected SS	303988	Corrected SS	294609.746
Coeff Variation	-564.47242	Std Error Mean	7.69919574

Basic Statistical Measures

Location		Variability	
Mean	-11.4930	Std Deviation	64.87458
Median	4.0000	Variance	4209
Mode	5.0000	Range	315.00000
		Interquartile Range	86.00000

Tests for Location: Mu0=0

Test	-Statistic-		-----p Value-----	
Student's t	t	-1.49275	Pr > |t|	0.1400
Sign	M	1.5	Pr >= |M|	0.8126
Signed Rank	S	-169.5	Pr >= |S|	0.3350

Tests for Normality

Test	---Statistic---		------p Value-----	
Shapiro-Wilk	W	0.965272	Pr < W	0.0466
Kolmogorov-Smirnov	D	0.109515	Pr > D	0.0343
Cramer-von Mises	W-Sq	0.087716	Pr > W-Sq	0.1657
Anderson-Darling	A-Sq	0.574876	Pr > A-Sq	0.1356

Quantiles (Definition 5)

Quantile	Estimate
100% Max	105
99%	105
95%	84
90%	66
75% Q3	34
50% Median	4
25% Q1	-52

How much did glucose change over time? Is the distribution of change over time approximately normal? Is there a significant difference in median glucose over time? Is there a significant difference in mean glucose over time?

12.9 Problems

1. A study is conducted comparing two competing medications for asthma. Sixteen subjects are involved in the investigation. The data shown reflect asthma symptom scores for patients randomly assigned to each treatment. Higher scores are indicative of worse asthma symptoms. Test the null hypothesis that there is no difference in asthma symptoms between medications. Run the Wilcoxon Rank Sum test using the normal approximation at a 5% level of significance.

Treatment A:	55	60	80	65	72	78	68	71
Treatment B:	80	82	86	89	76	81	90	76

2. We wish to evaluate a program designed to improve quality of life in older patients with coronary heart disease. Quality of life is measured on a scale of 0–100, with higher scores indicative of better quality of life. Quality-of-life measures are taken on each subject at baseline and then again after participating in the program. Based on the following data, is there evidence that the program significantly improves quality of life? Run the Wilcoxon Signed-Rank test using the normal approximation at a 5% level of significance.

Baseline:	80	55	63	76	88	45	65	77
Post-Program:	85	50	65	78	82	55	68	90

3. Data were collected from a random sample of eight patients currently undergoing treatment for hypertension. Each subject reported the average number of cigarettes smoked per day and was assigned a numerical value reflecting risk of cardiovascular disease (CVD). The risk assessments were computed by physicians and based on blood pressure, cholesterol level, and exercise status. The risk assessments ranged from 0 to 100, higher values indicating increased risk. Compute the Spearman correlation coefficient.

Number of Cigarettes:	0	2	6	8	12	0	2	20
Risk of CVD:		12	20	50	68	75	8	10	80

4. Suppose we are interested in whether there is a difference between the mean numbers of sick days taken by men and women in a local company. The numbers of sick days taken by men and women are shown here. Use the data to test the null hypothesis that there is no difference in sick days between men and women. Run the Wilcoxon Rank Sum test using the normal approximation at a 5% level of significance.

Men:	5	10	2	0	6	4	5	15
Women:	8	9	3	5	0	4	15	

5. A nutritionist is investigating the effects of a rigorous walking program on systolic blood pressure (SBP) in patients with mild hypertension.

Subjects who agree to participate have their systolic blood pressure measured at the start of the study and then after completing the 6-week walking program. The data are

Subject	Starting SBP	Ending SBP
1	140	128
2	130	125
3	150	140
4	160	162
5	135	137
6	128	130
7	142	135
8	151	140

Based on the data, is there evidence that SBP is significantly reduced by the walking program? Run the Wilcoxon Signed-Rank test using the normal approximation at a 5% level of significance.

6. An antismoking campaign is being evaluated prior to its implementation in high schools across the state. A pilot study involving six volunteers who smoke is conducted. Each volunteer reports the number of cigarettes smoked the day before enrolling in the study. Each is then subjected to the antismoking campaign, which involves educational material, support groups, formal programs designed to reduce or quit smoking, etc. After 4 weeks, each volunteer again reports the number of cigarettes smoked the day before. Based on the following pilot data, does it appear that the program is effective?

At Enrollment:	21	15	8	6	12	20
After Campaign:	12	10	10	6	10	20

Run the Wilcoxon Signed-Rank test using the normal approximation at a 5% level of significance.

SAS Problems

Use SAS to solve the following problems.

1. A study is conducted comparing two competing medications for asthma. Sixteen subjects are involved in the investigation. The data shown reflect asthma symptom scores for patients randomly assigned to each treatment. Higher scores are indicative of worse asthma symptoms. Test the null hypothesis that there is no difference in asthma symptoms between medications.

Treatment A:	55	60	80	65	72	78	68	71
Treatment B:	80	82	86	89	76	81	90	76

Use SAS Proc Univariate to run the Wilcoxon Signed-Rank test. Include the option to perform a test for normality.

2. We wish to evaluate a program designed to improve quality of life in older patients with coronary heart disease. Quality of life is measured on a scale of 0–100, with higher scores indicative of better quality of life. Quality-of-life measures are taken on each subject at baseline and then again after participating in the program. Based on the following data, is there evidence that the program significantly improves quality of life?

Baseline:	80	55	63	76	88	45	65	77
Post-Program:	85	50	65	78	82	55	68	90

Use SAS to perform a Wilcoxon Rank Sum test. Perform the test at a 5% level of significance.

3. A pharmaceutical company is interested in the effectiveness of a new preparation designed to relieve arthritis pain. Three variations of the compound have been prepared for investigation, which differ according to the proportion of the active ingredients: T15 contains 15% active ingredients, T40 contains 40% active ingredients, and T50 contains 50% active ingredients. A sample of 20 patients is selected to participate in a study comparing the three variations of the compound. A control compound, which is currently available over the counter, is also included in the investigation. Patients are randomly assigned to one of the four treatments (control, T15, T40, T50) and the time (in minutes) until pain relief is recorded on each subject. The data are

Control:	12	15	18	16	20
T15:	20	21	22	19	20
T40:	17	16	19	15	19
T50:	14	13	12	14	11

Use SAS to perform a Kruskal–Wallis test. Perform the test at a 5% level of significance.

4. Data were collected from a random sample of eight patients currently undergoing treatment for hypertension. Each subject reported the average number of cigarettes smoked per day and each was assigned a numerical value reflecting risk of cardiovascular disease (CVD). The risk assessments were computed by physicians and based on blood pressure, cholesterol level, and exercise status. The risk assessments ranged from 0 to 100, higher values indicating increased risk.

Number of Cigarettes:	0	2	6	8	12	0	2	20
Risk of CVD:		12	20	50	68	75	8	10	80

Use SAS to estimate the Spearman correlation coefficient. Test if the correlation is significant using a 5% level of significance.

Descriptive Statistics
(Ch. 2)

Probability
(Ch. 3)

Sampling Distributions
(Ch. 4)

Statistical Inference
(Chapters 5–13)

OUTCOME VARIABLE	GROUPING VARIABLE(S)/ PREDICTOR(S)	ANALYSIS	CHAPTER(S)
Continuous	—	Estimate μ; Compare μ to Known, Historical Value	5/12
Continuous	Dichotomous (2 groups)	Compare Independent Means (Estimate/Test $(\mu_1 - \mu_2)$) or the Mean Difference (μ_d)	6/12
Continuous	Discrete (>2 groups)	Test the Equality of k Means using Analysis of Variance $(\mu_1 = \mu_2 = \cdots = \mu_k)$	9/12
Continuous	Continuous	Estimate Correlation or Determine Regression Equation	10/12
Continuous	Several Continuous or Dichotomous	Multiple Linear Regression Analysis	10
Dichotomous	—	Estimate p; Compare p to Known, Historical Value	7
Dichotomous	Dichotomous (2 groups)	Compare Independent Proportions (Estimate/Test $(p_1 - p_2)$)	7/8
Dichotomous	Discrete (>2 groups)	Test the Equality of k Proportions (Chi-Square Test)	7
Dichotomous	Several Continuous or Dichotomous	Multiple Logistic Regression Analysis	11
Discrete	Discrete	Compare Distributions Among k Populations (Chi-Square Test)	7
Time to Event	Several Continuous or Dichotomous	Survival Analysis	13

13

Introduction to Survival Analysis

In Chapter 6 we presented estimation and statistical inference procedures for crude or unadjusted comparisons of two groups with respect to a continuous outcome variable. When the outcome variable in a prospective study or a clinical trial (i.e., a study in which the outcome is measured subsequent to treatment allocation) is continuous, the effect measure is the difference in means. The test of the effect of treatment is carried out using a two independent sample *t* test. To adjust for other variables when the outcome is continuous, multiple regression analysis can be used, as described in Chapter 10.

In Chapter 8 we presented estimation and statistical inference procedures for crude or unadjusted comparisons of two proportions and a technique for estimation and statistical inference adjusting for one categorical confounder. In Chapter 11 we presented logistic regression, which can be used to model the effect of independent variables on the risk of a dichotomous outcome. When the outcome variable in a prospective study or a clinical trial is dichotomous, the effect measure is the relative risk and the crude test of the effect of treatment is carried out using a chi-square test. If there are confounders to consider, the adjusted effect is assessed using the Cochran–Mantel–Haenszel chi-square statistic or with logistic regression analysis.

In this section we give a brief overview of survival analysis, which is used to compare groups with respect to a dichotomous outcome, as is logistic regression, but survival analysis techniques also takes into account different lengths of follow-up. Survival analysis techniques are used to estimate risks using all available data and are also used to estimate survival over time and to compare groups with respect to time to an event. Survival analysis techniques are beyond the scope of this book, but we do present a brief heuristic explanation of the theory.

13.1 Incomplete Follow-Up

In Chapters 8 and 11, we described procedures to compare proportions or risks between comparison groups. Some studies involve a long follow-up or observation period during which time each participant is measured for the occurrence or nonoccurrence of the event of interest. When the follow-up or observation period is long, subjects may withdraw from the study before the end of the observation period. Some might move or simply decide that they no longer wish to participate. These subjects are often termed "lost to follow-up." In addition, subjects may die during the study period. Subjects who are lost to follow-up or who die during the study period do not contribute to the overall counts of outcomes measured at the end of the study period, but their data should be included as much as possible in all analyses.

EXAMPLE 13.1   **Risk of Stroke**

Consider a very small study of five subjects in which the outcome of interest is stroke. Suppose that the study period is 5 years; that is, subjects are classified at the end of 5 years according to whether or not they had a stroke. Now suppose that among the five subjects in our study, two have strokes (after 2 and 3 years, respectively), one completes the 5-year period free of stroke, one subject dies after 1 year, and one subject drops out of the study after 4 years.

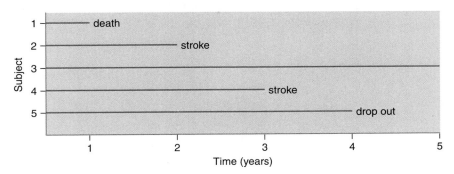

Based on these data, what can we say about the 5-year risk of stroke? We could restrict our analysis to those whose 5-year data are available, excluding the subject who died during the study period and the subject who dropped out. This would yield a 5-year risk estimate of $2/3 = 67\%$. However, the person who dropped out survived for 4 of the 5 years free of stroke, and the person who died survived for 1 year free of stroke. Thus, our estimate is probably too high. In fact, if we estimated 1-year, 2-year, 3-year, and 4-year risks of stroke using this method, we would obtain estimates of 0% (0/5), 25% (1/4), 50% (2/4), and 50% (2/4), respectively. Then, with no additional strokes, our 5-year estimate jumps to 67%! ▪

EXAMPLE 13.2   **Risk of Stroke Using Conditional Probabilities**

Suppose we sample a group of $n = 100$ individuals from a population and follow them for 2 years. The goal is to estimate the probability of surviving for 2 years. Twenty people die each year, and we estimate the 2-year survival probability as 0.60 (60/100).

Suppose that we then sample another group of $n = 100$ from the same population and follow them for 1 year. Seventy-five people survive. How can we use this additional information to better estimate the 2-year survival probability?

Recall the *conditional probability rule* from Chapter 3,

$$P(B \mid A) = \frac{P(A \text{ and } B)}{P(A)}$$

We can rewrite this as $P(A \text{ and } B) = P(A)P(B \mid A)$ and apply it to the example. Let A = survive year 1 and B = survive year 2. Then, using sample 1 only,

$$P(A) = P(\text{survive year 1}) = 80/100 = 0.80$$
$$P(B \mid A) = P(\text{survive year 2 given survival through year 1}) = 60/80 = 0.75$$
$$P(A \text{ and } B) = P(\text{survive both years}) = P(A)P(B \mid A) = (0.80)(0.75) = 0.60$$

Note that this is the correct survival probability.

Now we can use the combined data from the two samples to estimate year 1 survival by combining the two samples:

$$P(A) = P(\text{survive year 1 (both samples combined)})$$
$$= \frac{(80 + 75)}{(100 + 100)} = 155/200 = 0.775$$

$$P(A \text{ and } B) = P(\text{survive both years}) = P(A)P(B \mid A) = (0.775)(0.75) = 0.58$$

Notice that $P(A)$ is based on the combined sample and $P(B \mid A)$ is based on sample 1 only. Thus our estimate of 2-year survival is 0.60 if we only use sample 1 but is 0.58 if we include all available data. Survival analysis techniques allow us to do this. ■

13.2 Time to Event

Another application of survival analysis techniques is based on the date at which events occur, in addition to they simply do or do not occur.

EXAMPLE 13.3 **Risk of Stroke Using Time to Event Data**

Consider another very small study of five subjects in which the outcome of interest is stroke, also with a 5-year study period. Suppose that in this study we have complete data, and that two of the five participants had strokes during the study period. The estimated 5-year risk of stroke is thus $2/5 = 40\%$. Consider the following two graphs:

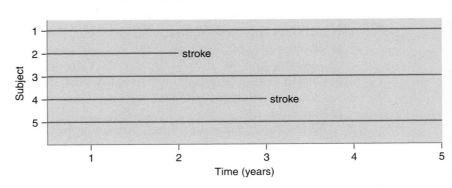

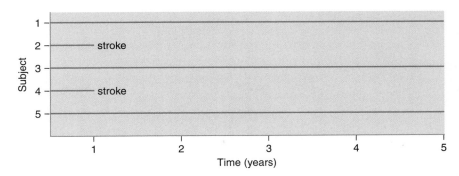

In both cases, there are two strokes among the five subjects. However, the strokes in the first graph occur much later than those in the second graph. Using a simple proportion to estimate risk yields does not allow us to distinguish these two scenarios. Survival analysis techniques take into account time to event in addition to the occurrence of the event.   ■

13.3 Survival Analysis Techniques

Survival analysis methods are used when the time to event is important and/or when there are withdrawals or losses to follow-up. The probability of survival through a specified time is calculated using (a) the probability of survival through the previous interval and (b) the conditional probability of surviving the current interval given survival through the previous interval.

The Kaplan–Meier method creates a new interval each time there is an event; the life table method uses prespecified intervals, such as months or years. Cox regression analysis allows the inclusion of potential confounders in survival analysis models. We will not present these techniques here, but we encourage the reader to explore them in more advanced texts.

Introduction to Statistical Computing Using SAS

A.1 Introduction to SAS

A *SAS program* is a list of commands in the SAS language. We use the SAS editor to create SAS programs and then execute them using the *submit* command. The components of a SAS program are outlined in the following sections. When a SAS program is executed, a *log* and *output* are produced. The program, log, and output, described in detail here, can be printed and/or saved in files on your computer (or computer account).

SAS can be implemented on a variety of operating platforms (e.g., personal computer, mainframe). The operating platform does not dramatically change the structure and operation of the program. SAS can also be implemented in several operational modes, including a mode in which the user enters SAS program code to perform a specific application as well as a menu-driven mode in which the user selects the desired statistical application from a list of options by pointing and clicking. In the following, we illustrate the use of SAS in the former mode, in all cases specifying the SAS code to perform specific analyses.

A.1.1 Components of a SAS Program

Each basic SAS program is made up of three components:

- The **Data Step,** which contains variable names and labels
- The **Raw Data Section,** or the actual observations considered for analysis

■ The **Procedure Section,** which contains the call statements for the appropriate statistical analysis (e.g., summary statistics, two-sample *t* test, analysis of variance); several procedures can be invoked in this section to perform the desired analyses

The following sample SAS program displays each component. The parts of the program presented in boldface represent those that are specific to each application and can be changed, as appropriate, by the user. The notes to the right of the SAS program (in blue) are for orientation and are not part of the program. In addition, the blank lines are there only to accommodate the notes. In practice, the SAS program will be single-spaced. Indentation is used solely for readability and does not influence processing.

Sample SAS Program

Notes

Sample SAS Program	Notes
`data` **`one;`**	Beginning of the Data Step. SAS allows the user to choose a data set name (e.g., **one**).
`input` **`x;`**	Specification of variables. Here we consider a single variable which we name **x**.
`cards;`	Beginning of the Raw Data section.
5	Actual observations—one observation (**x**) per subject.
6	
12	
`run;`	End of the Raw Data section.
`proc print;`	SAS Procedure that prints the data.
`var` **`x;`**	Specification of the variable to be printed (**x**).
`run;`	End of the Procedure call.
`proc means;`	SAS Procedure to generate summary statistics (e.g., mean, standard deviation).
`var` **`x;`**	Specification of the analytic variable (**x**).
`run;`	End of the Procedure call.

The data set called **one** is a temporary SAS data set and exists only for the duration of the program execution. It does not exist after the SAS session is over and it will not be saved. It is, however, possible to create permanent SAS data sets. At this point, our focus is on small, temporary data sets.

The statements that make up a SAS program are generally called the SAS code. The three components of SAS programs will be discussed in detail in subsequent sections.

The sample SAS program shown produces the following output. The notes to the right of the SAS output (in blue) are for orientation and are not part of the output. In addition, the blank lines are there only to accommodate the notes. In practice, the SAS output will be single-spaced.

Sample SAS Output

Notes

```
OBS  X
 1   5
 2   6
 3   12
```

Output from the Print Procedure:
SAS prints a column labeled "OBS"
   denoting the observation number, followed by each
   value of the variable x.

```
Analysis Variable: X
```

Output from the Means Procedure:
Summary statistics (See Chapter 3 for a complete discussion).

```
N      Mean      Std Dev     Minimum      Maximum
-------------------------------------------------

3      7.666     3.7859      5.0000       12.0000
-------------------------------------------------
```

A.1.2 Overview of the SAS System

SAS uses three windows to display information:

- The **PROGRAM,** or **PGM** Window (also called the Editor or Advanced Editor Window), which contains the SAS program code
- The **LOG** Window, which displays the SAS execution statements, notes, error messages, etc.
- The **OUTPUT,** or **OUT** Window, which displays the results of the statistical analysis

Throughout this book we present SAS programs and corresponding output. We do not illustrate the contents of the LOG Window. The information in the LOG Window is very useful, primarily to verify that the data are read correctly by SAS and that the procedure statements are entered and interpreted appropriately.

To view the contents of any window (i.e., PGM, LOG, or OUTPUT), simply click on any part of that window. The box in the top corner of each window (i.e., PGM, LOG, or OUTPUT) is used to maximize or minimize the window. Clicking on the box will enlarge or shrink the current window display.

Program creation, editing, and execution may be simplified by using the command line option within SAS. To move from one window to another, click on any part of that window or type <u>PGM</u>, <u>LOG</u>, or <u>OUTPUT</u> in the command line at the top of any window, followed by [enter] to move to the PROGRAM, LOG, and OUTPUT windows, respectively.

The following table displays some of the more commonly used SAS commands, a description of their functions, and the windows in which the commands are used. All commands are issued in the command line. Either the arrow keys or the [Home] key, which moves the cursor directly to the command line, can be used to move to the command line.

On some platforms, SAS also displays a toolbox window where commands can be issued to perform specific functions. Commands that are issued at the command line (see table) can also be issued in the appropriate space in the toolbox window. The toolbox also has some built-in functions that appear as buttons in the toolbox window (e.g., submit, cut, copy, paste). Specific functions can be performed using the buttons.

SAS COMMAND	*Function*	*Windows*
submit	executes SAS program	PGM
recall	recalls last program executed into the PGM window	PGM
file filename (ext[1])	saves the contents of window into the file named "filename"	PGM (use ext=SAS) LOG (use ext=LOG) OUTPUT (use ext=LST)
inc filename	includes a copy of the file named "filename.sas" in the PGM window	PGM
pgm	moves to the PROGRAM window	LOG OUTPUT
log	moves to the LOG window	PGM OUTPUT
out	moves to the OUTPUT window	PGM LOG
help	displays online help	PGM LOG OUTPUT
clear	clears the contents of the window	PGM LOG OUTPUT
bye	exits SAS	PGM LOG OUTPUT

[1] The extension (ext) is a three-character code used to distinguish between program files (extension 'SAS'), log files (extension 'LOG'), and output files (extension 'LST'). SAS *automatically* appends these extensions when you save code in a particular window.

A.1.3 Creating and Executing a SAS Program

The following is a step-by-step guide to creating and executing a SAS program. The guide can be applied in any statistical computing application presented in this book.

1. Start SAS (Type SAS).
2. Click on the PGM window (or enter PGM from LOG or OUTPUT command lines).
3. Enter the program code (statements) by typing directly into the SAS Program window. The SAS Program editor has line numbers in the left-hand margin. The program code is typed to the right of the line numbers. The column directly adjacent to the line numbers is reserved and cannot be used to enter data or program code. The arrow keys can be used to move around in the SAS Program editor to edit the program. Typing SAS commands into the SAS editor creates a *temporary* SAS program file, which you will save as a *permanent* program file after checking that it works correctly.
4. Once the program code is complete, execute the program. Move the cursor to the command line in the PGM window (use arrow keys or [Home] key). Enter <u>submit</u>.
5. Check the LOG for error messages and for documentation of desired procedure.
   If there are errors (in which case no output appears in the OUTPUT Window) or if the program did not execute correctly, do the following:

   a. Return to the PGM window (click on PGM window or type PGM followed by [enter] in command line of LOG window). Recall the SAS program by typing <u>recall</u> followed by [enter] in the command line of the PGM window.

   b. Edit the program code to fix the errors and/or modify the code to perform the desired analysis. Use the arrow keys to move around within the program window.

   c. Go to the LOG window (click on LOG window or enter LOG in command line of the PGM window). At the command line, type <u>clear</u> followed by [enter] to clear the contents of the window for the next program execution.

   d. Go to the OUTPUT window (click on OUTPUT window or enter OUT in command line of current window). At the command line, type <u>clear</u> followed by [enter] to clear the contents of the window for the next program execution.

e. Return to the PGM window (click on PGM window or type PGM followed by [enter] in command line of OUTPUT window).

f. Return to step 4 and continue the process.

If there are no errors, then continue to step 6.

6. Save the SAS PROGRAM code, the LOG, and the SAS OUTPUT into files by performing the following steps:

a. Return to the PGM window (click on PGM window or enter PGM in command line of current window).

Recall the SAS program by typing recall followed by [enter] in the command line.

At the command line, type file 'filename' followed by [enter], where filename is the selected name. The '.sas' extension is automatically appended to the filename.

b. Go to the LOG window (click on LOG window or enter LOG in command line of current window).

At the command line, type file 'filename' followed by [enter]. The '.log' extension is automatically appended to the filename.

c. Go to the OUTPUT window (click on OUTPUT window or enter OUTPUT in the command line of current window). At the command line, type file 'filename' followed by [enter]. The '.lst' extension is automatically appended to the filename.

** You have now saved three files on your computer or computer account called filename.sas, filename.log, and filename.lst.

7. Exit SAS by typing **bye** followed by [enter] in the command line of the current window.

8. Print hard copies of the three files (program, log, and output) using the appropriate print command on your system. For example, print filename.pgm [enter], print filename.log [enter], and print filename.out [enter]

9. Log off or sign off the system using the appropriate logout command.

A.2 The Data Step

The Data Step, the first component of a SAS program, contains (among other items) the variable names, specifications, and labels. We will illustrate a variety of programming statements that can be used in the Data Step.

SAS, like many computing languages, offers a variety of options for inputting and manipulating data. SAS can read and analyze both numeric and alphanumeric, or character, data. We present several different techniques for inputting and manipulating data in the following Data Step. Sample data sets are provided to illustrate each technique.

A.2.1 Inputting Data: Types of Data

In SAS, data are classified as numeric, alphanumeric (or character), or date variables (e.g., 01/15/1998). Numeric data include numbers, such as 48, 4.8, and 0.48. SAS expects to read and analyze numeric data and no special considerations are necessary to input numeric data. Alphanumeric data, or character data, include letters and symbols (and possibly numbers). These include data elements, such as male, female, M, or F. To input character data, you must inform SAS that the data are character as opposed to numeric. To do this, simply follow the variable name in the input statement with a "$" symbol, which denotes a character variable. The following data set includes age (in years) and gender (denoted M or F) recorded on each of four subjects:

```
20 F
32 M
24 F
31 M
```

The following SAS code will correctly input the data:

```
data one;
  input age gender $;
cards;
20 F
32 M
24 F
31 M
run;
proc print;
run;
```

The following output is produced by the Print procedure. Since no variables are specified (e.g., var age), SAS prints the values of all of the variables in the data set. Note that SAS inserts a column labeled "OBS," indicating the observation numbers:

OBS	AGE	GENDER
1	20	F
2	32	M
3	24	F
4	31	M

A.2.2 Inputting Data: Types of Input

Two of the more common techniques for inputting data are (1) list, or free, for mat, and (2) column, or fixed, format. (A third technique, formatted data, i described in Section A.2.4. "Advanced Data Input and Data Manipulation") To illustrate the different techniques, consider the following data set, which includes four variables (listed in the columns below) recorded on five subject (listed on each row):

10	12	11	1.4
22	12	99	4.3
15	12	64	3.1
12	5	3	8.9
99	45	66	0.5

A. LIST, OR FREE, FORMAT

As long as the data are separated by at least one space, the following SAS cod may be used to input the data. The data do not have to be lined up in columns only separated by one or more spaces on each line. Notice that four variables called x1, x2, x3 and x4, are input.

```
data one;
  input x1 x2 x3 x4;
cards;
10        12      11      1.4
22        12      99      4.3
15        12      64      3.1
12         5       3      8.9
99        45      66      0.5
run;
proc print;
run;
```

B. COLUMN, OR FIXED, FORMAT

If the data set is rectangular (i.e., the observations are lined up in columns and rows), then the following SAS code is used to input the data, where the num bers following each variable name denote the columns in which the actua data elements are located in the Raw Data section.

```
data one;
  input x1 1-2 x2 4-5 x3 7-8 x4 10-12;
cards;
10 12 11 1.4
22 12 99 4.3
```

```
15 12 64 3.1
12  5  3 8.9
99 45 66 0.5
run;
proc print;
run;
```

Both programs shown produce the following output:

OBS	X1	X2	X3	X4
1	10	12	11	1.4
2	22	12	99	4.3
3	15	12	64	3.1
4	12	5	3	8.9
5	99	45	66	0.5

A.2.3 Missing Values

Every effort should always be made to ensure that data are complete and accurate. However, even with intense effort on the part of investigators, it is not always possible to obtain values for every variable under study for each subject.

For example, suppose a study is conducted in which seven variables are measured on each of five subjects: height (in inches), weight (in pounds), systolic blood pressure (in mmHg), diastolic blood pressure (in mmHg), gender (M or F), age (in years), and race (Asian, Black, Hispanic, Other, White). Suppose that one subject does not have his weight measured and another does not report her race. We would not want to eliminate these subjects altogether since there are some variables collected on these subjects that are nonmissing and can be analyzed.

SAS can input and maintain missing data values. Missing values of numeric variables (e.g., sbp) are denoted by a period ".”; missing values of alphanumeric, or character, variables are denoted by a blank space " ". The following data set includes seven variables measured on five subjects and includes two missing values. Notice that the missing values are denoted with a period or a blank space (without quotation marks) for the numeric and alphanumeric variables, respectively.

```
63  145  135  70  F  32  black
67  132  120  60  F  31  hispanic
60  117  130  80  F  33
68  187  140  60  M  26  white
72  145   .   55  M  29  white
```

The following SAS code inputs seven variables using column formats:

```
data one;
  input height 1-2 weight 4-6 sbp 8-10 dbp 12-13
         gender $ 15 age 17-18 race $ 20-27;
cards;
63   145   135   70   F   32   black
67   132   120   60   F   31   hispanic
60   117   130   80   F   33
68   187   140   60   M   26   white
72   145    .    55   M   29   white
run;
proc print;
run;
```

The following output is produced by the Print procedure.

OBS	HEIGHT	WEIGHT	SBP	DBP	GENDER	AGE	RACE
1	63	145	135	70	F	32	black
2	67	132	120	60	F	31	hispanic
3	60	117	130	80	F	33	
4	68	187	140	60	M	26	white
5	72	.	145	55	M	29	white

A.2.4 Advanced Data Input and Data Manipulation*

*This section contains advanced statistical computing techniques. It is de
signed for more advanced users and can be omitted without disrupting the
progression of material.

This section covers inputting formatted data, the use of line pointers, and
the drop and keep functions.

INPUTTING FORMATTED DATA

If a data set is rectangular, the following SAS code may be used to input the
data, where the "@" symbol "points to" the starting column location of each
variable and the number following each variable name denotes the variable for
mat (e.g., 2.0 denotes a variable of length 2 with no decimal places, 3.1 denotes
a variable of length 3 with 1 decimal place). *Note:* 2. can be used in place of 2.0

```
data one;
  input @1 x1 2.0 @4 x2 2.0 @7 x3 2.0 @10 x4 3.1;
```

Notice that x1, x2, and x3 all have the same format (2.0). The following SAS code is equivalent:

```
data one;
  input (x1 x2 x3) (2. 2. 2.) @10 x4 3.1;
```

The following is also equivalent, where the "+1" moves the column pointer to the right 1 column after inputting x1, x2, and x3:

```
data one;
  input (x1-x3) (2. +1) @10 x4 3.1;
```

SAS allows the user to mix input options (e.g., formatted input and list, or free, format):

```
data one;
  input (x1-x3) (2. +1) x4;
```

INPUTTING DATA: LINE POINTERS

In addition to the column pointers, just illustrated, SAS allows the user to manipulate the rows, or lines, in a data set. For example, suppose we record total serum cholesterol values on a sample of five subjects at three different points in time. The data set consists of three lines (rows) per person, with exam 1 values for total cholesterol on the first line, exam 2 values on the second line, and exam 3 values on the third line. The data follow; the first entry on each line (row) is the exam number (i.e., 1, 2, or 3), the second entry is the subject identifier (sequential numbers), and the third entry is the observed total cholesterol value. A "." denotes a missing value.

1 1 180	exam number=1, subject identifier=1, cholesterol=180
2 1 160	exam number=2, subject identifier=1, cholesterol=160
3 1 177	exam number=3, subject identifier=1, cholesterol=177
1 2 240	exam number=1, subject identifier=2, cholesterol=240
2 2 220	
3 2 146	
1 3 .	
2 3 230	
3 3 210	
1 4 170	
2 4 200	
3 4 240	
1 5 180	
2 5 .	
3 5 190	exam number=3, subject identifier=5, cholesterol=190

The data are input as follows. The "#" symbol denotes the line number in the data set; the numbers following the variable names denote the columns in which the data are stored. Notice that the exam number (i.e., 1, 2, 3), stored in column 1 on each line, is ignored (i.e., not input).

```
data one;
  input #1 id 3 tc1 5-7
        #2 tc2 5-7
        #3 tc3 5-7;
cards;
1 1 180
2 1 160
3 1 177
1 2 240
2 2 220
3 2 146
1 3  .
2 3 230
3 3 210
1 4 170
2 4 200
3 4 240
1 5 180
2 5  .
3 5 190
run;
proc print;
run;
```

The Print procedure generates the following output:

```
OBS   ID   TC1   TC2   TC3
1     1    180   160   177
2     2    240   220   146
3     3     .    230   210
4     4    170   200   240
5     5    180    .    190
```

THE DROP FUNCTION

Suppose (for the same data set) we are only interested in the first two exams. The "drop" function can be used to remove variables from a data set. Note that the data are never deleted or removed permanently—a *variable* is simply omitted from a SAS data set:

```
data one;
  input #1 id 3 tc1 5-7
        #2 tc2 5-7
        #3 tc3 5-7;
  drop tc3;
cards;
1 1 180
2 1 160
3 1 177
1 2 240
2 2 220
3 2 146
1 3 .
2 3 230
3 3 210
1 4 170
2 4 200
3 4 240
1 5 180
2 5 .
3 5 190
run;
proc print;
run;
```

Or equivalently:

```
data one;
  input #1 id 3 tc1 5-7
        #2 tc2 5-7
        #3;
cards;
1 1 180
2 1 160
3 1 177
1 2 240
2 2 220
3 2 146
1 3 .
2 3 230
3 3 210
1 4 170
```

```
2 4 200
3 4 240
1 5 180
2 5 .
3 5 190
run;
proc print;
run;
```

NOTE: The #3 indicates that there are three lines of data per subject and is necessary so
that the correct observations are read from the appropriate lines in the data set.

Both programs shown produce the following output:

```
OBS        ID        TC1        TC2
1          1         180        160
2          2         240        220
3          3          .         230
4          4         170        200
5          5         180         .
```

Suppose we only want the second exam:

```
data one;
  input #1 id 3 tc1 5-7
        #2 tc2 5-7
        #3;
  drop tc1;
cards;
1 1 180
2 1 160
3 1 177
1 2 240
2 2 220
3 2 146
1 3 .
2 3 230
3 3 210
1 4 170
2 4 200
3 4 240
1 5 180
2 5 .
3 5 190
```

```
run;
proc print;
run;
```

The following program is equivalent and illustrates the use of line holders. The "@" symbol at the end of an input line holds the pointer at that line until the next input statement.

```
data one;
  input exam 1 @;
  if exam eq 2 then input id 3 tc2 5-7;
cards;
1 1 180
2 1 160
3 1 177
1 2 240
2 2 220
3 2 146
1 3 .
2 3 230
3 3 210
1 4 170
2 4 200
3 4 240
1 5 180
2 5 .
3 5 190
run;
proc print;
run;
```

Both programs shown produce the following output:

OBS	ID	TC1
1	1	160
2	2	220
3	3	230
4	4	200
5	5	.

Now, suppose that only lines with nonmissing data are in the data set. Again, suppose we are interested only in the exam 2 values. In this case, we no longer have exactly three lines per person. Instead, the data is as follows. Notice that subject 3 has only two lines of data.

```
1 1 180
2 1 160
3 1 177
1 2 240
2 2 220
3 2 146
2 3 230
3 3 210
1 4 170
2 4 200
3 4 240
1 5 180
3 5 190
```

To input only the second exam value from a data set that does not contain three lines per person, we must use the line holder:

```
data one;
  input exam 1 @;
  if exam eq 2 then input id 3 tc2 5-7;
cards;
1 1 180
2 1 160
3 1 177
1 2 240
2 2 220
3 2 146
2 3 230
3 3 210
1 4 170
2 4 200
3 4 240
1 5 180
3 5 190
run;
proc print;
run;
```

The program shown above produces the following output:

```
OBS       ID        TC2
1         1         160
2         2         220
```

3	3	230
4	4	200
5	5	.

Suppose we record data (a continuous variable) on 10 subjects and want descriptive statistics on that variable. The data could be entered in 10 rows, and SAS Proc Means (see Chapter 2) could be used to generate descriptive statistics:

```
data one;                  Data set name=one.
  input id x;              Two variables are input—id and x.
cards;                     Beginning of Raw Data Section.
1  23                      id=1, x=23
2  43                      id=2, x=43
3  66
4  31
5  28
6  73
7  92
8  19
9  33
10 55
run;
proc means;                Procedure call to generate summary
                                statistics.
  var x;                   Specification of analytic variable x.
run;
```

The same can be achieved using line holders:

```
data one;
  input id x @@;

cards;
1  23  2  43  3  66  4  31  5  28
6  73  7  92  8  19  9  33  10  55
run;

proc means;
  var x;
run;
```

NOTE: "@@" holds the line until all data have been read and then moves to the next line.

The following program is equivalent, only the id variable is created in the program instead of input:

```
data one;
  input x @@;                    Input variable x.
  id=id+1;                       Create the variable id by adding 1 for each subject.

  cards;
  23 43 66 31 28 73 92 19 33 55
  run;

  proc means;
   var x;
  run;
```

The three programs shown produce the following output:

Analysis Variable: X

N	Mean	Std Dev	Minimum	Maximum
10	46.300	25.2901	19.0000	92.0000

Statistical Tables

B.1 Statistical Tables

Table B.1 *Probabilities of the Binomial Distribution*

Table entries represent $P(X = x)$ for n trials and $P(\text{success}) = p$,
e.g., $P(X = 4 \mid n = 10, p = 0.2) = 0.0881$.

x	.10	.20	.30	.40	.50	.60	.70	.80	.90
0	0.8100	0.6400	0.4900	0.3600	0.2500	0.1600	0.0900	0.0400	0.0100
1	0.1800	0.3200	0.4200	0.4800	0.5000	0.4800	0.4200	0.3200	0.1800
2	0.0100	0.0400	0.0900	0.1600	0.2500	0.3600	0.4900	0.6400	0.8100
0	0.7290	0.5120	0.3430	0.2160	0.1250	0.0640	0.0270	0.0080	0.0010
1	0.2430	0.3840	0.4410	0.4320	0.3750	0.2880	0.1890	0.0960	0.0270
2	0.0270	0.0960	0.1890	0.2880	0.3750	0.4320	0.4410	0.3840	0.2430
3	0.0010	0.0080	0.0270	0.0640	0.1250	0.2160	0.3430	0.5120	0.7290
0	0.6561	0.4096	0.2401	0.1296	0.0625	0.0256	0.0081	0.0016	0.0001
1	0.2916	0.4096	0.4116	0.3456	0.2500	0.1536	0.0756	0.0256	0.0036
2	0.0486	0.1536	0.2646	0.3456	0.3750	0.3456	0.2646	0.1536	0.0486
3	0.0036	0.0256	0.0756	0.1536	0.2500	0.3456	0.4116	0.4096	0.2916
4	0.0001	0.0016	0.0081	0.0256	0.0625	0.1296	0.2401	0.4096	0.6561
0	0.5905	0.3277	0.1681	0.0778	0.0313	0.0102	0.0024	0.0003	0.0000
1	0.3280	0.4096	0.3601	0.2592	0.1562	0.0768	0.0284	0.0064	0.0005

n	x	.10	.20	.30	.40	p .50	.60	.70	.80	.90
	2	0.0729	0.2048	0.3087	0.3456	0.3125	0.2304	0.1323	0.0512	0.008:
	3	0.0081	0.0512	0.1323	0.2304	0.3125	0.3456	0.3087	0.2048	0.072!
	4	0.0005	0.0064	0.0283	0.0768	0.1563	0.2592	0.3601	0.4096	0.328:
	5	0.0000	0.0003	0.0024	0.0102	0.0313	0.0778	0.1681	0.3277	0.590!
6	0	0.5314	0.2621	0.1176	0.0467	0.0156	0.0041	0.0007	0.0001	0.000(
	1	0.3543	0.3932	0.3025	0.1866	0.0938	0.0369	0.0102	0.0015	0.000:
	2	0.0984	0.2458	0.3241	0.3110	0.2344	0.1382	0.0595	0.0154	0.001:
	3	0.0146	0.0819	0.1852	0.2765	0.3125	0.2765	0.1852	0.0819	0.014(
	4	0.0012	0.0154	0.0595	0.1382	0.2344	0.3110	0.3241	0.2458	0.098
	5	0.0001	0.0015	0.0102	0.0369	0.0938	0.1866	0.3025	0.3932	0.354:
	6	0.0000	0.0001	0.0007	0.0041	0.0156	0.0467	0.1176	0.2621	0.531
7	0	0.4783	0.2097	0.0824	0.0280	0.0078	0.0016	0.0002	0.0000	0.000(
	1	0.3720	0.3670	0.2471	0.1306	0.0547	0.0172	0.0036	0.0004	0.000(
	2	0.1240	0.2753	0.3177	0.2613	0.1641	0.0774	0.0250	0.0043	0.000:
	3	0.0230	0.1147	0.2269	0.2903	0.2734	0.1935	0.0972	0.0287	0.002(
	4	0.0026	0.0287	0.0972	0.1935	0.2734	0.2903	0.2269	0.1147	0.023(
	5	0.0002	0.0043	0.0250	0.0774	0.1641	0.2613	0.3177	0.2753	0.124(
	6	0.0000	0.0004	0.0036	0.0172	0.0547	0.1306	0.2471	0.3670	0.372(
	7	0.0000	0.0000	0.0002	0.0016	0.0078	0.0280	0.0824	0.2097	0.478:
8	0	0.4305	0.1678	0.0576	0.0168	0.0039	0.0007	0.0001	0.0000	0.000(
	1	0.3826	0.3355	0.1977	0.0896	0.0313	0.0079	0.0012	0.0001	0.000(
	2	0.1488	0.2936	0.2965	0.2090	0.1094	0.0413	0.0100	0.0011	0.000(
	3	0.0331	0.1468	0.2541	0.2787	0.2188	0.1239	0.0467	0.0092	0.000
	4	0.0046	0.0459	0.1361	0.2322	0.2734	0.2322	0.1361	0.0459	0.004(
	5	0.0004	0.0092	0.0467	0.1239	0.2188	0.2787	0.2541	0.1468	0.033:
	6	0.0000	0.0011	0.0100	0.0413	0.1094	0.2090	0.2965	0.2936	0.148
	7	0.0000	0.0001	0.0012	0.0079	0.0313	0.0896	0.1977	0.3355	0.382(
	8	0.0000	0.0000	0.0001	0.0007	0.0039	0.0168	0.0576	0.1678	0.430!
9	0	0.3874	0.1342	0.0404	0.0101	0.0020	0.0003	0.0000	0.0000	0.000(
	1	0.3874	0.3020	0.1556	0.0605	0.0176	0.0035	0.0004	0.0000	0.000(
	2	0.1722	0.3020	0.2668	0.1612	0.0703	0.0212	0.0039	0.0003	0.000(
	3	0.0446	0.1762	0.2668	0.2508	0.1641	0.0743	0.0210	0.0028	0.000:
	4	0.0074	0.0661	0.1715	0.2508	0.2461	0.1672	0.0735	0.0165	0.000:
	5	0.0008	0.0165	0.0735	0.1672	0.2461	0.2508	0.1715	0.0661	0.007
	6	0.0001	0.0028	0.0210	0.0743	0.1641	0.2508	0.2668	0.1762	0.044(
	7	0.0000	0.0003	0.0039	0.0212	0.0703	0.1612	0.2668	0.3020	0.172:
	8	0.0000	0.0000	0.0004	0.0035	0.0176	0.0605	0.1556	0.3020	0.387
	9	0.0000	0.0000	0.0000	0.0003	0.0020	0.0101	0.0404	0.1342	0.387

n	x	p .10	.20	.30	.40	.50	.60	.70	.80	.90
10	0	0.3487	0.1074	0.0282	0.0060	0.0010	0.0001	0.0000	0.0000	0.0000
	1	0.3874	0.2684	0.1211	0.0403	0.0098	0.0016	0.0001	0.0000	0.0000
	2	0.1937	0.3020	0.2335	0.1209	0.0439	0.0106	0.0014	0.0001	0.0000
	3	0.0574	0.2013	0.2668	0.2150	0.1172	0.0425	0.0090	0.0008	0.0000
	4	0.0112	0.0881	0.2001	0.2508	0.2051	0.1115	0.0368	0.0055	0.0001
	5	0.0015	0.0264	0.1029	0.2007	0.2461	0.2007	0.1029	0.0264	0.0015
	6	0.0001	0.0055	0.0368	0.1115	0.2051	0.2508	0.2001	0.0881	0.0112
	7	0.0000	0.0008	0.0090	0.0425	0.1172	0.2150	0.2668	0.2013	0.0574
	8	0.0000	0.0001	0.0014	0.0106	0.0439	0.1209	0.2335	0.3020	0.1937
	9	0.0000	0.0000	0.0001	0.0016	0.0098	0.0403	0.1211	0.2684	0.3874
	10	0.0000	0.0000	0.0000	0.0001	0.0010	0.0060	0.0282	0.1074	0.3487
11	0	0.3138	0.0859	0.0198	0.0036	0.0005	0.0000	0.0000	0.0000	0.0000
	1	0.3835	0.2362	0.0932	0.0266	0.0054	0.0007	0.0000	0.0000	0.0000
	2	0.2131	0.2953	0.1998	0.0887	0.0269	0.0052	0.0005	0.0000	0.0000
	3	0.0710	0.2215	0.2568	0.1774	0.0806	0.0234	0.0037	0.0002	0.0000
	4	0.0158	0.1107	0.2201	0.2365	0.1611	0.0701	0.0173	0.0017	0.0000
	5	0.0025	0.0388	0.1321	0.2207	0.2256	0.1471	0.0566	0.0097	0.0003
	6	0.0003	0.0097	0.0566	0.1471	0.2256	0.2207	0.1321	0.0388	0.0025
	7	0.0000	0.0017	0.0173	0.0701	0.1611	0.2365	0.2201	0.1107	0.0158
	8	0.0000	0.0002	0.0037	0.0234	0.0806	0.1774	0.2568	0.2215	0.0710
	9	0.0000	0.0000	0.0005	0.0052	0.0269	0.0887	0.1998	0.2953	0.2131
	10	0.0000	0.0000	0.0000	0.0007	0.0054	0.0266	0.0932	0.2362	0.3835
	11	0.0000	0.0000	0.0000	0.0000	0.0005	0.0036	0.0198	0.0859	0.3138
12	0	0.2824	0.0687	0.0138	0.0022	0.0002	0.0000	0.0000	0.0000	0.0000
	1	0.3766	0.2062	0.0712	0.0174	0.0029	0.0003	0.0000	0.0000	0.0000
	2	0.2301	0.2835	0.1678	0.0639	0.0161	0.0025	0.0002	0.0000	0.0000
	3	0.0852	0.2362	0.2397	0.1419	0.0537	0.0125	0.0015	0.0001	0.0000
	4	0.0213	0.1329	0.2311	0.2128	0.1208	0.0420	0.0078	0.0005	0.0000
	5	0.0038	0.0532	0.1585	0.2270	0.1934	0.1009	0.0291	0.0033	0.0000
	6	0.0005	0.0155	0.0792	0.1766	0.2256	0.1766	0.0792	0.0155	0.0005
	7	0.0000	0.0033	0.0291	0.1009	0.1934	0.2270	0.1585	0.0532	0.0038
	8	0.0000	0.0005	0.0078	0.0420	0.1208	0.2128	0.2311	0.1329	0.0213
	9	0.0000	0.0001	0.0015	0.0125	0.0537	0.1419	0.2397	0.2362	0.0852
	10	0.0000	0.0000	0.0002	0.0025	0.0161	0.0639	0.1678	0.2835	0.2301
	11	0.0000	0.0000	0.0000	0.0003	0.0029	0.0174	0.0712	0.2062	0.3766
	12	0.0000	0.0000	0.0000	0.0000	0.0002	0.0022	0.0138	0.0687	0.2824
13	0	0.2542	0.0550	0.0097	0.0013	0.0001	0.0000	0.0000	0.0000	0.0000
	1	0.3672	0.1787	0.0540	0.0113	0.0016	0.0001	0.0000	0.0000	0.0000

n	x					p				
		.10	.20	.30	.40	.50	.60	.70	.80	.90
	2	0.2448	0.2680	0.1388	0.0453	0.0095	0.0012	0.0001	0.0000	0.0000
	3	0.0997	0.2457	0.2181	0.1107	0.0349	0.0065	0.0006	0.0000	0.0000
	4	0.0277	0.1535	0.2337	0.1845	0.0873	0.0243	0.0034	0.0001	0.0000
	5	0.0055	0.0691	0.1803	0.2214	0.1571	0.0656	0.0142	0.0011	0.0000
	6	0.0008	0.0230	0.1030	0.1968	0.2095	0.1312	0.0442	0.0058	0.0001
	7	0.0001	0.0058	0.0442	0.1312	0.2095	0.1968	0.1030	0.0230	0.0008
	8	0.0000	0.0011	0.0142	0.0656	0.1571	0.2214	0.1803	0.0691	0.0055
	9	0.0000	0.0001	0.0034	0.0243	0.0873	0.1845	0.2337	0.1535	0.0277
	10	0.0000	0.0000	0.0006	0.0065	0.0349	0.1107	0.2181	0.2457	0.0997
	11	0.0000	0.0000	0.0001	0.0012	0.0095	0.0453	0.1388	0.2680	0.2448
	12	0.0000	0.0000	0.0000	0.0001	0.0016	0.0113	0.0540	0.1787	0.3672
	13	0.0000	0.0000	0.0000	0.0000	0.0001	0.0013	0.0097	0.0550	0.2542
14	0	0.2288	0.0440	0.0068	0.0008	0.0001	0.0000	0.0000	0.0000	0.0000
	1	0.3559	0.1539	0.0407	0.0073	0.0009	0.0001	0.0000	0.0000	0.0000
	2	0.2570	0.2501	0.1134	0.0317	0.0056	0.0005	0.0000	0.0000	0.0000
	3	0.1142	0.2501	0.1943	0.0845	0.0222	0.0033	0.0002	0.0000	0.0000
	4	0.0349	0.1720	0.2290	0.1549	0.0611	0.0136	0.0014	0.0000	0.0000
	5	0.0078	0.0860	0.1963	0.2066	0.1222	0.0408	0.0066	0.0003	0.0000
	6	0.0013	0.0322	0.1262	0.2066	0.1833	0.0918	0.0232	0.0020	0.0000
	7	0.0002	0.0092	0.0618	0.1574	0.2095	0.1574	0.0618	0.0092	0.0002
	8	0.0000	0.0020	0.0232	0.0918	0.1833	0.2066	0.1262	0.0322	0.0013
	9	0.0000	0.0003	0.0066	0.0408	0.1222	0.2066	0.1963	0.0860	0.0078
	10	0.0000	0.0000	0.0014	0.0136	0.0611	0.1549	0.2290	0.1720	0.0349
	11	0.0000	0.0000	0.0002	0.0033	0.0222	0.0845	0.1943	0.2501	0.1142
	12	0.0000	0.0000	0.0000	0.0005	0.0056	0.0317	0.1134	0.2501	0.2570
	13	0.0000	0.0000	0.0000	0.0001	0.0009	0.0073	0.0407	0.1539	0.3559
	14	0.0000	0.0000	0.0000	0.0000	0.0001	0.0008	0.0068	0.0440	0.2288
15	0	0.2059	0.0352	0.0047	0.0005	0.0000	0.0000	0.0000	0.0000	0.0000
	1	0.3432	0.1319	0.0305	0.0047	0.0005	0.0000	0.0000	0.0000	0.0000
	2	0.2669	0.2309	0.0916	0.0219	0.0032	0.0003	0.0000	0.0000	0.0000
	3	0.1285	0.2501	0.1700	0.0634	0.0139	0.0016	0.0001	0.0000	0.0000
	4	0.0428	0.1876	0.2186	0.1268	0.0417	0.0074	0.0006	0.0000	0.0000
	5	0.0105	0.1032	0.2061	0.1859	0.0916	0.0245	0.0030	0.0001	0.0000
	6	0.0019	0.0430	0.1472	0.2066	0.1527	0.0612	0.0116	0.0007	0.0000
	7	0.0003	0.0138	0.0811	0.1771	0.1964	0.1181	0.0348	0.0035	0.0000
	8	0.0000	0.0035	0.0348	0.1181	0.1964	0.1771	0.0811	0.0138	0.0003
	9	0.0000	0.0007	0.0116	0.0612	0.1527	0.2066	0.1472	0.0430	0.0019
	10	0.0000	0.0001	0.0030	0.0245	0.0916	0.1859	0.2061	0.1032	0.0105
	11	0.0000	0.0000	0.0006	0.0074	0.0417	0.1268	0.2186	0.1876	0.0428

					p					
n	x	.10	.20	.30	.40	.50	.60	.70	.80	.90
	12	0.0000	0.0000	0.0001	0.0016	0.0139	0.0634	0.1700	0.2501	0.1285
	13	0.0000	0.0000	0.0000	0.0003	0.0032	0.0219	0.0916	0.2309	0.2669
	14	0.0000	0.0000	0.0000	0.0000	0.0005	0.0047	0.0305	0.1319	0.3432
	15	0.0000	0.0000	0.0000	0.0000	0.0000	0.0005	0.0047	0.0352	0.2059
16	0	0.1853	0.0281	0.0033	0.0003	0.0000	0.0000	0.0000	0.0000	0.0000
	1	0.3294	0.1126	0.0228	0.0030	0.0002	0.0000	0.0000	0.0000	0.0000
	2	0.2745	0.2111	0.0732	0.0150	0.0018	0.0001	0.0000	0.0000	0.0000
	3	0.1423	0.2463	0.1465	0.0468	0.0085	0.0008	0.0000	0.0000	0.0000
	4	0.0514	0.2001	0.2040	0.1014	0.0278	0.0040	0.0002	0.0000	0.0000
	5	0.0137	0.1201	0.2099	0.1623	0.0667	0.0142	0.0013	0.0000	0.0000
	6	0.0028	0.0550	0.1649	0.1983	0.1222	0.0392	0.0056	0.0002	0.0000
	7	0.0004	0.0197	0.1010	0.1889	0.1746	0.0840	0.0185	0.0012	0.0000
	8	0.0001	0.0055	0.0487	0.1417	0.1964	0.1417	0.0487	0.0055	0.0001
	9	0.0000	0.0012	0.0185	0.0840	0.1746	0.1889	0.1010	0.0197	0.0004
	10	0.0000	0.0002	0.0056	0.0392	0.1222	0.1983	0.1649	0.0550	0.0028
	11	0.0000	0.0000	0.0013	0.0142	0.0667	0.1623	0.2099	0.1201	0.0137
	12	0.0000	0.0000	0.0002	0.0040	0.0278	0.1014	0.2040	0.2001	0.0514
	13	0.0000	0.0000	0.0000	0.0008	0.0085	0.0468	0.1465	0.2463	0.1423
	14	0.0000	0.0000	0.0000	0.0001	0.0018	0.0150	0.0732	0.2111	0.2745
	15	0.0000	0.0000	0.0000	0.0000	0.0002	0.0030	0.0228	0.1126	0.3294
	16	0.0000	0.0000	0.0000	0.0000	0.0000	0.0003	0.0033	0.0281	0.1853
17	0	0.1668	0.0225	0.0023	0.0002	0.0000	0.0000	0.0000	0.0000	0.0000
	1	0.3150	0.0957	0.0169	0.0019	0.0001	0.0000	0.0000	0.0000	0.0000
	2	0.2800	0.1914	0.0581	0.0102	0.0010	0.0001	0.0000	0.0000	0.0000
	3	0.1556	0.2393	0.1245	0.0341	0.0052	0.0004	0.0000	0.0000	0.0000
	4	0.0605	0.2093	0.1868	0.0796	0.0182	0.0021	0.0001	0.0000	0.0000
	5	0.0175	0.1361	0.2081	0.1379	0.0472	0.0081	0.0006	0.0000	0.0000
	6	0.0039	0.0680	0.1784	0.1839	0.0944	0.0242	0.0026	0.0001	0.0000
	7	0.0007	0.0267	0.1201	0.1927	0.1484	0.0571	0.0095	0.0004	0.0000
	8	0.0001	0.0084	0.0644	0.1606	0.1855	0.1070	0.0276	0.0021	0.0000
	9	0.0000	0.0021	0.0276	0.1070	0.1855	0.1606	0.0644	0.0084	0.0001
	10	0.0000	0.0004	0.0095	0.0571	0.1484	0.1927	0.1201	0.0267	0.0007
	11	0.0000	0.0001	0.0026	0.0242	0.0944	0.1839	0.1784	0.0680	0.0039
	12	0.0000	0.0000	0.0006	0.0081	0.0472	0.1379	0.2081	0.1361	0.0175
	13	0.0000	0.0000	0.0001	0.0021	0.0182	0.0796	0.1868	0.2093	0.0605
	14	0.0000	0.0000	0.0000	0.0004	0.0052	0.0341	0.1245	0.2393	0.1556
	15	0.0000	0.0000	0.0000	0.0001	0.0010	0.0102	0.0581	0.1914	0.2800
	16	0.0000	0.0000	0.0000	0.0000	0.0001	0.0019	0.0169	0.0957	0.3150
	17	0.0000	0.0000	0.0000	0.0000	0.0000	0.0002	0.0023	0.0225	0.1668

						p				
n	x	.10	.20	.30	.40	.50	.60	.70	.80	.90
18	0	0.1501	0.0180	0.0016	0.0001	0.0000	0.0000	0.0000	0.0000	0.0000
	1	0.3002	0.0811	0.0126	0.0012	0.0001	0.0000	0.0000	0.0000	0.0000
	2	0.2835	0.1723	0.0458	0.0069	0.0006	0.0000	0.0000	0.0000	0.0000
	3	0.1680	0.2297	0.1046	0.0246	0.0031	0.0002	0.0000	0.0000	0.0000
	4	0.0700	0.2153	0.1681	0.0614	0.0117	0.0011	0.0000	0.0000	0.0000
	5	0.0218	0.1507	0.2017	0.1146	0.0327	0.0045	0.0002	0.0000	0.0000
	6	0.0052	0.0816	0.1873	0.1655	0.0708	0.0145	0.0012	0.0000	0.0000
	7	0.0010	0.0350	0.1376	0.1892	0.1214	0.0374	0.0046	0.0001	0.0000
	8	0.0002	0.0120	0.0811	0.1734	0.1669	0.0771	0.0149	0.0008	0.0000
	9	0.0000	0.0033	0.0386	0.1284	0.1855	0.1284	0.0386	0.0033	0.0000
	10	0.0000	0.0008	0.0149	0.0771	0.1669	0.1734	0.0811	0.0120	0.0002
	11	0.0000	0.0001	0.0046	0.0374	0.1214	0.1892	0.1376	0.0350	0.0010
	12	0.0000	0.0000	0.0012	0.0145	0.0708	0.1655	0.1873	0.0816	0.0052
	13	0.0000	0.0000	0.0002	0.0045	0.0327	0.1146	0.2017	0.1507	0.0218
	14	0.0000	0.0000	0.0000	0.0011	0.0117	0.0614	0.1681	0.2153	0.0700
	15	0.0000	0.0000	0.0000	0.0002	0.0031	0.0246	0.1046	0.2297	0.1680
	16	0.0000	0.0000	0.0000	0.0000	0.0006	0.0069	0.0458	0.1723	0.2835
	17	0.0000	0.0000	0.0000	0.0000	0.0001	0.0012	0.0126	0.0811	0.3002
	18	0.0000	0.0000	0.0000	0.0000	0.0000	0.0001	0.0016	0.0180	0.1501
19	0	0.1351	0.0144	0.0011	0.0001	0.0000	0.0000	0.0000	0.0000	0.0000
	1	0.2852	0.0685	0.0093	0.0008	0.0000	0.0000	0.0000	0.0000	0.0000
	2	0.2852	0.1540	0.0358	0.0046	0.0003	0.0000	0.0000	0.0000	0.0000
	3	0.1796	0.2182	0.0869	0.0175	0.0018	0.0001	0.0000	0.0000	0.0000
	4	0.0798	0.2182	0.1491	0.0467	0.0074	0.0005	0.0000	0.0000	0.0000
	5	0.0266	0.1636	0.1916	0.0933	0.0222	0.0024	0.0001	0.0000	0.0000
	6	0.0069	0.0955	0.1916	0.1451	0.0518	0.0085	0.0005	0.0000	0.0000
	7	0.0014	0.0443	0.1525	0.1797	0.0961	0.0237	0.0022	0.0000	0.0000
	8	0.0002	0.0166	0.0981	0.1797	0.1442	0.0532	0.0077	0.0003	0.0000
	9	0.0000	0.0051	0.0514	0.1464	0.1762	0.0976	0.0220	0.0013	0.0000
	10	0.0000	0.0013	0.0220	0.0976	0.1762	0.1464	0.0514	0.0051	0.0000
	11	0.0000	0.0003	0.0077	0.0532	0.1442	0.1797	0.0981	0.0166	0.0002
	12	0.0000	0.0000	0.0022	0.0237	0.0961	0.1797	0.1525	0.0443	0.0014
	13	0.0000	0.0000	0.0005	0.0085	0.0518	0.1451	0.1916	0.0955	0.0069
	14	0.0000	0.0000	0.0001	0.0024	0.0222	0.0933	0.1916	0.1636	0.0266
	15	0.0000	0.0000	0.0000	0.0005	0.0074	0.0467	0.1491	0.2182	0.0798
	16	0.0000	0.0000	0.0000	0.0001	0.0018	0.0175	0.0869	0.2182	0.1796
	17	0.0000	0.0000	0.0000	0.0000	0.0003	0.0046	0.0358	0.1540	0.2852
	18	0.0000	0.0000	0.0000	0.0000	0.0000	0.0008	0.0093	0.0685	0.2852
	19	0.0000	0.0000	0.0000	0.0000	0.0000	0.0001	0.0011	0.0144	0.135

n	x					p				
		.10	.20	.30	.40	.50	.60	.70	.80	.90
20	0	0.1216	0.0115	0.0008	0.0000	0.0000	0.0000	0.0000	0.0000	0.0000
	1	0.2702	0.0576	0.0068	0.0005	0.0000	0.0000	0.0000	0.0000	0.0000
	2	0.2852	0.1369	0.0278	0.0031	0.0002	0.0000	0.0000	0.0000	0.0000
	3	0.1901	0.2054	0.0716	0.0123	0.0011	0.0000	0.0000	0.0000	0.0000
	4	0.0898	0.2182	0.1304	0.0350	0.0046	0.0003	0.0000	0.0000	0.0000
	5	0.0319	0.1746	0.1789	0.0746	0.0148	0.0013	0.0000	0.0000	0.0000
	6	0.0089	0.1091	0.1916	0.1244	0.0370	0.0049	0.0002	0.0000	0.0000
	7	0.0020	0.0545	0.1643	0.1659	0.0739	0.0146	0.0010	0.0000	0.0000
	8	0.0004	0.0222	0.1144	0.1797	0.1201	0.0355	0.0039	0.0001	0.0000
	9	0.0001	0.0074	0.0654	0.1597	0.1602	0.0710	0.0120	0.0005	0.0000
	10	0.0000	0.0020	0.0308	0.1171	0.1762	0.1171	0.0308	0.0020	0.0000
	11	0.0000	0.0005	0.0120	0.0710	0.1602	0.1597	0.0654	0.0074	0.0001
	12	0.0000	0.0001	0.0039	0.0355	0.1201	0.1797	0.1144	0.0222	0.0004
	13	0.0000	0.0000	0.0010	0.0146	0.0739	0.1659	0.1643	0.0545	0.0020
	14	0.0000	0.0000	0.0002	0.0049	0.0370	0.1244	0.1916	0.1091	0.0089
	15	0.0000	0.0000	0.0000	0.0013	0.0148	0.0746	0.1789	0.1746	0.0319
	16	0.0000	0.0000	0.0000	0.0003	0.0046	0.0350	0.1304	0.2182	0.0898
	17	0.0000	0.0000	0.0000	0.0000	0.0011	0.0123	0.0716	0.2054	0.1901
	18	0.0000	0.0000	0.0000	0.0000	0.0002	0.0031	0.0278	0.1369	0.2852
	19	0.0000	0.0000	0.0000	0.0000	0.0000	0.0005	0.0068	0.0576	0.2702
	20	0.0000	0.0000	0.0000	0.0000	0.0000	0.0000	0.0008	0.0115	0.1216
21	0	0.1094	0.0092	0.0006	0.0000	0.0000	0.0000	0.0000	0.0000	0.0000
	1	0.2553	0.0484	0.0050	0.0003	0.0000	0.0000	0.0000	0.0000	0.0000
	2	0.2837	0.1211	0.0215	0.0020	0.0001	0.0000	0.0000	0.0000	0.0000
	3	0.1996	0.1917	0.0585	0.0086	0.0006	0.0000	0.0000	0.0000	0.0000
	4	0.0998	0.2156	0.1128	0.0259	0.0029	0.0001	0.0000	0.0000	0.0000
	5	0.0377	0.1833	0.1643	0.0588	0.0097	0.0007	0.0000	0.0000	0.0000
	6	0.0112	0.1222	0.1878	0.1045	0.0259	0.0027	0.0001	0.0000	0.0000
	7	0.0027	0.0655	0.1725	0.1493	0.0554	0.0087	0.0005	0.0000	0.0000
	8	0.0005	0.0286	0.1294	0.1742	0.0970	0.0229	0.0019	0.0000	0.0000
	9	0.0001	0.0103	0.0801	0.1677	0.1402	0.0497	0.0063	0.0002	0.0000
	10	0.0000	0.0031	0.0412	0.1342	0.1682	0.0895	0.0176	0.0008	0.0000
	11	0.0000	0.0008	0.0176	0.0895	0.1682	0.1342	0.0412	0.0031	0.0000
	12	0.0000	0.0002	0.0063	0.0497	0.1402	0.1677	0.0801	0.0103	0.0001
	13	0.0000	0.0000	0.0019	0.0229	0.0970	0.1742	0.1294	0.0286	0.0005
	14	0.0000	0.0000	0.0005	0.0087	0.0554	0.1493	0.1725	0.0655	0.0027
	15	0.0000	0.0000	0.0001	0.0027	0.0259	0.1045	0.1878	0.1222	0.0112
	16	0.0000	0.0000	0.0000	0.0007	0.0097	0.0588	0.1643	0.1833	0.0377
	17	0.0000	0.0000	0.0000	0.0001	0.0029	0.0259	0.1128	0.2156	0.0998

n	x	.10	.20	.30	.40	p .50	.60	.70	.80	.90
	18	0.0000	0.0000	0.0000	0.0000	0.0006	0.0086	0.0585	0.1917	0.1996
	19	0.0000	0.0000	0.0000	0.0000	0.0001	0.0020	0.0215	0.1211	0.2837
	20	0.0000	0.0000	0.0000	0.0000	0.0000	0.0003	0.0050	0.0484	0.2553
	21	0.0000	0.0000	0.0000	0.0000	0.0000	0.0000	0.0006	0.0092	0.1094
22	0	0.0985	0.0074	0.0004	0.0000	0.0000	0.0000	0.0000	0.0000	0.0000
	1	0.2407	0.0406	0.0037	0.0002	0.0000	0.0000	0.0000	0.0000	0.0000
	2	0.2808	0.1065	0.0166	0.0014	0.0001	0.0000	0.0000	0.0000	0.0000
	3	0.2080	0.1775	0.0474	0.0060	0.0004	0.0000	0.0000	0.0000	0.0000
	4	0.1098	0.2108	0.0965	0.0190	0.0017	0.0001	0.0000	0.0000	0.0000
	5	0.0439	0.1898	0.1489	0.0456	0.0063	0.0004	0.0000	0.0000	0.0000
	6	0.0138	0.1344	0.1808	0.0862	0.0178	0.0015	0.0000	0.0000	0.0000
	7	0.0035	0.0768	0.1771	0.1314	0.0407	0.0051	0.0002	0.0000	0.0000
	8	0.0007	0.0360	0.1423	0.1642	0.0762	0.0144	0.0009	0.0000	0.0000
	9	0.0001	0.0140	0.0949	0.1703	0.1186	0.0336	0.0032	0.0001	0.0000
	10	0.0000	0.0046	0.0529	0.1476	0.1542	0.0656	0.0097	0.0003	0.0000
	11	0.0000	0.0012	0.0247	0.1073	0.1682	0.1073	0.0247	0.0012	0.0000
	12	0.0000	0.0003	0.0097	0.0656	0.1542	0.1476	0.0529	0.0046	0.0000
	13	0.0000	0.0001	0.0032	0.0336	0.1186	0.1703	0.0949	0.0140	0.0001
	14	0.0000	0.0000	0.0009	0.0144	0.0762	0.1642	0.1423	0.0360	0.0007
	15	0.0000	0.0000	0.0002	0.0051	0.0407	0.1314	0.1771	0.0768	0.0035
	16	0.0000	0.0000	0.0000	0.0015	0.0178	0.0862	0.1808	0.1344	0.0138
	17	0.0000	0.0000	0.0000	0.0004	0.0063	0.0456	0.1489	0.1898	0.0439
	18	0.0000	0.0000	0.0000	0.0001	0.0017	0.0190	0.0965	0.2108	0.1098
	19	0.0000	0.0000	0.0000	0.0000	0.0004	0.0060	0.0474	0.1775	0.2080
	20	0.0000	0.0000	0.0000	0.0000	0.0001	0.0014	0.0166	0.1065	0.2808
	21	0.0000	0.0000	0.0000	0.0000	0.0000	0.0002	0.0037	0.0406	0.2407
	22	0.0000	0.0000	0.0000	0.0000	0.0000	0.0000	0.0004	0.0074	0.0985
23	0	0.0886	0.0059	0.0003	0.0000	0.0000	0.0000	0.0000	0.0000	0.0000
	1	0.2265	0.0339	0.0027	0.0001	0.0000	0.0000	0.0000	0.0000	0.0000
	2	0.2768	0.0933	0.0127	0.0009	0.0000	0.0000	0.0000	0.0000	0.0000
	3	0.2153	0.1633	0.0382	0.0041	0.0002	0.0000	0.0000	0.0000	0.0000
	4	0.1196	0.2042	0.0818	0.0138	0.0011	0.0000	0.0000	0.0000	0.0000
	5	0.0505	0.1940	0.1332	0.0350	0.0040	0.0002	0.0000	0.0000	0.0000
	6	0.0168	0.1455	0.1712	0.0700	0.0120	0.0008	0.0000	0.0000	0.0000
	7	0.0045	0.0883	0.1782	0.1133	0.0292	0.0029	0.0001	0.0000	0.0000
	8	0.0010	0.0442	0.1527	0.1511	0.0584	0.0088	0.0004	0.0000	0.0000
	9	0.0002	0.0184	0.1091	0.1679	0.0974	0.0221	0.0016	0.0000	0.0000
	10	0.0000	0.0064	0.0655	0.1567	0.1364	0.0464	0.0052	0.0001	0.0000
	11	0.0000	0.0019	0.0332	0.1234	0.1612	0.0823	0.0142	0.0005	0.0000

					p				
n	x	.10	.20	.30	.40	.50	.60	.70	.80	.90
	12	0.0000	0.0005	0.0142	0.0823	0.1612	0.1234	0.0332	0.0019	0.0000
	13	0.0000	0.0001	0.0052	0.0464	0.1364	0.1567	0.0655	0.0064	0.0000
	14	0.0000	0.0000	0.0016	0.0221	0.0974	0.1679	0.1091	0.0184	0.0002
	15	0.0000	0.0000	0.0004	0.0088	0.0584	0.1511	0.1527	0.0442	0.0010
	16	0.0000	0.0000	0.0001	0.0029	0.0292	0.1133	0.1782	0.0883	0.0045
	17	0.0000	0.0000	0.0000	0.0008	0.0120	0.0700	0.1712	0.1455	0.0168
	18	0.0000	0.0000	0.0000	0.0002	0.0040	0.0350	0.1332	0.1940	0.0505
	19	0.0000	0.0000	0.0000	0.0000	0.0011	0.0138	0.0818	0.2042	0.1196
	20	0.0000	0.0000	0.0000	0.0000	0.0002	0.0041	0.0382	0.1633	0.2153
	21	0.0000	0.0000	0.0000	0.0000	0.0000	0.0009	0.0127	0.0933	0.2768
	22	0.0000	0.0000	0.0000	0.0000	0.0000	0.0001	0.0027	0.0339	0.2265
	23	0.0000	0.0000	0.0000	0.0000	0.0000	0.0000	0.0003	0.0059	0.0886
24	0	0.0798	0.0047	0.0002	0.0000	0.0000	0.0000	0.0000	0.0000	0.0000
	1	0.2127	0.0283	0.0020	0.0001	0.0000	0.0000	0.0000	0.0000	0.0000
	2	0.2718	0.0815	0.0097	0.0006	0.0000	0.0000	0.0000	0.0000	0.0000
	3	0.2215	0.1493	0.0305	0.0028	0.0001	0.0000	0.0000	0.0000	0.0000
	4	0.1292	0.1960	0.0687	0.0099	0.0006	0.0000	0.0000	0.0000	0.0000
	5	0.0574	0.1960	0.1177	0.0265	0.0025	0.0001	0.0000	0.0000	0.0000
	6	0.0202	0.1552	0.1598	0.0560	0.0080	0.0004	0.0000	0.0000	0.0000
	7	0.0058	0.0998	0.1761	0.0960	0.0206	0.0017	0.0000	0.0000	0.0000
	8	0.0014	0.0530	0.1604	0.1360	0.0438	0.0053	0.0002	0.0000	0.0000
	9	0.0003	0.0236	0.1222	0.1612	0.0779	0.0141	0.0008	0.0000	0.0000
	10	0.0000	0.0088	0.0785	0.1612	0.1169	0.0318	0.0026	0.0000	0.0000
	11	0.0000	0.0028	0.0428	0.1367	0.1488	0.0608	0.0079	0.0002	0.0000
	12	0.0000	0.0008	0.0199	0.0988	0.1612	0.0988	0.0199	0.0008	0.0000
	13	0.0000	0.0002	0.0079	0.0608	0.1488	0.1367	0.0428	0.0028	0.0000
	14	0.0000	0.0000	0.0026	0.0318	0.1169	0.1612	0.0785	0.0088	0.0000
	15	0.0000	0.0000	0.0008	0.0141	0.0779	0.1612	0.1222	0.0236	0.0003
	16	0.0000	0.0000	0.0002	0.0053	0.0438	0.1360	0.1604	0.0530	0.0014
	17	0.0000	0.0000	0.0000	0.0017	0.0206	0.0960	0.1761	0.0998	0.0058
	18	0.0000	0.0000	0.0000	0.0004	0.0080	0.0560	0.1598	0.1552	0.0202
	19	0.0000	0.0000	0.0000	0.0001	0.0025	0.0265	0.1177	0.1960	0.0574
	20	0.0000	0.0000	0.0000	0.0000	0.0006	0.0099	0.0687	0.1960	0.1292
	21	0.0000	0.0000	0.0000	0.0000	0.0001	0.0028	0.0305	0.1493	0.2215
	22	0.0000	0.0000	0.0000	0.0000	0.0000	0.0006	0.0097	0.0815	0.2718
	23	0.0000	0.0000	0.0000	0.0000	0.0000	0.0001	0.0020	0.0283	0.2127
	24	0.0000	0.0000	0.0000	0.0000	0.0000	0.0000	0.0002	0.0047	0.0798
25	0	0.0718	0.0038	0.0001	0.0000	0.0000	0.0000	0.0000	0.0000	0.0000
	1	0.1994	0.0236	0.0014	0.0000	0.0000	0.0000	0.0000	0.0000	0.0000

p

n	x	.10	.20	.30	.40	.50	.60	.70	.80	.90
	2	0.2659	0.0708	0.0074	0.0004	0.0000	0.0000	0.0000	0.0000	0.0000
	3	0.2265	0.1358	0.0243	0.0019	0.0001	0.0000	0.0000	0.0000	0.0000
	4	0.1384	0.1867	0.0572	0.0071	0.0004	0.0000	0.0000	0.0000	0.0000
	5	0.0646	0.1960	0.1030	0.0199	0.0016	0.0000	0.0000	0.0000	0.0000
	6	0.0239	0.1633	0.1472	0.0442	0.0053	0.0002	0.0000	0.0000	0.0000
	7	0.0072	0.1108	0.1712	0.0800	0.0143	0.0009	0.0000	0.0000	0.0000
	8	0.0018	0.0623	0.1651	0.1200	0.0322	0.0031	0.0001	0.0000	0.0000
	9	0.0004	0.0294	0.1336	0.1511	0.0609	0.0088	0.0004	0.0000	0.0000
	10	0.0001	0.0118	0.0916	0.1612	0.0974	0.0212	0.0013	0.0000	0.0000
	11	0.0000	0.0040	0.0536	0.1465	0.1328	0.0434	0.0042	0.0001	0.0000
	12	0.0000	0.0012	0.0268	0.1140	0.1550	0.0760	0.0115	0.0003	0.0000
	13	0.0000	0.0003	0.0115	0.0760	0.1550	0.1140	0.0268	0.0012	0.0000
	14	0.0000	0.0001	0.0042	0.0434	0.1328	0.1465	0.0536	0.0040	0.0000
	15	0.0000	0.0000	0.0013	0.0212	0.0974	0.1612	0.0916	0.0118	0.0001
	16	0.0000	0.0000	0.0004	0.0088	0.0609	0.1511	0.1336	0.0294	0.0004
	17	0.0000	0.0000	0.0001	0.0031	0.0322	0.1200	0.1651	0.0623	0.0018
	18	0.0000	0.0000	0.0000	0.0009	0.0143	0.0800	0.1712	0.1108	0.0072
	19	0.0000	0.0000	0.0000	0.0002	0.0053	0.0442	0.1472	0.1633	0.0239
	20	0.0000	0.0000	0.0000	0.0000	0.0016	0.0199	0.1030	0.1960	0.0646
	21	0.0000	0.0000	0.0000	0.0000	0.0004	0.0071	0.0572	0.1867	0.1384
	22	0.0000	0.0000	0.0000	0.0000	0.0001	0.0019	0.0243	0.1358	0.2265
	23	0.0000	0.0000	0.0000	0.0000	0.0000	0.0004	0.0074	0.0708	0.2659
	24	0.0000	0.0000	0.0000	0.0000	0.0000	0.0000	0.0014	0.0236	0.1994
	25	0.0000	0.0000	0.0000	0.0000	0.0000	0.0000	0.0001	0.0038	0.0718

Table B.2 *Probabilities of the Standard Normal Distribution Z*

Table entries represent $P(Z < Z_i)$, e.g., $P(Z < -1.96) = 0.0250$, $P(Z < 1.96) = 0.9750$.

Z_i	.00	.01	.02	.03	.04	.05	.06	.07	.08	.09
-3.0	0.0013	0.0013	0.0013	0.0012	0.0012	0.0011	0.0011	0.0011	0.0010	0.0010
-2.9	0.0019	0.0018	0.0018	0.0017	0.0016	0.0016	0.0015	0.0015	0.0014	0.0014
-2.8	0.0026	0.0025	0.0024	0.0023	0.0023	0.0022	0.0021	0.0021	0.0020	0.0019
-2.7	0.0035	0.0034	0.0033	0.0032	0.0031	0.0030	0.0029	0.0028	0.0027	0.0026
-2.6	0.0047	0.0045	0.0044	0.0043	0.0041	0.0040	0.0039	0.0038	0.0037	0.0036
-2.5	0.0062	0.0060	0.0059	0.0057	0.0055	0.0054	0.0052	0.0051	0.0049	0.0048
-2.4	0.0082	0.0080	0.0078	0.0075	0.0073	0.0071	0.0069	0.0068	0.0066	0.0064
-2.3	0.0107	0.0104	0.0102	0.0099	0.0096	0.0094	0.0091	0.0089	0.0087	0.0084
-2.2	0.0139	0.0136	0.0132	0.0129	0.0125	0.0122	0.0119	0.0116	0.0113	0.0110
-2.1	0.0179	0.0174	0.0170	0.0166	0.0162	0.0158	0.0154	0.0150	0.0146	0.0143

z_i	.00	.01	.02	.03	.04	.05	.06	.07	.08	.09
-2.0	0.0228	0.0222	0.0217	0.0212	0.0207	0.0202	0.0197	0.0192	0.0188	0.0183
-1.9	0.0287	0.0281	0.0274	0.0268	0.0262	0.0256	0.0250	0.0244	0.0239	0.0233
-1.8	0.0359	0.0351	0.0344	0.0336	0.0329	0.0322	0.0314	0.0307	0.0301	0.0294
-1.7	0.0446	0.0436	0.0427	0.0418	0.0409	0.0401	0.0392	0.0384	0.0375	0.0367
-1.6	0.0548	0.0537	0.0526	0.0516	0.0505	0.0495	0.0485	0.0475	0.0465	0.0455
-1.5	0.0668	0.0655	0.0643	0.0630	0.0618	0.0606	0.0594	0.0582	0.0571	0.0559
-1.4	0.0808	0.0793	0.0778	0.0764	0.0749	0.0735	0.0721	0.0708	0.0694	0.0681
-1.3	0.0968	0.0951	0.0934	0.0918	0.0901	0.0885	0.0869	0.0853	0.0838	0.0823
-1.2	0.1151	0.1131	0.1112	0.1093	0.1075	0.1056	0.1038	0.1020	0.1003	0.0985
-1.1	0.1357	0.1335	0.1314	0.1292	0.1271	0.1251	0.1230	0.1210	0.1190	0.1170
-1.0	0.1587	0.1562	0.1539	0.1515	0.1492	0.1469	0.1446	0.1423	0.1401	0.1379
-0.9	0.1841	0.1814	0.1788	0.1762	0.1736	0.1711	0.1685	0.1660	0.1635	0.1611
-0.8	0.2119	0.2090	0.2061	0.2033	0.2005	0.1977	0.1949	0.1922	0.1894	0.1867
-0.7	0.2420	0.2389	0.2358	0.2327	0.2296	0.2266	0.2236	0.2206	0.2177	0.2148
-0.6	0.2743	0.2709	0.2676	0.2643	0.2611	0.2578	0.2546	0.2514	0.2483	0.2451
-0.5	0.3085	0.3050	0.3015	0.2981	0.2946	0.2912	0.2877	0.2843	0.2810	0.2776
-0.4	0.3446	0.3409	0.3372	0.3336	0.3300	0.3264	0.3228	0.3192	0.3156	0.3121
-0.3	0.3821	0.3783	0.3745	0.3707	0.3669	0.3632	0.3594	0.3557	0.3520	0.3483
-0.2	0.4207	0.4168	0.4129	0.4090	0.4052	0.4013	0.3974	0.3936	0.3897	0.3859
-0.1	0.4602	0.4562	0.4522	0.4483	0.4443	0.4404	0.4364	0.4325	0.4286	0.4247
-0.0	0.5000	0.4960	0.4920	0.4880	0.4840	0.4801	0.4761	0.4721	0.4681	0.4641
0.0	0.5000	0.5040	0.5080	0.5120	0.5160	0.5199	0.5239	0.5279	0.5319	0.5359
0.1	0.5398	0.5438	0.5478	0.5517	0.5557	0.5596	0.5636	0.5675	0.5714	0.5753
0.2	0.5793	0.5832	0.5871	0.5910	0.5948	0.5987	0.6026	0.6064	0.6103	0.6141
0.3	0.6179	0.6217	0.6255	0.6293	0.6331	0.6368	0.6406	0.6443	0.6480	0.6517
0.4	0.6554	0.6591	0.6628	0.6664	0.6700	0.6736	0.6772	0.6808	0.6844	0.6879
0.5	0.6915	0.6950	0.6985	0.7019	0.7054	0.7088	0.7123	0.7157	0.7190	0.7224
0.6	0.7257	0.7291	0.7324	0.7357	0.7389	0.7422	0.7454	0.7486	0.7517	0.7549
0.7	0.7580	0.7611	0.7642	0.7673	0.7704	0.7734	0.7764	0.7794	0.7823	0.7852
0.8	0.7881	0.7910	0.7939	0.7967	0.7995	0.8023	0.8051	0.8078	0.8106	0.8133
0.9	0.8159	0.8186	0.8212	0.8238	0.8264	0.8289	0.8315	0.8340	0.8365	0.8389
1.0	0.8413	0.8438	0.8461	0.8485	0.8508	0.8531	0.8554	0.8577	0.8599	0.8621
1.1	0.8643	0.8665	0.8686	0.8708	0.8729	0.8749	0.8770	0.8790	0.8810	0.8830
1.2	0.8849	0.8869	0.8888	0.8907	0.8925	0.8944	0.8962	0.8980	0.8997	0.9015
1.3	0.9032	0.9049	0.9066	0.9082	0.9099	0.9115	0.9131	0.9147	0.9162	0.9177
1.4	0.9192	0.9207	0.9222	0.9236	0.9251	0.9265	0.9279	0.9292	0.9306	0.9319

Z_i	.00	.01	.02	.03	.04	.05	.06	.07	.08	.09
1.5	0.9332	0.9345	0.9357	0.9370	0.9382	0.9394	0.9406	0.9418	0.9429	0.9441
1.6	0.9452	0.9463	0.9474	0.9484	0.9495	0.9505	0.9515	0.9525	0.9535	0.9545
1.7	0.9554	0.9564	0.9573	0.9582	0.9591	0.9599	0.9608	0.9616	0.9625	0.9633
1.8	0.9641	0.9649	0.9656	0.9664	0.9671	0.9678	0.9686	0.9693	0.9699	0.9706
1.9	0.9713	0.9719	0.9726	0.9732	0.9738	0.9744	0.9750	0.9756	0.9761	0.9767
2.0	0.9772	0.9778	0.9783	0.9788	0.9793	0.9798	0.9803	0.9808	0.9812	0.9817
2.1	0.9821	0.9826	0.9830	0.9834	0.9838	0.9842	0.9846	0.9850	0.9854	0.9857
2.2	0.9861	0.9864	0.9868	0.9871	0.9875	0.9878	0.9881	0.9884	0.9887	0.9890
2.3	0.9893	0.9896	0.9898	0.9901	0.9904	0.9906	0.9909	0.9911	0.9913	0.9916
2.4	0.9918	0.9920	0.9922	0.9925	0.9927	0.9929	0.9931	0.9932	0.9934	0.9936
2.5	0.9938	0.9940	0.9941	0.9943	0.9945	0.9946	0.9948	0.9949	0.9951	0.9952
2.6	0.9953	0.9955	0.9956	0.9957	0.9959	0.9960	0.9961	0.9962	0.9963	0.9964
2.7	0.9965	0.9966	0.9967	0.9968	0.9969	0.9970	0.9971	0.9972	0.9973	0.9974
2.8	0.9974	0.9975	0.9976	0.9977	0.9977	0.9978	0.9979	0.9979	0.9980	0.9981
2.9	0.9981	0.9982	0.9982	0.9983	0.9984	0.9984	0.9985	0.9985	0.9986	0.9986
3.0	0.9987	0.9987	0.9987	0.9988	0.9988	0.9989	0.9989	0.9989	0.9990	0.9990

Table B.2A Z *Values for Confidence Intervals*

Confidence Level	$Z_{1-\alpha/2}$	α (Total Tail Area)
99.99%	3.819	0.0001
99.9%	3.291	0.001
99%	2.576	0.01
95%	1.960	0.05
90%	1.645	0.10
80%	1.282	0.20

Table B.2B Z *Values for Tests of Hypothesis*

Lower-Tailed Tests	α	Z_α	Decision Rule
$H_0: \mu = \mu_0$	0.0001	-3.719	Reject H_0 if $Z \leq Z_\alpha$
$H_1: \mu < \mu_0$	0.001	-3.090	
	0.005	-2.576	
	0.010	-2.326	
	0.025	-1.960	
	0.050	-1.645	
	0.100	-1.282	

Table B.2B *(continued)*

Upper-Tailed Tests	α	$Z_{1-\alpha}$	Decision Rule
$H_0: \mu = \mu_0$	0.0001	3.719	Reject H_0 if $Z \geq Z_{1-\alpha}$
$H_1: \mu > \mu_0$	0.001	3.090	
	0.005	2.576	
	0.010	2.326	
	0.025	1.960	
	0.050	1.645	
	0.100	1.282	

Two-Tailed Tests	α	$Z_{1-\alpha/2}$	Decision Rule
$H_0: \mu = \mu_0$	0.0001	3.819	Reject H_0 if $Z \leq -Z_{1-\alpha/2}$
$H_1: \mu \neq \mu_0$	0.001	3.291	or if $Z \geq Z_{1-\alpha/2}$
	0.010	2.576	
	0.050	1.960	
	0.100	1.645	
	0.200	1.282	

Table B.3 *Critical Values of the t Distribution*

Table entries represent values from t distribution with upper-tail area equal to α, e.g., $P(t_{df} > t) = \alpha$, $P(t_6 > 1.943) = 0.05$.

Confidence Level CL		80%	90%	95%	98%	99%
Two Sided α	α_2	.20	.10	.05	.02	.01
One Sided α	α	.10	.05	.025	.01	.005
	df					
	1	3.078	6.314	12.71	31.82	63.66
	2	1.886	2.920	4.303	6.965	9.925
	3	1.638	2.353	3.182	4.541	5.841
	4	1.533	2.132	2.776	3.747	4.604
	5	1.476	2.015	2.571	3.365	4.032
	6	1.440	1.943	2.447	3.143	3.707
	7	1.415	1.895	2.365	2.998	3.499
	8	1.397	1.860	2.306	2.896	3.355
	9	1.383	1.833	2.262	2.821	3.250
	10	1.372	1.812	2.228	2.764	3.169

Confidence Level	CL	80%	90%	95%	98%	99%
Two Sided α	α_2	.20	.10	.05	.02	.01
One Sided α	α	.10	.05	.025	.01	.005
	df					
	11	1.363	1.796	2.201	2.718	3.106
	12	1.356	1.782	2.179	2.681	3.055
	13	1.350	1.771	2.160	2.650	3.012
	14	1.345	1.761	2.145	2.624	2.977
	15	1.341	1.753	2.131	2.602	2.947
	16	1.337	1.746	2.120	2.583	2.921
	17	1.333	1.740	2.110	2.567	2.898
	18	1.330	1.734	2.101	2.552	2.878
	19	1.328	1.729	2.093	2.539	2.861
	20	1.325	1.725	2.086	2.528	2.845
	21	1.323	1.721	2.080	2.518	2.831
	22	1.321	1.717	2.074	2.508	2.819
	23	1.319	1.714	2.069	2.500	2.807
	24	1.318	1.711	2.064	2.492	2.797
	25	1.316	1.708	2.060	2.485	2.787
	26	1.315	1.706	2.056	2.479	2.779
	27	1.314	1.703	2.052	2.473	2.771
	28	1.313	1.701	2.048	2.467	2.763
	29	1.311	1.699	2.045	2.462	2.756
	30	1.310	1.697	2.042	2.457	2.750
	31	1.309	1.696	2.040	2.453	2.744
	32	1.309	1.694	2.037	2.449	2.738
	33	1.308	1.692	2.035	2.445	2.733
	34	1.307	1.691	2.032	2.441	2.728
	35	1.306	1.690	2.030	2.438	2.724
	36	1.306	1.688	2.028	2.434	2.719
	37	1.305	1.687	2.026	2.431	2.715
	38	1.304	1.686	2.024	2.429	2.712
	39	1.304	1.685	2.023	2.426	2.708
	40	1.303	1.684	2.021	2.423	2.704
	41	1.303	1.683	2.020	2.421	2.701
	42	1.302	1.682	2.018	2.418	2.698
	43	1.302	1.681	2.017	2.416	2.695

Confidence Level	CL	80%	90%	95%	98%	99%
Two Sided α	α_2	.20	.10	.05	.02	.01
One Sided α	α	.10	.05	.025	.01	.005
	df					
	44	1.301	1.680	2.015	2.414	2.692
	45	1.301	1.679	2.014	2.412	2.690
	46	1.300	1.679	2.013	2.410	2.687
	47	1.300	1.678	2.012	2.408	2.685
	48	1.299	1.677	2.011	2.407	2.682
	49	1.299	1.677	2.010	2.405	2.680
	50	1.299	1.676	2.009	2.403	2.678
	51	1.298	1.675	2.008	2.402	2.676
	52	1.298	1.675	2.007	2.400	2.674
	53	1.298	1.674	2.006	2.399	2.672
	54	1.297	1.674	2.005	2.397	2.670
	55	1.297	1.673	2.004	2.396	2.668
	56	1.297	1.673	2.003	2.395	2.667
	57	1.297	1.672	2.002	2.394	2.665
	58	1.296	1.672	2.002	2.392	2.663
	59	1.296	1.671	2.001	2.391	2.662
	60	1.296	1.671	2.000	2.390	2.660
	61	1.296	1.670	2.000	2.389	2.659
	62	1.295	1.670	1.999	2.388	2.657
	63	1.295	1.669	1.998	2.387	2.656
	64	1.295	1.669	1.998	2.386	2.655
	65	1.295	1.669	1.997	2.385	2.654
	66	1.295	1.668	1.997	2.384	2.652
	67	1.294	1.668	1.996	2.383	2.651
	68	1.294	1.668	1.995	2.382	2.650
	69	1.294	1.667	1.995	2.382	2.649
	70	1.294	1.667	1.994	2.381	2.648
	71	1.294	1.667	1.994	2.380	2.647
	72	1.293	1.666	1.993	2.379	2.646
	73	1.293	1.666	1.993	2.379	2.645
	74	1.293	1.666	1.993	2.378	2.644
	75	1.293	1.665	1.992	2.377	2.643
	∞	1.282	1.645	1.960	2.326	2.576

Table B.4A *Critical Values of the F Distribution with Upper-Tail Area = 0.05*

$P(F > F_{df1,df2}) = 0.05$, e.g., $P(F_{3,20} > 3.10) = 0.05$

denominator df (df2)	1	2	3	4	5	6	7	8	9	10	20	30	40	50
1	161.4	199.5	215.7	224.6	230.2	234.0	236.8	238.9	240.5	241.9	248.0	250.1	251.1	251.8
2	18.51	19.00	19.16	19.25	19.30	19.33	19.35	19.37	19.38	19.40	19.45	19.46	19.47	19.48
3	10.13	9.55	9.28	9.12	9.01	8.94	8.89	8.85	8.81	8.79	8.66	8.62	8.59	8.58
4	7.71	6.94	6.59	6.39	6.26	6.16	6.09	6.04	6.00	5.96	5.80	5.75	5.72	5.70
5	6.61	5.79	5.41	5.19	5.05	4.95	4.88	4.82	4.77	4.74	4.56	4.50	4.46	4.44
6	5.99	5.14	4.76	4.53	4.39	4.28	4.21	4.15	4.10	4.06	3.87	3.81	3.77	3.75
7	5.59	4.74	4.35	4.12	3.97	3.87	3.79	3.73	3.68	3.64	3.44	3.38	3.34	3.32
8	5.32	4.46	4.07	3.84	3.69	3.58	3.50	3.44	3.39	3.35	3.15	3.08	3.04	3.02
9	5.12	4.26	3.86	3.63	3.48	3.37	3.29	3.23	3.18	3.14	2.94	2.86	2.83	2.80
10	4.96	4.10	3.71	3.48	3.33	3.22	3.14	3.07	3.02	2.98	2.77	2.70	2.66	2.64
11	4.84	3.98	3.59	3.36	3.20	3.09	3.01	2.95	2.90	2.85	2.65	2.57	2.53	2.51
12	4.75	3.89	3.49	3.26	3.11	3.00	2.91	2.85	2.80	2.75	2.54	2.47	2.43	2.40
13	4.67	3.81	3.41	3.18	3.03	2.92	2.83	2.77	2.71	2.67	2.46	2.38	2.34	2.31
14	4.60	3.74	3.34	3.11	2.96	2.85	2.76	2.70	2.65	2.60	2.39	2.31	2.27	2.24
15	4.54	3.68	3.29	3.06	2.90	2.79	2.71	2.64	2.59	2.54	2.33	2.25	2.20	2.18
16	4.49	3.63	3.24	3.01	2.85	2.74	2.66	2.59	2.54	2.49	2.28	2.19	2.15	2.12
17	4.45	3.59	3.20	2.96	2.81	2.70	2.61	2.55	2.49	2.45	2.23	2.15	2.10	2.08
18	4.41	3.55	3.16	2.93	2.77	2.66	2.58	2.51	2.46	2.41	2.19	2.11	2.06	2.04
19	4.38	3.52	3.13	2.90	2.74	2.63	2.54	2.48	2.42	2.38	2.16	2.07	2.03	2.00
20	4.35	3.49	3.10	2.87	2.71	2.60	2.51	2.45	2.39	2.35	2.12	2.04	1.99	1.97
21	4.32	3.47	3.07	2.84	2.68	2.57	2.49	2.42	2.37	2.32	2.10	2.01	1.96	1.94
22	4.30	3.44	3.05	2.82	2.66	2.55	2.46	2.40	2.34	2.30	2.07	1.98	1.94	1.91
23	4.28	3.42	3.03	2.80	2.64	2.53	2.44	2.37	2.32	2.27	2.05	1.96	1.91	1.88
24	4.26	3.40	3.01	2.78	2.62	2.51	2.42	2.36	2.30	2.25	2.03	1.94	1.89	1.86
25	4.24	3.39	2.99	2.76	2.60	2.49	2.40	2.34	2.28	2.24	2.01	1.92	1.87	1.84
26	4.23	3.37	2.98	2.74	2.59	2.47	2.39	2.32	2.27	2.22	1.99	1.90	1.85	1.82
27	4.21	3.35	2.96	2.73	2.57	2.46	2.37	2.31	2.25	2.20	1.97	1.88	1.84	1.81
28	4.20	3.34	2.95	2.71	2.56	2.45	2.36	2.29	2.24	2.19	1.96	1.87	1.82	1.79
29	4.18	3.33	2.93	2.70	2.55	2.43	2.35	2.28	2.22	2.18	1.94	1.85	1.81	1.77
30	4.17	3.32	2.92	2.69	2.53	2.42	2.33	2.27	2.21	2.16	1.93	1.84	1.79	1.76
31	4.16	3.30	2.91	2.68	2.52	2.41	2.32	2.25	2.20	2.15	1.92	1.83	1.78	1.75
32	4.15	3.29	2.90	2.67	2.51	2.40	2.31	2.24	2.19	2.14	1.91	1.82	1.77	1.74
33	4.14	3.28	2.89	2.66	2.50	2.39	2.30	2.23	2.18	2.13	1.90	1.81	1.76	1.72
34	4.13	3.28	2.88	2.65	2.49	2.38	2.29	2.23	2.17	2.12	1.89	1.80	1.75	1.71
35	4.12	3.27	2.87	2.64	2.49	2.37	2.29	2.22	2.16	2.11	1.88	1.79	1.74	1.70
36	4.11	3.26	2.87	2.63	2.48	2.36	2.28	2.21	2.15	2.11	1.87	1.78	1.73	1.69
37	4.11	3.25	2.86	2.63	2.47	2.36	2.27	2.20	2.14	2.10	1.86	1.77	1.72	1.68
38	4.10	3.24	2.85	2.62	2.46	2.35	2.26	2.19	2.14	2.09	1.85	1.76	1.71	1.68
39	4.09	3.24	2.85	2.61	2.46	2.34	2.26	2.19	2.13	2.08	1.85	1.75	1.70	1.67
40	4.08	3.23	2.84	2.61	2.45	2.34	2.25	2.18	2.12	2.08	1.84	1.74	1.69	1.66
41	4.08	3.23	2.83	2.60	2.44	2.33	2.24	2.17	2.12	2.07	1.83	1.74	1.69	1.65
42	4.07	3.22	2.83	2.59	2.44	2.32	2.24	2.17	2.11	2.06	1.83	1.73	1.68	1.65
43	4.07	3.21	2.82	2.59	2.43	2.32	2.23	2.16	2.11	2.06	1.82	1.72	1.67	1.64
44	4.06	3.21	2.82	2.58	2.43	2.31	2.23	2.16	2.10	2.05	1.81	1.72	1.67	1.63
45	4.06	3.20	2.81	2.58	2.42	2.31	2.22	2.15	2.10	2.05	1.81	1.71	1.66	1.63

denominator df (df2)	numerator df (df1)													
	1	2	3	4	5	6	7	8	9	10	20	30	40	50
46	4.05	3.20	2.81	2.57	2.42	2.30	2.22	2.15	2.09	2.04	1.80	1.71	1.65	1.62
47	4.05	3.20	2.80	2.57	2.41	2.30	2.21	2.14	2.09	2.04	1.80	1.70	1.65	1.61
48	4.04	3.19	2.80	2.57	2.41	2.29	2.21	2.14	2.08	2.03	1.79	1.70	1.64	1.61
49	4.04	3.19	2.79	2.56	2.40	2.29	2.20	2.13	2.08	2.03	1.79	1.69	1.64	1.60
50	4.03	3.18	2.79	2.56	2.40	2.29	2.20	2.13	2.07	2.03	1.78	1.69	1.63	1.60
75	3.97	3.12	2.73	2.49	2.34	2.22	2.13	2.06	2.01	1.96	1.71	1.61	1.55	1.52
100	3.94	3.09	2.70	2.46	2.31	2.19	2.10	2.03	1.97	1.93	1.68	1.57	1.52	1.48
125	3.92	3.07	2.68	2.44	2.29	2.17	2.08	2.01	1.96	1.91	1.66	1.55	1.49	1.45
150	3.90	3.06	2.66	2.43	2.27	2.16	2.07	2.00	1.94	1.89	1.64	1.54	1.48	1.44
175	3.90	3.05	2.66	2.42	2.27	2.15	2.06	1.99	1.93	1.89	1.63	1.52	1.46	1.42
200	3.89	3.04	2.65	2.42	2.26	2.14	2.06	1.98	1.93	1.88	1.62	1.52	1.46	1.41

Table B.4B *Critical Values of the F Distribution with Upper Tail Area* $= 0.025$

$P(F > F_{df1,df2}) = 0.025$, e.g., $P(F_{3,20} > 3.86) = 0.025$

denominator df (df2)	numerator df (df1)													
	1	2	3	4	5	6	7	8	9	10	20	30	40	50
1	647.8	799.5	864.2	899.6	921.8	937.1	948.2	956.7	963.3	968.6	993.1	1001	1006	1008
2	38.51	39.00	39.17	39.25	39.30	39.33	39.36	39.37	39.39	39.40	39.45	39.46	39.47	39.48
3	17.44	16.04	15.44	15.10	14.88	14.73	14.62	14.54	14.47	14.42	14.17	14.08	14.04	14.01
4	12.22	10.65	9.98	9.60	9.36	9.20	9.07	8.98	8.90	8.84	8.56	8.46	8.41	8.38
5	10.01	8.43	7.76	7.39	7.15	6.98	6.85	6.76	6.68	6.62	6.33	6.23	6.18	6.14
6	8.81	7.26	6.60	6.23	5.99	5.82	5.70	5.60	5.52	5.46	5.17	5.07	5.01	4.98
7	8.07	6.54	5.89	5.52	5.29	5.12	4.99	4.90	4.82	4.76	4.47	4.36	4.31	4.28
8	7.57	6.06	5.42	5.05	4.82	4.65	4.53	4.43	4.36	4.30	4.00	3.89	3.84	3.81
9	7.21	5.71	5.08	4.72	4.48	4.32	4.20	4.10	4.03	3.96	3.67	3.56	3.51	3.47
10	6.94	5.46	4.83	4.47	4.24	4.07	3.95	3.85	3.78	3.72	3.42	3.31	3.26	3.22
11	6.72	5.26	4.63	4.28	4.04	3.88	3.76	3.66	3.59	3.53	3.23	3.12	3.06	3.03
12	6.55	5.10	4.47	4.12	3.89	3.73	3.61	3.51	3.44	3.37	3.07	2.96	2.91	2.87
13	6.41	4.97	4.35	4.00	3.77	3.60	3.48	3.39	3.31	3.25	2.95	2.84	2.78	2.74
14	6.30	4.86	4.24	3.89	3.66	3.50	3.38	3.29	3.21	3.15	2.84	2.73	2.67	2.64
15	6.20	4.77	4.15	3.80	3.58	3.41	3.29	3.20	3.12	3.06	2.76	2.64	2.59	2.55
16	6.12	4.69	4.08	3.73	3.50	3.34	3.22	3.12	3.05	2.99	2.68	2.57	2.51	2.47
17	6.04	4.62	4.01	3.66	3.44	3.28	3.16	3.06	2.98	2.92	2.62	2.50	2.44	2.41
18	5.98	4.56	3.95	3.61	3.38	3.22	3.10	3.01	2.93	2.87	2.56	2.44	2.38	2.35
19	5.92	4.51	3.90	3.56	3.33	3.17	3.05	2.96	2.88	2.82	2.51	2.39	2.33	2.30
20	5.87	4.46	3.86	3.51	3.29	3.13	3.01	2.91	2.84	2.77	2.46	2.35	2.29	2.25
21	5.83	4.42	3.82	3.48	3.25	3.09	2.97	2.87	2.80	2.73	2.42	2.31	2.25	2.21
22	5.79	4.38	3.78	3.44	3.22	3.05	2.93	2.84	2.76	2.70	2.39	2.27	2.21	2.17
23	5.75	4.35	3.75	3.41	3.18	3.02	2.90	2.81	2.73	2.67	2.36	2.24	2.18	2.14
24	5.72	4.32	3.72	3.38	3.15	2.99	2.87	2.78	2.70	2.64	2.33	2.21	2.15	2.11
25	5.69	4.29	3.69	3.35	3.13	2.97	2.85	2.75	2.68	2.61	2.30	2.18	2.12	2.08
26	5.66	4.27	3.67	3.33	3.10	2.94	2.82	2.73	2.65	2.59	2.28	2.16	2.09	2.05
27	5.63	4.24	3.65	3.31	3.08	2.92	2.80	2.71	2.63	2.57	2.25	2.13	2.07	2.03
28	5.61	4.22	3.63	3.29	3.06	2.90	2.78	2.69	2.61	2.55	2.23	2.11	2.05	2.01
29	5.59	4.20	3.61	3.27	3.04	2.88	2.76	2.67	2.59	2.53	2.21	2.09	2.03	1.99
30	5.57	4.18	3.59	3.25	3.03	2.87	2.75	2.65	2.57	2.51	2.20	2.07	2.01	1.97

denominator						numerator df (df1)							
df	1	2	3	4	5	6	7	8	9	10	20	30	40	50
(df2)													
31	5.55	4.16	3.57	3.23	3.01	2.85	2.73	2.64	2.56	2.50	2.18	2.06	1.99	1.95
32	5.53	4.15	3.56	3.22	3.00	2.84	2.71	2.62	2.54	2.48	2.16	2.04	1.98	1.93
33	5.51	4.13	3.54	3.20	2.98	2.82	2.70	2.61	2.53	2.47	2.15	2.03	1.96	1.92
34	5.50	4.12	3.53	3.19	2.97	2.81	2.69	2.59	2.52	2.45	2.13	2.01	1.95	1.90
35	5.48	4.11	3.52	3.18	2.96	2.80	2.68	2.58	2.50	2.44	2.12	2.00	1.93	1.89
36	5.47	4.09	3.50	3.17	2.94	2.78	2.66	2.57	2.49	2.43	2.11	1.99	1.92	1.88
37	5.46	4.08	3.49	3.16	2.93	2.77	2.65	2.56	2.48	2.42	2.10	1.97	1.91	1.87
38	5.45	4.07	3.48	3.15	2.92	2.76	2.64	2.55	2.47	2.41	2.09	1.96	1.90	1.85
39	5.43	4.06	3.47	3.14	2.91	2.75	2.63	2.54	2.46	2.40	2.08	1.95	1.89	1.84
40	5.42	4.05	3.46	3.13	2.90	2.74	2.62	2.53	2.45	2.39	2.07	1.94	1.88	1.83
41	5.41	4.04	3.45	3.12	2.89	2.74	2.62	2.52	2.44	2.38	2.06	1.93	1.87	1.82
42	5.40	4.03	3.45	3.11	2.89	2.73	2.61	2.51	2.43	2.37	2.05	1.92	1.86	1.81
43	5.39	4.02	3.44	3.10	2.88	2.72	2.60	2.50	2.43	2.36	2.04	1.92	1.85	1.80
44	5.39	4.02	3.43	3.09	2.87	2.71	2.59	2.50	2.42	2.36	2.03	1.91	1.84	1.80
45	5.38	4.01	3.42	3.09	2.86	2.70	2.58	2.49	2.41	2.35	2.03	1.90	1.83	1.79
46	5.37	4.00	3.42	3.08	2.86	2.70	2.58	2.48	2.41	2.34	2.02	1.89	1.82	1.78
47	5.36	3.99	3.41	3.07	2.85	2.69	2.57	2.48	2.40	2.33	2.01	1.89	1.82	1.77
48	5.35	3.99	3.40	3.07	2.84	2.69	2.56	2.47	2.39	2.33	2.01	1.88	1.81	1.77
49	5.35	3.98	3.40	3.06	2.84	2.68	2.56	2.46	2.39	2.32	2.00	1.87	1.80	1.76
50	5.34	3.97	3.39	3.05	2.83	2.67	2.55	2.46	2.38	2.32	1.99	1.87	1.80	1.75
75	5.23	3.88	3.30	2.96	2.74	2.58	2.46	2.37	2.29	2.22	1.90	1.76	1.69	1.65
100	5.18	3.83	3.25	2.92	2.70	2.54	2.42	2.32	2.24	2.18	1.85	1.71	1.64	1.59
125	5.15	3.80	3.22	2.89	2.67	2.51	2.39	2.30	2.22	2.15	1.82	1.68	1.61	1.56
150	5.13	3.78	3.20	2.87	2.65	2.49	2.37	2.28	2.20	2.13	1.80	1.67	1.59	1.54
175	5.11	3.77	3.19	2.86	2.64	2.48	2.36	2.27	2.19	2.12	1.79	1.65	1.57	1.52
200	5.10	3.76	3.18	2.85	2.63	2.47	2.35	2.26	2.18	2.11	1.78	1.64	1.56	1.51

Table B.5 *Critical Values of the χ^2 Distribution*

Table entries represent values from χ^2 distribution with upper-tail area equal to α.
$P(\chi^2 > \chi^2_{df}) = \alpha$, e.g., $P(\chi^2_3 > 7.81) = 0.05$

df	α				
	.10	.05	.025	.01	.005
1	2.71	3.84	5.02	6.63	7.88
2	4.61	5.99	7.38	9.21	10.60
3	6.25	7.81	9.35	11.34	12.84
4	7.78	9.49	11.14	13.28	14.86
5	9.24	11.07	12.83	15.09	16.75
6	10.64	12.59	14.45	16.81	18.55
7	12.02	14.07	16.01	18.48	20.28
8	13.36	15.51	17.53	20.09	21.95

df	α .10	.05	.025	.01	.005
9	14.68	16.92	19.02	21.67	23.59
10	15.99	18.31	20.48	23.21	25.19
11	17.28	19.68	21.92	24.72	26.76
12	18.55	21.03	23.34	26.22	28.30
13	19.81	22.36	24.74	27.69	29.82
14	21.06	23.68	26.12	29.14	31.32
15	22.31	25.00	27.49	30.58	32.80
16	23.54	26.30	28.85	32.00	34.27
17	24.77	27.59	30.19	33.41	35.72
18	25.99	28.87	31.53	34.81	37.16
19	27.20	30.14	32.85	36.19	38.58
20	28.41	31.41	34.17	37.57	40.00
21	29.62	32.67	35.48	38.93	41.40
22	30.81	33.92	36.78	40.29	42.80
23	32.01	35.17	38.08	41.64	44.18
24	33.20	36.42	39.36	42.98	45.56
25	34.38	37.65	40.65	44.31	46.93
26	35.56	38.89	41.92	45.64	48.29
27	36.74	40.11	43.19	46.96	49.64
28	37.92	41.34	44.46	48.28	50.99
29	39.09	42.56	45.72	49.59	52.34
30	40.26	43.77	46.98	50.89	53.67
40	51.81	55.76	59.34	63.69	66.77
50	63.17	67.50	71.42	76.15	79.49
60	74.40	79.08	83.30	88.38	91.95
70	85.53	90.53	95.02	100.4	104.2
80	96.58	101.9	106.6	112.3	116.3
90	107.6	113.1	118.1	124.1	128.3
100	118.5	124.3	129.6	135.8	140.2

Table B.6 *Critical Values of the Studentized Range Distribution, $\alpha = 0.05$*

	k = Number of treatments (groups) being compared							
df_{error} (df_{within})	3	4	5	6	7	8	9	10
5	4.60	5.22	5.67	6.03	6.33	6.58	6.80	6.99
6	4.34	4.90	5.30	5.63	5.90	6.12	6.32	6.49
7	4.16	4.68	5.06	5.36	5.61	5.82	6.00	6.16

df$_{error}$ (df$_{within}$)	$k = $ Number of treatments (groups) being compared							
	3	4	5	6	7	8	9	10
8	4.04	4.53	4.89	5.17	5.40	5.60	5.77	5.9
9	3.95	4.41	4.76	5.02	5.24	5.43	5.59	5.7
10	3.88	4.33	4.65	4.91	5.12	5.30	5.46	5.6
11	3.82	4.26	4.57	4.82	5.03	5.20	5.35	5.4
12	3.77	4.20	4.51	4.75	4.95	5.12	5.27	5.3
13	3.73	4.15	4.45	4.69	4.88	5.05	5.19	5.3
14	3.70	4.11	4.41	4.64	4.83	4.99	5.13	5.2
15	3.67	4.08	4.37	4.59	4.78	4.94	5.08	5.2
16	3.65	4.05	4.33	4.56	4.74	4.90	5.03	5.1
17	3.63	4.02	4.30	4.52	4.70	4.86	4.99	5.1
18	3.61	4.00	4.28	4.49	4.67	4.82	4.96	5.0
19	3.59	3.98	4.25	4.47	4.65	4.79	4.92	5.0
20	3.58	3.96	4.23	4.45	4.62	4.77	4.90	5.0
30	3.49	3.85	4.10	4.30	4.46	4.60	4.72	4.8
40	3.44	3.79	4.04	4.23	4.39	4.52	4.63	4.7
60	3.40	3.74	3.98	4.16	4.31	4.44	4.55	4.6
120	3.36	3.68	3.92	4.10	4.24	4.36	4.47	4.5
∞	3.31	3.63	3.86	4.03	4.17	4.29	4.39	4.4

B.2 SAS[1] Programs Used to Generate Table Entries

Table B.1 Probabilities of the Binomial Distribution

```
options ps=55 ls=80;
data in;
k=1;
file 'c:\sas\btable.out' noprint notitle;
do n=2 to 25 by 1;
x=0;
 do while (x le n);
 put +4 x 2.0 @@;
  do pi=0.1 to 0.9 by 0.10;
```

[1]SAS Institute Inc. *SAS® User's Guide: Basics, Version 6, Edition 8.* Cary, NC: SAS Institute Inc., 1985.

```
   if x=0 then p=probbnml(pi,n,x);
   else if x^=0 then p=probbnml(pi,n,x)-probbnml(pi,n,x-1);
   output;
   if mod(k,9) ^= 0 then put +2 p 6.4 @@;
   else if mod(k,9) = 0 then put +2 p 6.4 /;
   k+1;
  end;
 x+1;
 end;
end;
run;
```

Table B.2 Probabilities of the Standard Normal Distribution

```
options ps=55 ls=80;
data in;
k=1;
file 'c:\sas\ztable.out' noprint notitle;
do i=-3.09 to 3.09 by 0.01;
 p=probnorm(i);
 output;
 if mod(k,10) ^= 0 then put +2 p 6.4 @@;
 else if mod(k,10) = 0 then put +2 p 6.4 /;
 k+1;
end;
run;
```

Table B.3 Critical Values of the *t* Distribution

```
options ps=55 ls=80;
data in;
k=1;
file 'c:\sas\ttable.out' noprint notitle;
do df=1 to 75 by 1;
 do a=0.10,0.05,0.025,0.01,0.005;
 t=abs(tinv(a,df));
 output;
 if mod(k,5) ^= 0 then put +2 t 5.3 @@;
 else if mod(k,5) = 0 then put +2 t 5.3 /;
 k+1;
 end;
end;
run;
```

Table B.4 Critical Values of the *F* Distribution

```
options ps=55 ls=80;
data in;
k=1;
file 'c:\sas\ftable.out' noprint notitle;
do df2=1 to 49,50 to 200 by 25;
 do df1=1 to 9 by 1,10 to 50 by 10;
 f=finv(0.95,df1,df2);
 output;
 if mod(k,14) ^= 0 then put +2 f 5.2 @@;
 else if mod(k,14) = 0 then put +2 f 5.2 /;
 k+1;
 end;
end;
run;
```

Table B.5 Critical Values of the χ^2 Distribution

```
options ps=55 ls=80;
data in;
k=1;
file 'c:\sas\ctable.out' noprint notitle;
do df=1 to 29,30 to 100 by 10;
 do a=0.10,0.05,0.025,0.01,0.005;
 c=cinv(1-a,df);
 output;
 if mod(k,5) ^= 0 then put +2 c 5.2 @@;
 else if mod(k,5) = 0 then put +2 c 5.2 /;
 k+1;
 end;
end;
run;
```

Framingham Heart Study Longitudinal Data Documentation

The authors wish to thank Paul Sorlie, Ph.D., Leader of Analytical Resources Scientific Group, and Sean Coady, M.A., Health Statistician at the National Heart, Lung, and Blood Institute for preparing the Framingham Heart Study Data and Documentation.

The Framingham Heart Study is a long-term prospective study of the etiology of cardiovascular disease among a population of adults living in the community of Framingham, Massachusetts. The Framingham Heart Study was a landmark study in epidemiology in that it was the first prospective study of cardiovascular disease and identified the concept of risk factors and their joint effects. Beginning in 1948, the study initially enrolled 5209 subjects. Participants have been examined biennially since the inception of the study, and all subjects are continuously followed through regular surveillance for cardiovascular outcomes. Clinic examination data has included cardiovascular disease risk factors and markers of disease, such as blood pressure, blood chemistry, lung function, smoking history, health behaviors, ECG tracings, echocardiography, and medication use. Through regular surveillance of area hospitals, participant contact, and death certificates, the Framingham Heart Study reviews and adjudicates events for the occurrence of angina pectoris, myocardial infarction, heart failure, and cerebrovascular disease.

The enclosed data set is a subset of the data collected as part of the Framingham study and includes laboratory, clinic, questionnaire, and adjudicated event data on 4434 participants. Participant clinic data were collected during three examination periods, approximately 6 years apart, from roughly 1956 to 1968. Each participant was followed for a total of

24 years for the outcome of the following events: angina pectoris, my ocardial infarction, atherothrombotic infarction or cerebral hemorrhage (stroke), or death. (*Note:* **Although the enclosed data set contains Framingham data "as collected" by Framingham investigators, specific methods were employed to ensure an anonymous data set that protects patient confidentiality; therefore, this data set is inappropriate for publication purposes.**)

The data is provided in longitudinal form. Each participant has 1 to 3 observations depending on the number of exams the subject attended, and as a result there are 11,627 observations on the 4434 participants. Event data for each participant have been added without regard for prevalent disease status or when examination data were collected. For example, consider the following participant:

RANDID	age	SEX	time	period	prevchd	mi_fchd	timemifc
95148	52	2	0	1	0	1	3607
95148	58	2	2128	2	0	1	3607
95148	64	2	4192	3	1	1	3607

Participant 95148 entered the study (time = 0 or period = 1) free of prevalent coronary heart disease (prevchd = 0 at period = 1); however, during follow up, an MI event occurred at day 3607 following the baseline examination. The MI occurred after the second exam the subject attended (period = 2 or time = 2128 days), but before the third attended exam (period = 3 or time = 4192 days). Since the event occurred prior to the third exam, the subject was prevalent for CHD (prevchd = 1) at the third examination. Note that the event data (mi_fchd, timemifc) covers the entire follow-up period and does not change according to exam.

The following characteristics or risk factor data are provided in the data set. Missing values in the data set are indicated by a period (.). In SAS, missing values are numerically the smallest possible values (for example, < 0 or < −99999999).

Variable	Description	Units	Range or Count
RANDID	Unique identification number for each participant		2448–9999312
SEX	Participant sex	1 = Men 2 = Women	$n = 5022$ $n = 6605$
PERIOD	Examination cycle	1 = Period 1 2 = Period 2 3 = Period 3	$n = 4434$ $n = 3930$ $n = 3263$

Variable	Description	Units	Range or Count
TIME	Number of days since baseline exam		0–4854
AGE	Age at exam (years)		32–81
SYSBP	Systolic blood pressure (mean of last two of three measurements) (mmHg)		83.5–295
DIABP	Diastolic blood pressure (mean of last two of three measurements) (mmHg)		30–150
BPMEDS	Use of antihypertensive medication at exam	0 = Not currently used 1 = Current use	$n = 10090$ $n = 944$
CURSMOKE	Current cigarette smoking at exam	0 = Not current smoker 1 = Current smoker	$n = 6598$ $n = 5029$
CIGPDAY	Number of cigarettes smoked each day	0 = Not current smoker 1–90 cigarettes per day	
TOTCHOL	Serum total cholesterol (mg/dL)		107–696
HDLC	High-density lipoprotein cholesterol (mg/dL)	Available for period 3 only	10–189
LDLC	Low-density lipoprotein cholesterol (mg/dL)	Available for period 3 only	20–565
BMI	Body mass index, weight in kilograms/height meters squared		14.43–56.8
GLUCOSE	Casual serum glucose (mg/dL)		39–478
DIABETES	Diabetic according to criteria of first exam treated or first exam with casual glucose of 200 mg/dL or more	0 = Not a diabetic 1 = Diabetic	$n = 11097$ $n = 530$
HEARTRTE	Heart rate (ventricular rate) in beats/min		37–220
PREVAP	Prevalent angina pectoris at exam	0 = Free of disease 1 = Prevalent disease	$n = 11000$ $n = 627$
PREVCHD	Prevalent coronary heart disease defined as preexisting angina pectoris, myocardial infarction (hospitalized, silent or unrecognized), or coronary insufficiency (unstable angina)	0 = Free of disease 1 = Prevalent disease	$n = 10785$ $n = 842$
PREVMI	Prevalent myocardial infarction	0 = Free of disease 1 = Prevalent disease	$n = 11253$ $n = 374$
PREVSTRK	Prevalent stroke	0 = Free of disease 1 = Prevalent disease	$n = 11475$ $n = 152$
PREVHYP	Prevalent hypertensive. Subject was defined as hypertensive if treated or if second exam at which mean systolic was >= 140 mmHg or mean diastolic >=90 mmHg	0 = Free of disease 1 = Prevalent disease	$n = 6283$ $n = 5344$

For each participant the following event data is provided. For each type of event, '0' indicates the event did not occur during follow-up, and '1' indicates an event did occur during follow-up. Only the first event occurring during the interval of baseline (PERIOD = 1) to end of follow-up is provided:

Variable Name	Description
ANGINA	Angina pectoris
HOSPMI	Hospitalized myocardial infarction
MI_FCHD	Hospitalized myocardial infarction or fatal coronary heart disease
ANYCHD	Angina pectoris, myocardial infarction (hospitalized and silent or unrecognized), coronary insufficiency (unstable angina), or fatal coronary heart disease
STROKE	Atherothrombotic infarction, cerebral embolism, intracerebral hemorrhage, or subarachnoid hemorrhage or fatal cerebrovascular disease
CVD	Myocardial infarction (hospitalized and silent or unrecognized), fatal coronary heart disease, atherothrombotic infarction, cerebral embolism, intracerebral hemorrhage, or subarachnoid hemorrhage or fatal cerebrovascular disease
HYPERTEN	Hypertensive. Defined as the first exam treated for high blood pressure or second exam in which either systolic is ≥ 140 mmHg or diastolic ≥ 90 mmHg
DEATH	Death from any cause
TIMEAP	Number of days from baseline exam to first angina during the follow-up or number of days from baseline to censor date. Censor date may be end of follow-up, death, or last known contact date if subject is lost to follow-up
TIMEMI	Defined as above for the first HOSPMI event during follow-up
TIMEMIFC	Defined as above for the first MI_FCHD event during follow-up
TIMECHD	Defined as above for the first ANYCHD event during follow-up
TIMESTRK	Defined as above for the first STROKE event during follow-up
TIMECVD	Defined as above for the first CVD event during follow-up
TIMEHYP	Defined as above for the first HYPERTEN event during follow-up
TIMEDTH	Number of days from baseline exam to death if occurring during follow-up or number of days from baseline to censor date. Censor date may be end of follow-up or last known contact date if subject is lost to follow-up.

Note that defining hypertensive requires exam participation and bias can therefore occur. Subjects attending exams regularly have a greater opportunity to be defined as hypertensive. Subjects not attending exams would be assumed to be free of hypertension. Since hypertension is highly prevalent, this misclassification could potentially be large.

Defining Incident Events

Frequently, epidemiologists need to define the population at risk for some disease or event outcome, and individuals who have previously had an event need to be excluded from the analysis so that only new or first events are counted. Incidence or first event rates can be calculated using any of the three examinations as a baseline exam. The variables PREVAP, PREVMI, PREVCHD, PREVSTRK, and PREVHYP will define the population at risk for the outcome of interest. For example, assume we are interested in incident hospitalized myocardial infarction or fatal coronary heart disease. Consider again participant 95148 and participants 477082 and 1140225, whose data are given below.

RANDID	age	SEX	time	period	prevchd	mi_fchd	timemifc
95148	52	2	0	1	0	1	3607
95148	58	2	2128	2	0	1	3607
95148	64	2	4192	3	1	1	3607
477082	38	1	0	1	0	1	1718
477082	44	1	2119	2	1	1	1718
1140225	58	2	0	1	0	0	8766
1140225	64	2	2172	2	0	0	8766
1140225	69	2	4287	3	0	0	8766

Participants are often enrolled in an observational study without regard to past medical history. The study investigators will review the medical record to determine if the participant had any preexisting disease at the time of the first study examination. If preexisting disease is found, then the data for that subject will reflect prevalent disease at the first exam; however, the subject will continue to be followed for any new events. All participants, regardless of their prevalent disease status, will continue to be followed and events recorded until the study ends, the participant dies, or the participant cannot be contacted to ascertain status (lost to follow-up). For participants who enter the study free of disease, the incident events are used to determine prevalent disease status at later exams. For the three participants here, none entered the study with prevalent disease, and using period 1 as the baseline exam, the population at risk could be defined using code similiar to the following SAS code:

```
data work;
 set frmgham;
 if period=1 and prevchd=0;
run;
```

The data would appear as the following:

RANDID	age	SEX	time	period	prevchd	mi_fchd	timemifc
95148	52	2	0	1	0	1	3607
477082	38	1	0	1	0	1	1718
1140225	58	2	0	1	0	0	8766

The population at risk consists of all three participants (prevchd = 0), and follow-up time for the event of hospitalized MI or fatal CHD would be the time indicated under TIMEMIFC. The first two participants (95148 and 477082) would be regarded as having an incident event during follow-up.

Likewise, the second examination, or period = 2, could also be used as a baseline exam. The full data set can be subset to include only those at risk at the start of the second period. For example,

```
data work;
  set frmgham;
  if period=2 and prevchd=0;
run;
```

Since time to event is provided as days since the first visit, a new time variable would need to be created so that number of days under study extends from the second exam until the end of follow-up:

```
newtime=timemifc-time;
```

The revised data set that includes the population at risk beginning at period = 2 and extends until the end of follow-up would be

RANDID	age	SEX	time	period	prevchd	mi_fchd	timemifc	newtime
95148	58	2	2128	2	0	1	3607	1479
1140225	64	2	2172	2	0	0	8766	6594

The population at risk (those free of prevalent disease) now includes only participants 95148 and 1140225. The variable NEWTIME correctly reflects the number of days of follow-up from the second exam, or period = 2, until the first event or a censor point.

The same procedure can be used to define the third exam, or period = 3, as the baseline exam.

For more complex analyses, such as time-dependent analysis, or a counting process style of input, the user would have to subset the population to those free of disease at all exams, and event data would have to be modified to reflect when the event occurred relative to the examinations. Consider the following SAS code, which would modify the data set to a counting process style of input for an analysis on the Hospitalized MI-Fatal CHD endpoint. The variable NEWEVNT is modified from MI_FCHD so that the event indicator is '1' only once for each participant. The variables TIME and END-TIME define the interval the subject is at risk.

```
data analysis;
 set work;
 if prevchd=0;
run;

proc sort data=analysis;
 by randid descending period;
run;

data analysis;
 set analysis;
 by randid;

newevnt=mi_fchd;
 retain exmtime;
 if first.randid then do;
    endtime=timemifc; exmtime=time;
  end;
  else do;
    newevnt=0;
    endtime=exmtime;
    exmtime=time;
  end;
run;

proc sort data=analysis;
 by randid period;
run;
```

The data would appear, for example, as follows for three participants:

RANDID	age	SEX	period	time	endtime	newevnt	mi_fchd	timemifc
11263	43	2	1	0	2178	0	1	5719
11263	49	2	2	2178	4351	0	1	5719
11263	55	2	3	4351	5719	1	1	5719
12629	63	2	1	0	8766	0	0	8766
9069458	42	2	1	0	4362	0	0	8766
9069458	54	2	3	4362	8766	0	0	8766

SAS PROC CONTENTS PROCEDURE ON FRAMINGHAM LONGITUDINAL DATASET

The CONTENTS Procedure

Data Set Name: WORK.FRMGHAM	Observations:	11627
Member Type: DATA	Variables:	38
Engine: V8	Indexes:	0
Created: 14:50 Tuesday, March 2, 2004	Observation Length:	304
Last Modified: 14:50 Tuesday, March 2, 2004	Deleted Observations:	0
Protection:	Compressed:	NO
Data Set Type:	Sorted:	NO
Label:		

-----Engine/Host Dependent Information-----

Data Set Page Size: 16384
Number of Data Set Pages: 220
First Data Page: 1
Max Obs per Page: 53
Obs in First Data Page: 35
Number of Data Set Repairs: 0
Release Created: 8.0202M0
Host Created: WIN_PRO

The CONTENTS Procedure

-----Variables Ordered by Position-----

#	Variable	Type	Len	Label
1	SEX	Num	4	SEX
2	RANDID	Num	8	Random ID
3	totchol	Num	8	Serum Cholesterol mg/dL
4	age	Num	8	Age (years) at examination
5	sysbp	Num	8	Systolic BP mmHg
6	diabp	Num	8	Diastolic BP mmHg
7	cursmoke	Num	8	Current Cig Smoker Y/N
8	cigpday	Num	8	Cigarettes per day
9	bmi	Num	8	Body Mass Index (kg/(M*M)
10	diabetes	Num	8	Diabetic Y/N
11	bpmeds	Num	8	Anti-hypertensive meds Y/N
12	heartrte	Num	8	Ventricular Rate (beats/min)
13	glucose	Num	8	Casual Glucose mg/dL
14	prevchd	Num	8	Prevalent CHD (MI,AP,CI)
15	prevap	Num	8	Prevalent Angina
16	prevmi	Num	8	Prevalent MI (Hosp,Silent)
17	prevstrk	Num	8	Prevalent Stroke (Infarct,Hem)

18	prevhyp	Num	8	Prevalent Hypertension
19	time	Num	8	Days since Index Exam
20	period	Num	8	Examination cycle
21	hdlc	Num	8	HDL Cholesterol mg/dL
22	ldlc	Num	8	LDL Cholesterol mg/dL
23	death	Num	8	Death indicator
24	angina	Num	8	Incident Angina Pectoris
25	hospmi	Num	8	Incident Hospitalized MI
26	mi_fchd	Num	8	Incident Hosp MI-Fatal CHD
27	anychd	Num	8	Incident Hosp MI, AP, CI, Fatal CHD
28	stroke	Num	8	Incident Stroke Fatal/non-fatal
29	cvd	Num	8	Incident Hosp MI or Stroke, Fatal or Non
30	hyperten	Num	8	Incident Hypertension
31	timeap	Num	8	Days Baseline-Inc Angina
32	timemi	Num	8	Days Baseline-Inc Hosp MI
33	timemifc	Num	8	Days Baseline-Inc MI-Fatal CHD
34	timechd	Num	8	Days Baseline-Inc Any CHD
35	timestrk	Num	8	Days Baseline-Inc Stroke
36	timecvd	Num	8	Days Baseline-Inc CVD
37	timedth	Num	8	Days Baseline-Death
38	timehyp	Num	8	Days Baseline-Inc Hypertension

Distributions of selected variables by period and sex

Examination cycle 1

Means selected Risk factors	N	NMiss	Mean	Std	Min	P25	Median	P75	Max
Men									
Days since Index Exam	1944	0	0.00	0.00	0.00	0.00	0.00	0.00	0.00
Age (years) at examination	1944	0	49.79	8.72	33.00	42.00	49.00	57.00	69.00
Body Mass Index (kg/(M*M)	1939	5	26.17	3.41	15.54	23.97	26.08	28.32	40.38
Systolic BP mmHg	1944	0	131.74	19.44	83.50	118.00	129.00	141.50	235.00
Diastolic BP mmHg	1944	0	83.71	11.44	48.00	76.00	82.00	90.00	136.00
Serum Cholesterol mg/dL	1937	7	233.58	42.36	113.00	206.00	231.00	259.00	696.00
HDL Cholesterol mg/dL	0	1944	.	.	.	.	.	.	.
LDL Cholesterol mg/dL	0	1944	.	.	.	.	.	.	.
Casual Glucose mg/dL	1824	120	82.32	24.72	40.00	71.00	78.00	87.00	394.00
Cigarettes per day	1928	16	13.23	13.78	0.00	0.00	10.50	20.00	70.00
Ventricular Rate (beats/min)	1943	1	74.40	11.90	44.00	66.00	75.00	80.00	130.00
Women									
Days since Index Exam	2490	0	0.00	0.00	0.00	0.00	0.00	0.00	0.00
Age (years) at examination	2490	0	50.03	8.64	32.00	43.00	49.00	57.00	70.00
Body Mass Index (kg/(M*M)	2476	14	25.59	4.56	15.96	22.54	24.83	27.82	56.80
Systolic BP mmHg	2490	0	133.82	24.46	83.50	116.00	128.50	146.50	295.00
Diastolic BP mmHg	2490	0	82.60	12.50	50.00	74.00	81.00	89.00	142.50
Serum Cholesterol mg/dL	2445	45	239.68	46.22	107.00	206.00	237.00	269.00	600.00
HDL Cholesterol mg/dL	0	2490	.	.	.	.	.	.	.
LDL Cholesterol mg/dL	0	2490	.	.	.	.	.	.	.
Casual Glucose mg/dL	2213	277	82.07	24.14	40.00	72.00	78.00	86.00	394.00
Cigarettes per day	2474	16	5.65	8.96	0.00	0.00	0.00	10.00	50.00
Ventricular Rate (beats/min)	2490	0	77.06	12.15	46.00	69.00	75.00	85.00	143.00

Means selected Risk factors	N	NMiss	Mean	Std	Min	P25	Median	P75	Max
Examination cycle 2									
Men									
Days since Index Exam	1691	0	2173.67	72.44	1577.00	2142.00	2174.00	2205.00	2520.00
Age (years) at examination	1691	0	55.10	8.51	39.00	48.00	54.00	62.00	75.00
Body Mass Index (kg/(M*M)	1685	6	26.23	3.40	16.24	24.05	26.09	28.23	39.46
Systolic BP mmHg	1691	0	135.48	19.90	88.00	120.00	132.00	148.00	216.00
Diastolic BP mmHg	1691	0	84.61	10.91	53.00	78.00	84.00	91.00	124.00
Serum Cholesterol mg/dL	1666	25	241.82	42.14	115.00	214.00	240.00	266.00	614.00
HDL Cholesterol mg/dL	0	1691	.	.	.	.	.	.	.
LDL Cholesterol mg/dL	0	1691	.	.	.	.	.	.	.
Casual Glucose mg/dL	1518	173	82.24	23.31	40.00	70.00	77.00	88.00	362.00
Cigarettes per day	1682	9	12.23	15.04	0.00	0.00	2.00	20.00	90.00
Ventricular Rate (beats/min)	1691	0	75.92	12.66	42.00	68.00	75.00	83.00	130.00
Women									
Days since Index Exam	2239	0	2176.22	76.20	1633.00	2144.00	2175.00	2207.00	2765.00
Age (years) at examination	2239	0	55.66	8.56	39.00	48.00	55.00	62.00	76.00
Body Mass Index (kg/(M*M)	2229	10	25.65	4.58	15.33	22.54	24.88	27.85	56.80
Systolic BP mmHg	2239	0	138.06	24.30	88.00	121.00	134.00	151.00	282.00
Diastolic BP mmHg	2239	0	83.57	11.79	47.00	76.00	82.00	90.00	150.00
Serum Cholesterol mg/dL	2121	118	255.67	47.53	122.00	223.00	252.00	285.00	638.00
HDL Cholesterol mg/dL	0	2239	.	.	.	.	.	.	.
LDL Cholesterol mg/dL	0	2239	.	.	.	.	.	.	.
Casual Glucose mg/dL	1931	308	81.76	21.32	39.00	71.00	78.00	87.00	420.00
Cigarettes per day	2215	24	5.97	10.00	0.00	0.00	0.00	10.00	60.00
Ventricular Rate (beats/min)	2238	1	78.36	12.76	45.00	70.00	75.00	85.00	220.00
Examination cycle 3									
Men									
Days since Index Exam	1387	0	4353.75	97.74	3748.00	4312.00	4361.00	4403.00	4816.00
Age (years) at examination	1387	0	60.35	8.19	45.00	53.00	60.00	67.00	80.00
Body Mass Index (kg/(M*M)	1380	7	26.22	3.49	14.43	24.02	26.09	28.25	45.41
Systolic BP mmHg	1387	0	139.26	21.15	91.00	123.00	136.00	152.00	225.00
Diastolic BP mmHg	1387	0	82.55	11.29	30.00	75.00	81.50	90.00	123.00
Serum Cholesterol mg/dL	1312	75	225.74	41.13	130.00	198.00	222.00	252.00	413.00
HDL Cholesterol mg/dL	1304	83	43.71	13.30	10.00	35.00	42.00	51.00	138.00
LDL Cholesterol mg/dL	1304	83	170.55	44.66	34.00	140.00	167.50	199.00	376.00
Casual Glucose mg/dL	1163	224	91.17	28.99	49.00	77.00	85.00	97.00	423.00
Cigarettes per day	1380	7	8.70	13.51	0.00	0.00	0.00	20.00	80.00
Ventricular Rate (beats/min)	1387	0	75.88	12.73	43.00	66.00	75.00	85.00	150.00
Women									
Days since Index Exam	1876	0	4353.61	93.13	3919.00	4313.00	4362.00	4402.50	4854.00
Age (years) at examination	1876	0	60.87	8.37	44.00	54.00	60.00	67.00	81.00
Body Mass Index (kg/(M*M)	1866	10	25.65	4.45	14.53	22.59	24.80	27.94	56.80
Systolic BP mmHg	1876	0	140.92	24.14	86.00	123.00	138.00	156.00	267.00
Diastolic BP mmHg	1876	0	81.23	11.23	46.00	73.00	80.00	88.00	130.00
Serum Cholesterol mg/dL	1737	139	245.00	45.08	112.00	214.00	242.00	270.00	625.00
HDL Cholesterol mg/dL	1723	153	53.64	15.90	11.00	43.00	52.00	62.00	189.00
LDL Cholesterol mg/dL	1722	154	180.95	48.00	20.00	149.00	177.00	208.00	565.00
Casual Glucose mg/dL	1538	338	88.72	27.48	46.00	76.00	84.00	95.00	478.00
Cigarettes per day	1869	7	5.35	9.78	0.00	0.00	0.00	8.00	60.00
Ventricular Rate (beats/min)	1872	4	78.45	12.20	37.00	70.00	77.00	85.00	130.00

Examination cycle

| | 1 | | | | 2 | | | | 3 | | | |
| | Men | | Women | | Men | | Women | | Men | | Women | |
	N	Percent	N	Percent	N	Percent	N	Percent	N	Percent	N	Percent
Total	1944	100.00	2490	100.00	1691	100.00	2239	100.00	1387	100.00	1876	100.00
Current Cig Smoker Y/N												
No	769	39.56	1484	59.60	811	47.96	1392	62.17	848	61.14	1294	68.98
Yes	1175	60.44	1006	40.40	880	52.04	847	37.83	539	38.86	582	31.02
Diabetic Y/N												
No	1885	96.97	2428	97.51	1617	95.62	2158	96.38	1267	91.35	1742	92.86
Yes	59	3.03	62	2.49	74	4.38	81	3.62	120	8.65	134	7.14
Anti-hypertensive meds Y/N												
Missing	22	1.13	39	1.57	37	2.19	49	2.19	189	13.63	257	13.70
No	1880	96.71	2349	94.34	1553	91.84	1920	85.75	1060	76.42	1328	70.79
Yes	42	2.16	102	4.10	101	5.97	270	12.06	138	9.95	291	15.51
Prevalent CHD (MI,AP,CI)												
No	1820	93.62	2420	97.19	1516	89.65	2126	94.95	1187	85.58	1716	91.47
Yes	124	6.38	70	2.81	175	10.35	113	5.05	200	14.42	160	8.53
Prevalent MI (Hosp,Silent)												
No	1874	96.40	2474	99.36	1588	93.91	2212	98.79	1272	91.71	1833	97.71
Yes	70	3.60	16	0.64	103	6.09	27	1.21	115	8.29	43	2.29
Prevalent Angina												
No	1852	95.27	2435	97.79	1564	92.49	2146	95.85	1254	90.41	1749	93.23
Yes	92	4.73	55	2.21	127	7.51	93	4.15	133	9.59	127	6.77
Prevalent Stroke (Infarct,Hem)												
No	1930	99.28	2472	99.28	1675	99.05	2204	98.44	1357	97.84	1837	97.92
Yes	14	0.72	18	0.72	16	0.95	35	1.56	30	2.16	39	2.08
Prevalent Hypertension												
No	1313	67.54	1691	67.91	841	49.73	1130	50.47	542	39.08	766	40.83
Yes	631	32.46	799	32.09	850	50.27	1109	49.53	845	60.92	1110	59.17

Event Counts by sex

Counts of Endpoints by Sex	SEX			
	Men		Women	
	N	Percent	N	Percent
All	1944	100.00	2490	100.00
Incident Hypertension				
No	540	27.78	642	25.78
Yes	1404	72.22	1848	74.22
Incident Angina Pectoris				
No	1561	80.30	2148	86.27
Yes	383	19.70	342	13.73
Incident Hospitalized MI				
No	1624	83.54	2356	94.62
Yes	320	16.46	134	5.38
Incident Hosp MI-Fatal CHD				
No	1453	74.74	2250	90.36
Yes	491	25.26	240	9.64
Incident Stroke Fatal/non-fatal				
No	1751	90.07	2268	91.08
Yes	193	9.93	222	8.92
Incident Hosp MI, AP, CI, Fatal CHD				
No	1234	63.48	1960	78.71
Yes	710	36.52	530	21.29
Incident Hosp MI or Stroke, Fatal or Non				
No	1258	64.71	2019	81.08
Yes	686	35.29	471	18.92
Death indicator				
No	1101	56.64	1783	71.61
Yes	843	43.36	707	28.39

Distributions of Time to Event by sex

Time to Event	N	NMiss	Mean	Std	Min	P25	Median	P75	Max
Men									
Days Baseline-Inc Hypertension	1944	0	3313	3391	0	0	2156	6491	8766
Days Baseline-Inc Angina	1944	0	6507	2929	0	4572	8486	8766	8766
Days Baseline-Inc Hosp MI	1944	0	6736	2771	0	5006	8766	8766	8766
Days Baseline-Inc MI-Fatal CHD	1944	0	6655	2816	0	4822	8743	8766	8766
Days Baseline-Inc Stroke	1944	0	7003	2509	0	5608	8766	8766	8766
Days Baseline-Inc Any CHD	1944	0	6156	3067	0	3853	7653	8766	8766
Days Baseline-Inc CVD	1944	0	6274	3015	0	4009	7895	8766	8766
Days Baseline-Death	1944	0	7194	2386	26	6047	8766	8766	8766
Women									
Days Baseline-Inc Hypertension	2490	0	3532	3496	0	0	2219	7340	8766
Days Baseline-Inc Angina	2490	0	7209	2559	0	6132	8766	8766	8766
Days Baseline-Inc Hosp MI	2490	0	7634	2154	0	7541	8766	8766	8766
Days Baseline-Inc MI-Fatal CHD	2490	0	7600	2197	0	7452	8766	8766	8766
Days Baseline-Inc Stroke	2490	0	7540	2262	0	7283	8766	8766	8766
Days Baseline-Inc Any CHD	2490	0	7065	2656	0	5618	8766	8766	8766
Days Baseline-Inc CVD	2490	0	7243	2549	0	6241	8766	8766	8766
Days Baseline-Death	2490	0	7749	2037	34	8016	8766	8766	8766

Age Specific Angina and Hospitalized MI-Fatal CHD Incidence Rates by Sex

	Angina				Hospitalized MI - Fatal CHD			
	N*	Person Years	Events	Rate/ 1,000PY	N*	Person Years	Events	Rate/ 1,000PY
Men								
35-44	649	3,053	12	3.9	644	3,037	8	2.6
45-54	1,278	9,587	52	5.4	1,269	9,498	67	7.1
55-64	1,646	12,241	135	11.0	1,629	12,274	154	12.5
65-74	1,115	7,488	78	10.4	1,125	7,623	117	15.3
75-84	416	2,165	13	6.0	432	2,210	43	19.5
85+	52	93	1	10.8	54	97	6	62.0
Women								
35-44	783	3,765	3	0.8	783	3,769	2	0.5
45-54	1,634	12,316	26	2.1	1,631	12,400	12	1.0
55-64	2,229	17,261	123	7.1	2,238	17,675	60	3.4
65-74	1,640	11,679	98	8.4	1,705	12,421	78	6.3
75-84	707	3,815	35	9.2	769	4,262	55	12.9
85+	106	287	2	7.0	121	316	7	22.1

N* - Number of persons contributing person years to that age group. Incidence rates are calculated using derived age at time of event.

Age Specific Stroke and Cardiovascular Disease (Fatal and Non-Fatal) Incidence Rates by Sex

	Stroke				Cardiovascular Disease (CVD)			
	N*	Person Years	Events	Rate/ 1,000PY	N*	Person Years	Events	Rate/ 1,000PY
Men								
35-44	655	3,082	1	0.3	643	3,010	13	4.3
45-54	1,313	9,921	14	1.4	1,260	9,353	95	10.2
55-64	1,743	13,293	42	3.2	1,588	11,769	202	17.2
65-74	1,256	8,471	74	8.7	1,058	6,920	185	26.7
75-84	477	2,402	44	18.3	378	1,839	75	40.8
85+	50	97	4	41.1	41	65	9	138.0
Women								
35-44	782	3,761	2	0.5	781	3,759	5	1.3
45-54	1,638	12,420	10	0.8	1,621	12,282	31	2.5
55-64	2,283	17,932	47	2.6	2,209	17,180	133	7.7
65-74	1,760	12,713	83	6.5	1,631	11,588	148	12.8
75-84	774	4,230	52	12.3	695	3,737	85	22.7
85+	124	322	10	31.0	103	264	15	56.8

N* - Number of persons contributing person years to that age group. Incidence rates are calculated using derived age at time of event.
For CVD endpoint, population at risk defined by PREVCHD=0 AND PREVSTRK=0

Index